Down Syndrome
Living and Learning in the Community

Down Syndrome
Living and Learning in the Community

Edited by
Lynn Nadel
and
Donna Rosenthal

ND
SS

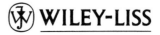 **WILEY-LISS**

A JOHN WILEY & SONS, INC., PUBLICATION

NEW YORK • CHICHESTER • BRISBANE • TORONTO • SINGAPORE

Address All Inquiries to the Publisher
Wiley-Liss, Inc., 605 Third Avenue, New York, NY 10158-0012

Copyright © 1995 Wiley-Liss, Inc.

Printed in the United States of America.

Library of Congress Cataloging-in-Publication Data

Down syndrome : living and learning in the community / editors, Lynn
  Nadel, Donna Rosenthal.
      p. cm.
    Proceedings of the Fifth International Down Syndrome Conference
  held in Orlando, Florida, 1993.
    Includes bibliographical references and index.
    ISBN 0-471-02192-X. — ISBN 0-471-02201-2 (paper). — ISBN
  0-471-02201-2 (pbk.)
      1. Down's syndrome—Congresses. I. Nadel, Lynn. II. Rosenthal,
  Donna. III. International Down Syndrome Conference (5th : 1993 :
  Orlando, Fla.)
  RC571.D684 1994
  616.85'8842—dc20   94-37595
                                                                    CIP

The text of this book is printed on acid-free paper.

10 9 8 7 6 5 4

Contents

Foreword

My name is Chris Burke and I live an exciting and happy life. That's because I am living my dreams. I love entertaining people and being an actor, and I like to help my fellow handi-capables.

Many people recognize me from my role as Corky Thatcher on "Life Goes On," an ABC-TV series for many years. Corky has Down syndrome and so do I. Only I call it Up syndrome, because having Down syndrome has never made me feel down. I'm always up. One reason it is uplifting is because of the tremendous support I have received from my family and all the people in my life. My teachers, my friends, and the people I have worked with are very important to me, just like I am important to them.

Being part of a community is important for all people, whether they have Down syndrome or not. Everybody likes to be included. That's why I think it's great that people are now understanding what life is about. It's about ability, not disability.

This was especially clear at the International Down Syndrome Conference in Orlando, Florida organized by the National Down Syndrome Society. The conference was really special. It brought together people with Down syndrome as well as everybody else. It was exciting to talk to parents and professionals from all over the world and share with them, too. It gave me a chance to try out my new role as a leader at the National Down Syndrome Society, giving encouragement to families and young people that all people can succeed in achieving their dreams. There were people from 47 different countries at the conference. And even though we didn't all speak the same language, we communicated well, and learned a lot. We learned that we all have goals and ideas. We have jobs. We have a place in the larger community. But most of all, we have dreams, and we live them every day.

Christopher Burke

Preface

This book is a direct result of the Fifth International Down Syndrome Conference. The purpose of this conference was to bring together families and professionals from every part of the world to meet one another, and to acquire state of the art knowledge about Down syndrome and the programs and services that are evolving to help people with this genetic disorder achieve their full potential in community life.

In the past twenty years, our knowledge about the health care, education, living arrangements, socialization and employment of people with Down syndrome has changed rapidly and substantially. Living at home within the community is now the norm. Growing up with one's peers at school and at play, working side by side, dating and living independently, and growing old now present opportunities and new vistas to conquer for people with Down syndrome.

Addressing these challenges and achieving goals and success are the focus of this book. Each section opens with a commentary written by a young adult with Down syndrome who describes in his or her own words feelings and accomplishments, and offers advice.

The book is divided into seven sections. Section I focuses on personal observations by four parents on the theme of empowerment and independence.

Section II discusses behavior, an area of increasing interest and concern. As people with Down syndrome become fully included in community life, they experience challenges and demands and high expectations. Behavior reflects these challenges and, like everyone else, people with Down syndrome are affected by the myriad of stresses and frustrations they encounter. Documenting behavioral changes in people with Down syndrome is in the beginning phase and this book sets forth initial studies in this critical area.

The family is, of course, the integral entity that shapes the life of the person with Down syndrome. In Section III of the book, the topics of family support, siblings, respite, and planning for the future are addressed in detail.

Down syndrome is synonymous with mental challenge. The exploration of cognitive development and language acquisition in Section IV is critical. Acquisition of language and cognitive development are now known to continue well into adulthood, and this knowledge impacts importantly on education.

Section V, which focuses on education, explores important concepts such as: inclusive rather than separate learning experiences, and continuity of learning from early intervention of six weeks of age into the adult years.

Health care advances discussed in Section VI have opened new doors for people with Down syndrome. Today individuals with this genetic disorder live an average of 55 years, and some people with Down syndrome are reaching age 70 and beyond. Increased medical knowledge and successful treatment are enabling people with Down syndrome to take an active role in sports and recreational activities, to fully participate in school and at work and to grow into old age.

In the final part of the book, Section VII, we look at two areas which are very important for people living longer and healthier lives: independent living arrangements in the community and meaningful employment opportunities and achievement within the work force.

It is an exciting time for people with Down syndrome. New opportunities, new challenges and new successes are constantly being charted. Of course, no one can function alone. It is only when people with Down syndrome, their families, professionals, concerned individuals and the community at large interact together that the ultimate goals and dreams of people with Down syndrome will be achieved.

Lynn Nadel, Ph.D.
Donna Rosenthal, M.S.

Acknowledgments

The Fifth International Down Syndrome Conference, held at the Walt Disney World Swan Hotel in Orlando, Florida, was sponsored by the National Down Syndrome Society (NDSS) in cooperation with the European Down Syndrome Association (EDSA). The organization of the conference was handled by the staff of the Society, whose efforts made this international congress a memorable meeting.

The National Down Syndrome Society is deeply appreciative of the very generous support of: Ivory Soap/The Procter & Gamble Company, Barnes & Noble, Inc., Barnett Banks Inc., Consolidated-Tomoka Land Company, Woolworth Corporation, The Industrial Bank of Japan, Limited, Mr. and Mrs. Stuart D. Watson, Mr. and Mrs. James R. Maher, Mr. and Mrs. J. Barton Goodwin, Wick and Christine Allison, Mr. and Mrs. Jeffrey B. Haines, Martha Roby Stephens and Jane Cowles, Mr. and Mrs. Anthony Moulton, Canadian Down Syndrome Society, Rita and Tom O'Neill, The Eden Foundation, Association for Children with Down Syndrome, Inc., Fannie and Edward Baker, Kathleen Hanlon and John Cloyes, Down Syndrome Parent Group of Western New York, Inc., Constance McCashin and Sam Weisman, Mr. and Mrs. Craig Safan, Mrs. Charlotte Simmons, and Mr. and Mrs. Derk Zimmerman. Their contributions have made the conference and this book of proceedings a reality.

Course credits for this important program were provided by Columbia University School of Social Work; University of Arizona College of Education and Faculty of Social and Behavioral Sciences; and The University of California, Irvine, College of Medicine.

A very special thanks to Janet S. Brown, MSW, for her help and assistance with the book.

Additional information may be obtained from the National Down Syndrome Society, 666 Broadway, New York, NY 10012-2317. The telephone numbers for the Society are (212) 460-9330 and (800) 221-4602, and the fax number is (212) 979-2873.

I. Personal Observations

A Vision of the Future

Emily Perl Kingsley

The only way to have a view of the future is to take a really good look at the past. Then we can, perhaps, see where we've been, where we are now, and, maybe, where we want to go from here. When it has to do with young people who have Down syndrome, the future, in my view, can be expressed in two words: "expectations" and "opportunity."

My husband Charles and I started in this "Down syndrome business" 19 years ago, the day that our son Jason was born. We were given no expectations whatsoever. Some of you know this story and I hope you'll bear with me if you do. Sadly, this is not an unfamiliar story to a lot of you.

Our obstetrician took my husband aside and told him that this was a child who was never going to accomplish anything. This was a child who, he said, would probably never sit up, stand, walk, talk, or have any meaningful thoughts whatsoever. He would never recognize us as his parents. He would never be able to distinguish us from any other adults who were halfway nice to him. And the recommendation that he gave Charles was to institutionalize the child immediately and go home and tell our friends and family that the baby had died in childbirth.

This is about as rock-bottom a beginning as you can get. The expectations he gave us were nil. After the obstetrician gave Charles this terribly gloomy advice, Charles said one of his most brilliant lines ever. He said to the obstetrician "Okay, maybe my son will never grow up to be a brain surgeon. Maybe all he'll ever be is an obstetrician!"

I am not exactly sure what it took to disregard the advice of this man, but whatever it was, we summoned it up and decided to bring Jason home. And we brought him home with, as I say, no expectations for his future. Some time later, we were told by another doctor, "Well, it wouldn't hurt to talk to him a lot and stimulate him and surround him with color and music and input and so on," and see if we might not get some small accomplishments from this child. I didn't know what you say to a two-day old child who doesn't know any language yet, but they told me to just keep talking to him, so I tried to think up things to say. For example, I kept describing his wallpaper to him. As I was changing his diaper I would say, "Look at the flowers. See the flowers?"

3

This was a new wallpaper that we had put up that had gigantic red and purple flowers. In the interest of having maximum stimulation and color and input, we tore down the old, bland, pastel-colored baby wallpaper we had originally chosen and replaced it with wallpaper that had huge, brilliant, red and purple flowers. I kept saying to him, over and over, "See the flower, see the flower." Frankly, I didn't know what else to say. Then one day, when he was about four months old, I said, again, "See the flower," and he turned and put his little hand right in the middle of a big red flower. Now, I don't know whether this was totally accidental, whether he was just stretching, but to me, it was a message. It seemed to me as if he had internalized what I had been saying to him all those months and he was saying to me, "Yeah, Mom, I get it already. I know this is a flower. Let's go on to something else, huh?"

In any case, I went crazy. I jumped up and down and I started to cry and I ran to the phone and I called up Charles and I said, "This kid can learn! There's something in there! This is not a vegetable! This is a person! This is a person who can learn!" And that was the first day that, emotionally, I made the commitment to my own child. Up to that point, I was "going through the motions." But that was the day when I started to recognize that perhaps my son was a human being. Perhaps he was a person and an individual.

So, starting that very day, we intensified the stimulation and input and became almost obsessive about it. And Jason did very well. When he was about four years old, he was beginning to decode. He was able to recognize words that were printed on a page, spell them out, and occasionally even be able to put them together and pronounce them. This was pretty impressive stuff!

At that time, we were considering buying a home in a different town in our county. So we went to the head of the Special Education department of that town and we said, "We've got this kid. He's got Down syndrome. He's four years old and he's starting to read. What kind of classes and what kind of educational program do you provide for a kid like that?" The man, the head of Special Education, laughed and said, (and you have to forgive me, I'm about to use terminology which I swore would never come out of my lips again, but I only tell you this in historical context) "Don't be silly. In my 23 years of experience I've never yet seen a Mongoloid who could read."

At that point, Charles had another wonderful retort. He stood up and he said to this man, this "educator," "Listen, we're not looking for a guy with 23 years of experience. We're looking for a guy with three years of experience who's up to date!" And we turned on our heels and walked out. Obviously we did not buy the house in that particular town. I have to tell you that now, fifteen years later, this particular man has been "reborn." He advocates full inclusion and now chairs a task force on inclusive education! How this transformation was accomplished, I have no idea . . . but we are grateful for it.

At that time, 15 years ago, there were people who were adamantly taking the position that kids with Down syndrome were ineducable by definition. They maintained that it was not worth their time, effort, and money to educate these children. They would never need any education because the kids would never be able to accomplish anything anyway. And we've heard that story over and over again through the years. Sadly, I have heard that story in the last couple of days right here at this conference. And that's certainly one of the attitudes we all must work the hardest to overcome.

Our next step was to attempt to get Jason into a Montessori school. Even though the Montessori method had originally been designed for children with developmental disabilities, in America it had become a system that was very much in vogue for gifted and talented children. So to attempt to enroll a child with Down syndrome in a regular Montessori school was considered very revolutionary. We would take Jason to some of these Montessori schools and they were very impressed with him. He used the materials beautifully, had some very impressive skills, but, frankly, they were concerned mostly about the reactions of other parents. They were very nervous about how other people would react to having one of "our" kids in with their "typical, regular, ordinary" kids. One of the schools told us that they would love to have Jason come to their school, but they would have to charge us triple tuition "just in case he needed a little extra supervision." We thought that this was their not-too-subtle way of telling us, "Thanks, but no thanks."

Fortunately, we did find another Montessori school that was willing to take Jason. They had quite the reverse attitude, which was "Wow, what an opportunity! This is exciting! Let's see what we can do with this kid!" Which was exactly what we were looking for. Some time later, we found out that the parents of the other children in this school literally held a meeting trying to see if they could get Jason thrown out! I don't know whether they thought Down syndrome was "catching," that it was going to rub off. Perhaps they feared that the presence of a child with Down syndrome would adversely stigmatize their children "by association," the implication being that a class that contained a child who had Down syndrome would have to be a "retard class." I don't know exactly what their problem was. Whatever it was, it was based in fear, prejudice, and stereotype.

One day, when we were standing outside the school to pick up our kids, one of the mothers turned to me and said, in a terribly patronizing way, "I admire you so much. I spent nine months of my pregnancy praying that I wouldn't have a child like yours." Meanwhile, *my* kid was running rings around her kid academically!

Many of the things that we were fighting so hard for in those early days are now taken for granted. You don't have to fight for early intervention anymore. You don't have to fight for infant stimulation. It's not only taken for granted, it's the law. And we're beginning to see the trend towards inclusive education. We're hearing success stories about kids being educated in their regular neighborhood schools with their brothers and sisters, friends, and neighbors. This is becoming the accepted way—not everywhere yet—but for those of you who are on the threshold of these new movements, it's very exciting.

Those of us who missed that phase will always regret that we didn't have those opportunities. But, as I say, I am talking about "expectations" and "opportunities." And the opportunities for kids with Down syndrome these days are expanding and increasing tremendously. It can only get better and better.

Take a look at those six remarkable young people who spoke at the opening of the International Down Syndrome Conference. What an incredible display of ability and poise. And these are youngsters from a whole generation ago, historically speaking, kids from Jason's generation and, even older, who probably had battles to fight that were even more intense than the ones he had. And look at what was produced.

We will be dazzled by your kids, who are little now, growing up with the kind of programs that have recently been put in place. Of course, nothing is guaranteed. Each child is an individual and each child has his own profile, his own abilities, deficits, challenges, and raw material to work with. But if the opportunities are there, and if the expectations are there, then two thirds of the battle are over. All children, and especially our children, will do better if we work with them, educate them, and give them opportunities to grow, learn, and develop.

I've spent a lot of my life working in the media. I'll never forget the feelings that I had the night that Jason was born, when I looked at the television, sitting there, all by myself, after everybody had gone home after visiting hours. I felt as if I had fallen off the end of the earth. People like us didn't exist anymore. Everybody on TV was so "normal," they were so beautiful and healthy and perfect and superperfect. I think at that moment I realized that there are a whole lot of us out here who are not being spoken to.

At that time, I had been working for Sesame Street for a couple of years. We started examining the curriculum for its applicability to "children with special needs" and what were called "slow learners." So the impetus to incorporate people with all kinds of disabilities into Sesame Street actually began before Jason was born.

I was going to those meetings while I was pregnant, which is a kind of interesting irony. But when Jason was actually born, needless to say, what was previously an academic interest became a personal crusade. At Sesame Street, I am considered a great nuisance because I am constantly reminding them to remember to "get some kids with disabilities into that film, get the kids with disabilities onto the Street . . . ," etc.

But I am pleased to tell you that the people at Sesame Street are tremendously responsive to all of this. I can safely say that, until *Life Goes On,* Sesame Street was the only regularly scheduled program on television that regularly cast people with physical and mental disabilities on a regular basis without regard to their disabilities. And we are extremely proud of that.

Sesame Street is very committed to regular casting of kids with all kinds of disabilities including, of course, Down syndrome. The executive producer has promised me that kids with disabilities will appear on the show no fewer than two to three times every week. I encourage you, once this starts happening, to take a moment and jot a note to Sesame Street telling them that it's been noticed and it's been appreciated. I very strongly believe that we parents must write to people when they disappoint us, and we also must write to people when they do things for which we are grateful.

Parenthetically, Charles and I went off to the Epcot Center the other night. We went in to see the Captain Eo movie at the Kodak pavilion. The Captain Eo movie has a preshow while you are waiting for the movie to begin. They entertain you with a slide show from Kodak. And it is absolutely delightful, sort of.

It's from Kodak, so the photographic quality is superb. It consists of a series of photographs of "Americana." It starts with babies and then little kids, and the little kids grow up to be middle-size kids and then big kids and teenagers. They fall in love and they get married. All of the stages of life are captured in these photographs. They worked very hard to make sure that these photographs are ethnically and racially balanced, gender balances, all that kind of thing. But there is not one person with any kind of physical or mental disability in that entire slide show. It was disgusting.

People with mental and physical disabilities are the largest minority group in this country. They outnumber blacks, they outnumber Latinos, they greatly outnumber Asians. We are an enormous group that has not yet gotten our act together in terms of advocacy and communicating the kind of economic clout that we have.

I have a form letter in my computer that is a complaint letter about things like this—catalogs that come in that don't depict any kids or adults with disabilities, for example. Now, for the first time, we are beginning to see people with disabilities showing up in advertising catalogs. Macy's, Nieman Marcus, Target, K-Mart, and Walmart are now beginning to show an occasional person in a wheelchair, an occasional kid with Down syndrome. It's a pittance, but it's beginning. They are beginning to recognize that we are out there, in considerable numbers. Maybe the Americans With Disabilities Act has had something to do with this. I'm not sure. But the advertisers are beginning to realize that we are a sizable proportion of their consumer body. When I receive a large catalog that shows absolutely no people with disabilities whatsoever, I pull this letter out of my computer, print it out and send it off. All I have to do is insert the name of the offending company. I urge you to do the same.

If fifty of you go home and write a note to Kodak and Disney, and say, "It was a charming show, but where was the representation of America's largest minority group? It is an outrage for us to be totally excluded from a portrayal of Americana. We are part of America. We are entitled to see ourselves and it is an absolute insult for you to have left us out so completely. This only perpetuates erroneous stereotypes about our differentness, our strangeness. We insist that you begin to represent this enormous group of people as the ordinary, participating American citizens that they are! And remember, there are tremendous numbers of us and we can buy Kodak film or we can buy somebody else's film!"

This is an area where progress has been made, but not nearly enough. I urge all of you to write letters or postcards. It doesn't take long, and I promise you those letters are read and taken seriously.

When Procter and Gamble did the first Ivory Soap commercial that had a little kid with Down syndrome in it, we spoke to groups very much like this, and urged people to send thanks to Procter and Gamble. And in fact, here's another brilliant thing that Charles came up with. He encouraged people to send their thanks on the inside of an Ivory Soap wrapper. Wasn't that smart? What we were communicating to Procter and Gamble was that not only were we grateful for the commercials, but we actually went out and bought the product! The account executive for Ivory Soap said that that commercial generated more mail and more response than any commercial they had done in the history of Procter and Gamble! And, she said, "Do you know that people actually wrote to us on the inside of a soap wrapper!"

We can make things happen. We can change things. People with disabilities are America's largest minority group and, if we all spoke with one voice, we could make anything happen we wanted to. We have a lot of people in this room and we could do it. So I urge you, when you see something that you like, write a note. And when you see something you don't like, write a note.

To just wind up the "media section," we all have to pay homage to the extraordinary and unprecedented impact of Chris Burke on changing the way the world sees our kids! There are no words to adequately express our gratitude for the improvement in public awareness and attitudes that this one charming and talented young man has accomplished.

Back to our story. As Jason grew older, we had other obstacles to overcome, such as getting him into summer camps that were designated for kids with Learning Disabilities. We once had the director of a camp tell us, "Oh we don't take children with Down syndrome." When I asked, "Why is that?" he replied, "Well, we like our kids to be able to socialize." I said, "Yeah, so? That's exactly what we want for our kid." And he said, "Oh yeah, hmm . . . well . . . uh."

As it turns out, Jason did end up going to that camp, over the trepidations of this particular camp director. Of course, it turned out to be a huge success and everybody loved him and he integrated perfectly. And afterwards, they came to us and said, "This was wonderful. This was a triumph. We're really embarrassed that we were so concerned about this."

So, again, you have to be working on your expectations of yourself, of your kids, of the world around you. And give the children the opportunities—*make* the opportunities, force them if you need to—because once the opportunities are there and the kids are fully participating, the kids take over and everything is absolutely fine.

The most wonderful thing about what's happened over the last 19 years is that perhaps we are beginning, or the world is beginning, to see our kids as individuals. This is so significant. In the past, our kids were seen as members of a group rather than as individual people: "Oh, Down syndrome kids, they do this."

And speaking of "Down syndrome kids," one of the important improvements and one of the real indications of progress has been People First Terminology, which we certainly didn't see in the early days when Jason was little. Now it is pretty much taken for granted that we don't say "Down syndrome people" any more. Although I must say that there were a couple of times, in this very convention (those of you who are still using that terminology know who you are) that we continued to hear the old terminology.

I am here to remind you that the new common practice is that we refer to the *person first,* and the *disability second.* The Down syndrome does not define our children or adults. It is not their identity. It is only one thing about them. So I urge those of you who are not using people first terminology to start talking about "people with Down syndrome" rather than "Down syndrome people." I think there has been quite a bit of progress over the last several years in this area, and I think that will continue to improve in the future. But, as I was saying, we are now starting to see these kids as individual people, who are developing their own talents, their own interests, their own abilities, and this is very significant.

In our county we have a kid named TJ who's received a brown belt or an orange belt in karate. He's fabulous. He's competing against regular karate students and holding his own very beautifully.

Jason's gotten very interested in oil painting. He's doing some really nice oil paintings. He also had a couple of years studying the violin. Many of these opportunities might not have been made available to kids with Down syndrome before.

Mitchell Levitz has played competitive town soccer. There is a kid named Elisa who does beautiful needlepoint. All of these talents and interests are being encouraged.

We are beginning to listen to our kids. To ask them what they like to do, instead of just shuffling them off to activities that we think are appropriate for them. We're beginning to ask them what they want to do. To give them the opportunities to develop their own styles, their own interests, their own tastes, giving them choices. This is essential. You can't just determine that you know best what your kid likes to do, or that any professional automatically knows what's best for the kid.

This is a kind of deep philosophical issue. For example, what kind of work does your son or daughter want to do? People have traditionally taken the position that any job is an okay job; that we should be so grateful to have our kids working in any job at all; that it really doesn't matter what kind of job it is. Well, our kids have preferences and things that they're good at and not so good at, as well as things they prefer to do. Leisure-time decisions represent the same kind of concept. They may not all want to go bowling Friday night—some others might like to do something else.

As parents we have to give them opportunities for growth, and with that, needless to say, comes a tremendous amount of risk. And this is the scary part. In our family, we're working very hard to train Jason to use public transportation. In our county, if he wants to take a train from our town to Chappaqua to White Plains, it's no big deal. He can go the five stops to White Plains, get off, walk to the mall or wherever he wants to go. However, if anything goes wrong, if he falls asleep, or if he is daydreaming, if he doesn't get off at White Plains for any reason, the next stop is *New York City*, Grand Central Station. It's not where you want your child to be when he has Down syndrome and he's all by himself, until such time as you've trained him to handle that trip.

So what we did is this: took the train with him down to Grand Central Station in New York City. We had a very intensive lesson on where the police are and where the phones are and where the emergency Information Booth is and so on. But I understand that we're going to have to do that trip about ten more times until he totally understands it. At this point, I'm not ready yet for him to take the train down to New York City by himself, but I haven't written it off for the future.

I'm willing to recognize that this is something that I want him to accomplish. As difficult and painful and scary as it is, I am going to have to make the opportunity for him to experience this growth. The way you do that is to work very hard at building in good judgment skills, decision-making skills, and strategies for dealing with the unexpected.

This is one of the things that we often leave unexplored with our kids. That is, we teach them so well to do the things that they are supposed to do that they can do them in their sleep. What we don't often remember is to teach our kids how to deal with things when everything goes topsy turvy. For example, if you teach your kid how to ride on a bus, you also must teach your kid what to do if the bus goes some other way, or if the bus breaks down and they let everybody out.

They need strategies to handle the unexpected. This is really difficult, but we have to be very careful not to limit our kid's growth because of our own fears. A certain amount of that fear is reasonable and what we parents live with all the time. But we have to take that into consideration if our kids are going to grow and progress and become independent, which is what they want to do and what they have the right to do, and, ultimately, what we want for them.

Talking about opportunities for independent growth, I have to tell you about a young couple whom we counseled. The young couple was from Russia. They were living in New York. They had a tiny baby with Down syndrome and they came to our house to talk about what it was going to be like to raise a child with Down syndrome.

This young man told me afterwards that the most important thing that he was told in the afternoon that we spent together, the thing that really turned him around and made this a workable situation for him, was that I said to him, "I'm sorry you can't meet Jason. He's off traveling in Spain with a bunch of teenagers." The fact that Jason was able to travel to Spain on a teen tour was all he had to hear in order to know that this was a manageable thing for him and his family.

We were pretty nervous for that whole week that Jason was in Spain. And, yes, he did get lost once in Seville. He went off in a different direction from the rest of the group. But he found somebody and he asked for help and whoever it was got him back together with the group and it had a happy ending. And we were three thousand miles away. There wasn't a thing we could do. We didn't even know about it until after it happened. He survived it. He grew from it. We all survived it, somehow.

I can't overestimate the importance of parent-to-parent support—to be there for each other, to reach out for each other, to share knowledge and experience, feelings, our set-backs, triumphs, easier times. What we are doing is not easy, this adventure that we all share, this road we all travel. As all of you know, it often takes several steps backward to make one step forward. Fortunately, the steps forward ultimately do outnumber the steps backward. But, you know, there are really bad days sometimes, and these "bad days" are made easier when we share them with each other.

The steps toward independence for our kids have to start very early. This is something that we didn't always realize. Jason is now 19 and he talks about wanting to be independent, to be on his own. We're now starting to teach him independent skills which we probably should have started long ago.

I know this will sound familiar to you. You're trying to get out of the house. The kid's jacket needs to be buttoned up. You say to the kid, "Button your jacket." The kid starts fiddling with his buttons. He's not very good at it, and you end up saying, "Oh for Pete's sake, I'll do it for you so we can get out of here!" Your own impatience to get going overcomes your better judgment, which is to let the kid struggle with it and learn to do it himself. This is just one example of a million different things where we need to let our kids have the experience of doing things for themselves, all through their lives. If we don't let them learn these things for themselves, they don't have a prayer of ever becoming independent.

The bottom line is that we basically want the same things for our kids with Down syndrome that we want for our other children and for ourselves. We want them to have choices in life. We want them to have opportunities to realize those choices. All of this leads to a better quality of life. And I want to emphasize—and re-emphasize—that it doesn't matter how far they ultimately go. That's not what is important.

We are extraordinarily proud of the six young people who presented papers at the conference. Not all of our kids are going to reach those levels. The important, crucial thing, the only thing that matters, is that your kid has the opportunities needed to maximize whatever is in him or her. And that no kid is ever denied opportunities based on a label or a diagnosis. Every child has a right to develop as an individual to whatever level is "in" that child. It's up to all of us to create the opportunities, to insist on them, to battle, to go head to head against people who have negative attitudes and who don't provide the opportunities for our kids to learn and grow.

What's come from all this growth and progress and all of this ability to see our kids as individuals is that we are beginning to recognize that along with their individual skills and individual aptitudes, our kids also have emotions. They have feelings. They have the same range of feelings as everybody else. In the past, people assumed that our kids were very nice, very placid, very affectionate, very pliable. Well, you know, they not only have the same range of feelings, they are able to love, to give, to feel things very very deeply. But beyond that, they are grappling with an increasing awareness of their own situation, and their own disability. This means that they are increasingly susceptible to feelings of disappointment or even depression.

Our kids have a complicated and difficult challenge, coming to some kind of acceptance of the fact that they have a developmental disability. Think of yourself in a similar position. Would this make you sad and discouraged?

We can't shelter them from these feelings and we must be available to help them work through these complicated feelings. Interestingly, our kids can benefit from psychotherapy. This is something which has not really been made available to them all that much. But they've got some serious emotional challenges, especially when they come into adolescence and adulthood, that need to be dealt with.

I think we cannot look away from this. Because this area is so challenging and difficult, too many parents pretend that it doesn't exist and say, "Oh, he's happy, she's content." But it is important to be there and pick up the indications that our kids have more awareness than we thought they did, and that they are struggling with it. We really need to be there for them, to help them with their self-esteem, with their identity, because this is some really serious stuff.

The other thing that has grown up recently that we didn't have in the past, and this can only grow and increase in the future, is the whole Self-Advocacy Movement. The kids are beginning to speak for themselves! They are beginning to tell us what they like, what they want, what they need, what they're interested in. And it is important for us to listen to them and to encourage them in their efforts towards expression of their feelings and ideas.

I suppose all of you are aware that Jason and his friend, Mitchell Levitz, have written a book which is called *Count Us In: Growing Up With Down Syndrome,* published by Harcourt, Brace & Company. This book is part of the Self-Advocacy Movement. It is entirely, 100% in their own words. It has not been edited for grammar or syntax. It is exactly the way they dictated it, and their rather charming idiosyncratic way of speaking is preserved in the book.

In the book, Jason and Mitchell share with us their deepest, innermost feelings and hopes, dreams, thoughts, and goals. I think it is going to be a rare opportunity for the rest of the world to get a "window" into the souls of two young people with Down syndrome, and to appreciate the fact that they have all these feelings. One thing that's wonderful about the book is that these two young men come out as very distinctly individual personalities. It's really quite fascinating, so I encourage you to take a look at the book.

So, what have I learned in these 19 years? I've learned not to limit or put a ceiling on my expectations for Jason, to have dreams and goals for him, to do everything I can to guarantee the opportunities that will help to realize those expectations. And we are being pleasantly surprised every day. Whenever I am in doubt, I always try to ask an expert. And in this case, the expert is Jason himself.

Jason wrote a small section in *Count Us In* that I would like to read to you because it crystalizes what he wants people to know about himself. This is the message that he wants sent out to the world. In this little segment, which he dictated to me, he actually conceptualized a face-to-face meeting with that original obstetrician. Think about that. He imagined what he would like to say to the man who told him, on the day of his birth, that he had no future, that he'd never amount to anything. These are his own words:

> When I was born, the obstetrician said that I cannot learn, never see my mom and dad, and never learn anything, and send me to an institution, which I think it was wrong. If I could see my obstetrician and talk to him, here are the things I would say to the obstetrician.
>
> I would say, "People with disabilities *can* learn. Then I would tell the obstetrician how smart I am. Like learning new languages, going to other foreign nations, going to teen groups and teen parties. Becoming in-

dependent, being a lighting board operator, an actor, the backstage crew and going to cast parties."

I would talk about history, math, English, algebra, business math and global studies. One thing I forgot to tell the obstetrician is, I plan to get an academic diploma when I pass my RCT exams [New York State Regents Competency Tests]. I am studying hard to pass my RCT's.

I performed on TV in "The Fall Guy." And even I wrote this book. He never imagined how I could write a book. I will send him a copy of this book so he'll know.

I will tell him that I play the violin, that I make relationships with other people. I make oil paintings, I play the piano. I can sing. I am competing in sports, in the drama group, that I have many friends and I have a full life.

So I want the obstetrician will never say that to any parent to have a baby with a disability any more. If you send a baby with a disability to an institution, the baby will miss all the opportunities to grow and to learn in a full life, and also to receive a diploma. The baby will miss relationships and love and independent living skills.

Give a baby with a disability a chance to grow a full life, to experience a half-full glass instead of a half-empty glass. And think of your abilities, not your disability.

I am glad that we didn't listen to the obstetrician. If we tell the obstetrician about this, he will responded differently to all other families with a baby with a disability. And when he does that, then we will listen to him again.

We will send a copy of the book to the obstetrician. We will say, "See page 27." I wonder what he will say. I wonder if he will come to us and call us and what is his response, and we would hope he would say he made a mistake. His emotional feelings is feeling sorry, depressed and mistaken of people with disabilities. He will never discriminate with people with disabilities again.

And then he will be a better doctor.

I get overwhelmed every time I read that, not only because he has such a wonderful message of hope and self-affirmation in this piece, but because he is so entirely without bitterness. He's not angry at this doctor. I haven't forgiven this doctor yet, but, somehow, *he* is able to forgive. And all of this is in the interest of making this man a better doctor. So there is a generosity of spirit in this piece which I find very moving.

So what's in the future? We have new generations of kids who are being raised and being educated alongside their peers who don't have disabilities, who are being given opportunities to experience all of life's options, who are going to have the opportunity to develop emotional depth and a richness in their lives, who are going to have the support of Federal law in many important areas of their life in guaranteeing education and employment, who are going to have advocates like the National Down Syndrome Society, for example, who are working tirelessly to improve public understanding and awareness of our kids.

I think our kids are going to be seen, increasingly, as the individuals they are, with individual abilities that are going to be nurtured and enhanced. I think we are going to see that our children have individual talents that are going to be encouraged and nurtured. I think we are going to recognize that they have individual personalities to be appreciated, individual life styles to be lived fully and with gusto, just like everybody else. And, frankly, I can't wait!

Fostering Independence from Early Childhood

Montserrat Trueta

All children, including children with mental handicaps, must have access to a series of favorable conditions from birth onwards if they are to develop a positive self-image and independence.

Affective and educative needs must be met, understanding these as a need for normality—a principle easy to understand but very difficult to administer when we consider the condition of the child and the difficulties these inflict on the family, especially on the mother–child relationship. If the symbiosis between the mother and child is broken or cannot emerge, the child will not receive normal attention from the mother and the lack of close understanding between mother and child (sometimes due to the timing of reactions, which in the child with mental handicaps may be much slower) will hinder the process of individualization and the development of the child's sense of identity. This can result in the child developing distorted defense mechanisms, which can at times be more crippling than the actual mental handicap and can mark the life of the person far more than the organic condition of Down syndrome. The parent must have access to support services, which should provide care for the mother so that she, in her turn, can understand and provide care for the child.

When parents receive the news that their child has Down syndrome it is usually unexpected and provokes sadness, grief, and insecurity. The act of communicating the diagnosis to the parents requires a high level of sensitivity and tact. The doctor faces an especially delicate dilemma, and the form in which he communicates the diagnosis—when, where, to whom and how—will influence the environment in which the child is to grow.

Parents usually experience a deep feeling of grief for the loss of the child they were expecting and idealized during pregnancy. Before the birth the mother feels that she knows the child she is carrying. Instead, she is confronted with a complete stranger; at the same time she mourns the loss of the expected child.

The form in which the news is broken to the parents will have a decisive influence on their attitude and their subsequent adaptation to the situation. Three things are necessary for the parents to resolve their psychological crisis:

15

1. Correct cognitive perception of the circumstances.
2. The handling of affectivity through adequate verbalization and expression of feelings and sentiments.
3. The search for and utilization of help and support.

It is recommended that the communication take place as soon as possible after birth, with the two parents together and, when possible, in the presence of the child. Information inadequately given without tact or sensitivity will make the parent's process of adaptation to the new situation far more difficult and can have lasting negative effects on the child and the whole family.

Normalization—that principle so difficult to practice—is the key in progress, development, and integration, and implies a change in the general attitudes derived from preconceived ideas so profoundly rooted in the minds and traditions of our society.

For some parents, denial, defense mechanisms, and other personal, unresolved, problems come into conflict, and as a result parents can overprotect the child and show lack of confidence and expectations in regard to the child's development. Their anxiety makes them wish their child could always remain a child and, thus, they do not allow him or her to grow up.

The child or young person with Down syndrome is like any other person of his own age without Down syndrome, with the same expectations, necessities, and worries. As an adolescent, he or she goes through the same physical and emotional changes as any other adolescent. In order to give them the best opportunity to develop we must treat them as we would treat anyone else of the same age. This is easier said than done but is extremely important, as it means receiving normal treatment versus treatment that is abnormal, and therefore, distorting. We must ensure that the child receives an adequate upbringing and that behavior is managed from a very early age. As a piece of practical advice, I recommend that when in doubt as to how we should react to any given situation, we should ask ourselves: "If this concerned another son or daughter, how would I react? What would I expect? What would I do?"

For a child to develop normally we must have confidence in him and show expectations regarding the possibilities of his development. This implies allowing him the opportunity to learn by experience even though this might mean taking risks. Only by personal experience and practice can we grow and develop self-confidence. The child must be encouraged to choose and take part in all aspects of the situations that concern him. When children are young, parents normally control them and influence their decisions. As the child grows older, parental supervision becomes more lax. For the parent of the child with a mental handicap, it is more difficult to relax that supervision. This can hinder the development of the child's independence.

Another very important factor in the development of the person with Down syndrome is the self-knowledge of his or her personal condition. The child with an intellectual disability can begin to realize that he or she has difficulties from a very early age, and when school starts the difficulties become apparent as comparison with other children becomes inevitable. When the child starts to ask questions it can be very stressful for the parents, as it reminds them, once again, of their child's condition. They can become concerned as to how this stress will affect the child. Parents should be truthful and encourage the child to talk about his or her feelings, sensations, limitations, worries, and fears. They must answer naturally and they should help the child try to understand and adjust to his or her condition. For most parents it is a difficult task and, once again, they may need help. Some prefer to change the subject with the excuse that they do not want to hurt the child. Actually it is their own anxiety at having to discuss something that still hurts them that is the deterrent. For the child, it is a relief to be able to talk freely and openly of his or her worries, and if they get open answers it is far more reassuring and helps them construct a positive self-image. From the very beginning, it is important to be sincere, listen to, and speak to the child. It is the time to explain that he has Down syndrome and that this causes some problems that make learning more difficult. At the same time he must understand that his parents are proud of him and have confidence in him. But none of this is possible if parents do not love their child. Above all, they must show that they love and accept him for what he is, not for what they would have liked him to be.

For the young person with Down syndrome to achieve a positive self-image and a sense of identity that will lead to independence, he or she must have an active role in the adult world. This is the ultimate goal. If the child's personal development has been along normal chronological-age-appropriate lines, the development of a social role will also proceed naturally. In the more frequent cases where care has not been adequate during the two most crucial periods of life—early childhood and adolescence—then the assignment of a social role in the working world is the ultimate "therapy." According to Montobbio (1992), the role acquired in a vocational project exercises "contention" through which the person with a mental handicap is accepted for what he really is. It could be the first time that the person is confronted with a reliable, normal program, which, in the long run can calm his fears and his need for protection. He must learn to work in programmed progressive steps over the years, work that gradually becomes more difficult until "he will be what he is, at least in his working life" (Montobbio, 1992).

Throughout all this long process there must be a close collaboration between the parents, the helping professionals, and the person with Down syndrome. It is the responsibility of the parents and the helping organizations to promote the necessary services and other resources to support the families and to enable the person with Down syndrome to optimize his development so that he can demonstrate his capabilities and participate in society, thus becoming an active and productive member of the community.

I should like to end by saying that although in 1986 I graduated in psychology, no one has been a better teacher than my son, Andy.

REFERENCE

1. E. Montobbio (1992): "Il Falsose nell' handicap mentale." Edizioni del Cerro. Nov.

Inspiring Self-Esteem:
A Parent's Perspective

Marian Burke

I write as a parent, not an expert, to share with you my experience and those of my family in raising my son, Chris Burke.

In 1965 when Chris was born, there was very little outside assistance available to our family. My husband, Frank, our two daughters, Ellen and Anne, our older son, J.R. and I therefore bonded together to set a certain tone for his behavior, appearance, and manners if he were to join us in all aspects of family life.

Very few of us, and we were no exception, are aware of or give any thought to the world of the challenged, until we are plunged into it. Mainstreaming and inclusion were not even a thought when Chris was a child. Therefore, it was difficult to make the nonchallenged world aware of a person like Chris, who needs to be recognized and understood the same as anyone else, and for him to feel comfortable in the presence of all facets of society. So, in our own way we subtly pursued our own program. I remember Anne, our younger daughter, doing a science report on Down syndrome. It fascinated her classmates and made them aware that this was not a perfect world and that there were people who required our understanding, encouragement, and love.

Ellen, our older daughter, wrote a memorable poem in her English class, apprising the other students and the teacher of how her brother would not be Chris if he were not just as he was.

J.R., our older son, was Chris' sports coach for all his early years and as a result the average youngster in the playground realized there were more similarities than dissimilarities between them and Chris, as Chris learned to dribble a basketball and shoot baskets, hit a hockey puck, kick a football, and hit a mean baseball.

Frank and I made it a point to travel near and far with him. By near I mean to restaurants, Broadway shows, movies, sports events, concerts, church, and the Philharmonic. The exposure enriched him and introduced him to a cross section of society and that society to him.

By far I mean travelling to historical sites such as Williamsburg, Virginia, Gettysburg, and Washington D.C.; resort areas, including Key West, Disney World, Cape

Cod, and Nashville. Since Chris was a devotee of "The Love Boat," cruises in the Caribbean were a must. We even included foreign countries in order to visit Ellen and her husband, Jack, who is in the foreign service. So, Chris traveled to Bogota, Medellin, and Cartagena in Colombia, Poland (during martial law), and Vancouver, Canada. We had a wonderful time seeing so much through his eyes.

These were just a few ventures, but it was a beginning and it gave all of us a sense of purpose, direction, love, pride, and understanding, which I feel we transferred to Chris. We felt very comfortable with Chris and thus he felt at ease with the world we introduced him to.

It is interesting how well some things in life work out. Our daughter Anne married when Chris was only five and lived in the same housing development we were in, in New York City. Chris obtained his first lessons in mobility training as a result. Each of our apartments overlooked a common playground so when Chris wanted to visit Anne, a mere phone call put her on the alert and she would watch for his arrival and we would do it in reverse when he was coming home. It was a simple venture, but one that gave him a feeling of independence and accomplishment.

When it came to education, we were very fortunate that we found the schools we felt would give Chris the direction, discipline, freedom, and corresponding responsibility we had set the tone for at home. I felt it is so important that each child be placed in the most comfortable situation his or her parents can find. In Chris' case, the Special Ed schools he attended gave him the opportunity to become comfortable in the role of leader, and I believe he is the better man for it today.

Since both of Chris' schools were located out of town, the second phase of mobility training went into action. Most times, when Chris came home for weekends or vacations, he traveled on the Boston–New York shuttle. Of course, arrangements were made at the Boston end to get him to and from school, and we would be there to greet him or send him off at the New York end. He became quite an adept traveler at an early age.

When he transferred to the Don Guanella School in the Philadelphia area, his brother J.R. would put him on an Amtrak train and we would meet him at Penn Station in New York City. Somehow, comedian that he was, he would always manage to slip by Frank and me, go to the Station Master's office and have a message announced. "Mr. and Mrs. Francis D. Burke, your party is waiting for you at the S.M. Office." He just loved the excitement of putting one over on us.

Getting back to the actual education, we realized that opting for Special Ed schools is not a universally popular concept. But, there were two very important considerations when Chris was being educated. 1) The education offered us for Chris in the public sector was just as *ex*clusive, if not more so, than what we found at Kennedy Child Study Center, Cardinal Cushing School, and Don Guanella School. 2) We were as concerned about after-school activities for Chris as we were about academics, and this problem was resolved at the aforementioned schools. Sports and field trips were an every day part of the curriculum.

Integration and inclusion had to be and were accomplished in the social aspect of his life and in the community-based programs we sought out, such as bible classes, recreation programs, and library reading hours that were offered both in New York and at our vacation home on Long Island.

We have to make life as normal as possible for our special children. They are willing recipients of all the help they receive. We must make certain that parents, educators, legislators, and service organizations work together to continue this mission in life to assist our challenged children so they can enjoy a normal and productive life.

What gives us tremendous pleasure is to know that what we started as a simple family project has been enhanced by the role Chris has played in "Life Goes On." As a result, the world has been made to stop, take stock, and reevaluate the value of the developmentally delayed and other challenged citizens.

To see ordinary people in an airport pay homage to Chris is exhilarating for Frank and me, not because of the celebrity aspect but because it shows he has proven his worth and the worth of all his peers and he has opened minds, hearts, and doors to acceptability of our children for whom and what they are.

To sum it up, I truly believe we must accept our children as they are presented to us, then work hard on all facets of their education—at home, in the community, and at school—so they can be independent. We do this for our other children, why not for our children who happen to have Down syndrome?

The Magic of Family Empowerment

Patricia McGill Smith

I was absolutely delighted when I was invited by the International Down Syndrome Conference to write on this subject because of my newly adopted grandson, who is now 4 years old. My son and daughter-in-law chose to adopt Sean, who has Down syndrome, and our family just thought that it was just the greatest thing that ever happened.

I often address groups about empowerment of parents of children with disabilities. However, it's clear that everyone, not just his parents, was affected in some way by Sean's entrance into our family. And so, in this chapter I want to focus on family empowerment. By the time I get done you're going to have a whole new definition of family. Because when you embark on this work, or when you have a child with Down syndrome or any other disability, you enter into a family that you didn't know you had. At the conference, for instance, I sat down with people from Norway, Italy, Japan, the United States. We were from different cultures and countries, yet we all felt and shared a common bond. The bond of disability brought us together and held us close. The greatest things that we have in our families are the ties and the bonds that bind us together. I found this great big family after my daughter was labeled as disabled. I didn't understand it at the time, but when I went to work for an ARC in Omaha, Nebraska I had no idea of the sort of wonderland that I was entering. Because I mean to tell you we've got more adopted people in my family than you can shake a stick at. For instance, five of Jane's teachers are still a part of our family. They're a part of us. Dr. Cordelia Robinson, who was one of Jane's first teachers, is now the head of the University Affiliated Program for Persons with Developmental Disabilities in Denver. Every time she comes to Washington, D.C. she stays at my house. She spends time with Jane, my other children, and me. We really are a part of one another. So, when I talk about families, please know that professionals are also family members.

Over the years of my career, I have been so concerned about the care and feeding of fathers. I have thought so often that fathers were left out of this wonderful extended family. I lived through the period of time when the birthing of children was strictly a woman's business. Later, it became more of a joint activity of a husband and wife. Now we know how important it is for a father to be a part of that whole experience.

21

I have seen a great difference in the involvement of fathers and I credit some of that to the fact that the fathers now are a part of the birthing experience. I also get very concerned about brothers and sisters. They will, more than likely, outlive their parents and, in some cases, that means that they'll live with the disability of their brother or sister longer than anyone else in the family. I'll talk a lot about my family because they're the ones who have taught me. My daughter and now my grandson are the people who have taught me the most.

When Jane was born she had 6 older brothers and sisters. I often tell people that I have a Ph.D. in Baby because I held and nurtured so many babies. Things with Jane didn't seem to be just right from her first week of life. I started asking questions like "Can she see?" "Can she hear?" She didn't respond to noise, didn't roll, and didn't grasp.

Finding out about this child with a disability unfolded over a period of time. That was a long and lonely year. When that disability diagnosis came it was devastating. By the time it arrived I was already searching for answers. I was searching for someone to tell me about Jane. The doctors kept telling me that she was within the normal range. While it was comforting to hear that, I knew she should sit up but didn't. I knew she should roll over but didn't. I knew she should do all these things (and more) and so I kept asking questions.

When she was 7 or 8 months old we went to a specialist and he said Jane was "developmentally delayed." That meant nothing to me. I thought, "What's that?" I am so pleased that today if you have a child 7 to 8 months old that has been labeled "developmentally delayed" you get help. In 1970–71 the best they could do was promise me that when Jane was about a year old they could tell me more.

So, I took her to the doctor on her first birthday and he told me nothing. I was so upset at that time that I just went to the telephone book and looked up pediatricians. I eventually found this person that I knew was the pediatrician of pediatricians. It took me 2 months to see him so you know that he was really good. I remember he was as tall as I am because I stood very close to him to hold Jane as he checked her over. It took him only 12–14 minutes. He looked me right in the face and he said, "Mother, this is simple. This child is retarded."

I guess in some ways I was ready for that diagnosis because I was seeking so hard to find an answer. However, when the diagnosis came it felt like a black sack came down over my head. You feel like someone cut you off at the knees or something. I don't remember driving home. I don't remember anything more of that day.

The following day we were supposed to go to a wedding. We're Irish Catholics and we have a lot of kids, cousins, relatives, and friends. What did I do? I did what my mother taught me long ago. When a crisis hits, just do whatever you were supposed to do. Therefore, we all went to the wedding.

It was a pretty distressful day for us. Nobody wanted to talk or look at us. I can remember some of the people touching me and I remember talking to my mother. I remember her saying that it was good that Jane didn't look retarded.

My family and friends were all worried about money. I always laughed because we never had any money. Whatever expenses Jane brought with her, we would be no worse off than before. They worried about lots of things but no one really worried about Jane. They were all worrying about me and Jane's daddy. The memory of that day is sort of a blur. I bet that everyone of you can remember a day that was a blur, or 2, 4, 10, 20, or more.

During the reception my brother came to me and said, "There's a man in the corner over there that would like to talk to you. His name is Joe Friend. Why don't you go and talk to him. He has a son with retardation. He's in a state institution but Joe thinks he can help you." I went over to that corner and I've always been so grateful ever since. The Friends were the first people that gave me hope. They talked to me about programs. They talked to me about people who could help us. They talked to me about the future. They even had the audacity to say that the day would come when we would be grateful for Jane's birth.

Joe Friend didn't tell me that day that he was President of a local ARC. He didn't have me sign up for membership. We didn't have to sell honey. We didn't have to do anything. They just helped us unconditionally. They treated us like family.

In the weeks that followed our family grew. A woman named Fran Porter called me and kept saying, "Get help! Get help!" But we were in the rock and rot stage. We just stayed home and rocked a while and did nothing. About 4 weeks later two or three other parents contacted me and, like Fran, implored me to "go and get help!"

I kept calling the doctor back. All he said was that Jane could grow and she could learn but not to do anything till she was four or five. I wanted help now! Finally, in desperation, I walked into a University Affiliated Program called Meyers Childrens Rehabilitation Center and just said "I need help." We have been getting help ever since. My new family members helped me take that first step.

Jane is now 23 years of age. I started talking to groups when Jane was four. I had little choice in the matter. My husband was ill and we needed food, so I applied for a job as the Coordinator of Pilot Parents in Omaha, Nebraska. I didn't think I would get it but I did. Like many of you, I moved from being a parent at home at my kitchen table to being a parent/professional at a desk. I began working, although I knew so little of what I was trying to do. However, I knew a few things and the few things I knew that day I know today. I know that it is absolutely imperative for the parents of children with any type of disability to get help at the earliest moment possible. The help of another parent is crucial.

I met a woman from Canada, and I asked her if they had Pilot Parents of Canada in her town. She replied, "Oh yes! The day after my baby was born a Pilot Parent came to my hospital and talked to me." I smiled and said, "I know about that."

The Pilot Parent movement started in the early 1970s in Omaha, Nebraska. I didn't think it up, but I was the lucky one to be hired as the executive at that time to try to help it grow. Just like Joe and Jenny Friend were able to help me that day, I had the privilege of helping many other parents to join the disability "family."

I could spend this entire chapter discussing what happened to me that first day, that first month, that first year, and those first times when you turn someone around. But for a moment I would like to focus on my belief that the longer parents languish in isolation, and are not helped through contact with other parents, the more damage occurs to them. Some of you may have met such parents. They may even be older than myself and yet, they are still bitter, angry and hurt over having a child with a disability.

Just as parents can be isolated, so can families. As I said before, Jane has six older brothers and sisters. The first four are boys. Those four boys, from the very beginning, were very protective of Jane, just as they were protective of their other sisters. There is a 15 year spread between these seven children and so the older ones have always looked out for the younger ones.

When I started to work outside the home, Jane was three and a half or four years of age. I never really had asked the children how they felt about being Jane's brothers and sisters. So one day when I was working on a sibling program, I came home and I started asking each one of my children, "What happened to you when Jane arrived on the scene?" My young son Paul, who is now an attorney in Atlanta, said "Well mom, I hate to give you the bad flash but I was 14 years old and all I could think of is who needs it and who wants it and what are we going to do with her?" He said, "I hated it. I was starting high school. Who wants to have a sister who's retarded?" I wish you could see his family empowerment and advocacy for her today. When I'm gone, he's going to take care of everything that's legal, like wills and money. Another of Jane's brothers, Mark, is a psychologist. He was 15 at the time. He wasn't paying much attention to the family, but he didn't like her much either. One day when he was in the depth of his own problems and I was trying to take care of Jane, someone said to me, "You've got to think of something positive about this older son of yours." I said, "I can't think of anything positive about him." His psychologists said, "Yes you can! Think of one thing that he does well." I thought for a long time and I said, "He's good with Jane." They said "Good! Start there. Every time he does something good with her, reinforce that." Mark taught her to give me five! He taught her to count raisins. Today, Mark is the father of my grandson Sean, the young man who has Down syndrome.

Family empowerment works! It starts with the immediate family. The way the immediate family treats the person with a disability is how the world is going to perceive him or her. When Jane was diagnosed the doctor said, "Oh that big family, they're going to be wonderful!" and I thought to myself, boy, is this guy stupid! This family is a millstone around my neck. All I could think of was how am I going to take care of Jane and meet the needs of six other children.

I learned then that family members key off of the parent(s) in the family. Through another extended family member, Dr. Rounos Simenson, I became empowered to believe that I could change Jane's situation. Dr. Simenson was just starting his career at the time, and had developed a program for Jane. Through his efforts, Jane learned to respond to verbal requests such as "touch your ear." I did everything he told me. It seemed that I never had time enough to really work with Jane. Her brothers and sisters were running me around in circles. Jane was progressing anyway. She could touch her nose, clap her hands, and do other things when asked.

I sat down to work with her one day and heard her babbling ma-ma-ma-da-da-da-da. I suddenly, very badly, wanted her to say ma-ma and know that was me. This need drove me to teach Jane by rewarding ma-ma, every time she said it, with Cheerios. She picked up on ma-ma quickly and we went on to other names. By the next time we went to the doctor, Jane could say Mama, Daddy, Mark, Paul, Jeanne, and Tricia.

This was the first time I designed a program for Jane. Through her success, Jane empowered me. Through my program, Jane was empowered. Over time, the empowerment spread. One day I looked around my living room and saw the neighborhood kids all in a circle playing with Jane. All of these children were part of Jane's teaching team. I used to laugh and say they were like a bunch of miniature speech therapists. By now, everyone in my ever-growing family was teaching Jane something. That's how we began. It's been going on at our house ever since.

I've tried to reflect on things and figure out how it happens. There are the bonds of love, but some of the lessons are hard to learn. Learning about the dignity of risk was hard. We just had to let Jane go and grow. We learned that teaching doesn't just happen. It takes dedicated time and dedicated people. Over time, the empowerment that started with me spread throughout most, if not all of the people who came to know Jane.

My family is empowered. My family includes blood relatives, siblings, parents, professionals, paraprofessionals, and now Jane's work colleagues. We are all part of the same family. Let's get about the business of empowering each other. There's no time to lose.

.

II. Behavior

Perspective

David McFarland

I've been asked to tell you about myself, what I do, my dreams and goals, and any advice I wish to give you.

As you know, I have lived with Down syndrome all my life. The living part is great, but changing attitudes is tough going. After I completed my education in segregated schools, I decided to try a regular high school system. Math, English, and science were taught. But I graduated with my secondary school diploma. Some people thought that I would be a senior citizen by the time I was finished. I also completed a cooking course at Joyce Brown College. Acting has been my main employment. It's difficult to find roles, since most stories do not include people with disabilities. The roles that are most challenging for me are the roles in which the person has very limited abilities. It's challenging because I want to make sure I portray the person with dignity. My second source of employment has been a regular guest speaker at two universities. I speak about four times a year at each university to students and the faculties of education and social services. A small portion of my income comes from my financial portfolio. I became interested in my own finances through the ads at my bank and the recessions of the 1980s.

Physical fitness is important to me. I play hockey with special sticks and I also swim. My swim specialties are free style, back stroke, breast stroke, and a butterfly. Sometimes I figure skate with the university skating club, and I am working on ballroom dances. I am also an amateur coach with the club. I use the university athletic complex for fitness, swim, and ballroom dancing.

I voted since I was 18 and have had the uneasy experience of being summoned for jury duty twice in three years. The first time, I read the summons. Some of the questions: "Are you blind?" I wondered how someone who was blind could read that form. There was another question that said, "Do you have a mental handicap?" I don't know. I have Down syndrome. I appeared for jury selection both times. I wasn't chosen, but the lawyers had to acknowledge me. As an advocate on behalf of the Metropolitan Toronto Association for Community Living, I had the opportunity to be a witness at an inquest. A person with Down syndrome was killed in a traffic accident. And some people in the community felt that people with disabilities should use only special buses. The inquest jury supported my testimony

27

that people with handicaps do and should have the right to use public transportation. Since 1981, I have been meeting with a group of young adults who have Down syndrome. We're part of the National FAA, the Future Adult Advisors. We've been working on improving our social and problem-solving skills. We've also been learning how to attend conferences. The major concerns are employment, housing, and further education. As far as my goals are concerned, I have already achieved many of them. My dreams are a little more difficult. I visualize the time when my friends and I are capable of choosing the right careers and have the skills to maintain the environment, and also to be able to manage our own lives. We need your understanding and skills to do this. We need to be given the time and the chance required to achieve our dreams.

You know what? Sometimes I wondered what it's like not to have Down syndrome. I wondered what I would look like. I wondered if I'd be a scientist studying the 47 chromosomes that affect my appearance and slow my rate of learning. Ladies and gentlemen, we both have a lot to learn, and let's learn from each other. Thank you very much.

Understanding Behavior in Its Developmental Context

Ian G. Manion

> When she is good she is very good, but when she is bad she is horrid!

This quote may well have originated from a famous English writer, but was used more recently by a primary school principal to describe the behavior of a 6-year-old child with Down syndrome. In many ways it captures the variability in behavior that can be seen both within and across children with Down syndrome, the myths and prejudices that can exist regarding such behavior, and the consequences that behavioral difficulties can have in all aspects of the child's life. It is important to improve our understanding of the behavior of children with Down syndrome as it has a direct impact on our attitudes towards the disorder, the way that we respond to these children in our roles as parents, professionals, and members of the community, as well as on the educational and social opportunities that are available to them.

This chapter focuses on the behavior of children with Down syndrome from birth to puberty. The goal is to place behavior into a developmental context while looking at specific behavioral strengths, deficits, and excesses that may be associated with Down syndrome. The key role that parents and significant others play and the importance of having developmentally age-appropriate expectations for the child with Down syndrome are stressed.

UNDERSTANDING BEHAVIOR

Definition of Behavior

The term behavior can have different meanings for different people. In this chapter the term is used in the broadest sense to encompass the behavioral, emotional, and social functioning of individuals across environments and situations as well as over time.

Behavior problems are typically described in terms of behavioral deficits and excesses. Deficits refer to those behaviors that a child should be able to do, but does so inconsistently, with varying degrees of difficulty, or not at all. Potential behavioral deficits that have been described in certain individuals with Down syndrome include:

29

self-help skills (e.g., eating, toileting), academic skills, language, social skills, appropriate play, motor skills, short-term memory, auditory–motor processing, attention span, problem solving, and safety discrimination. Excesses refer to those behaviors that are considered to be inappropriate due to their nature, frequency, or the circumstances in which they occur; they typically are disturbing to others and/or dangerous to the child. Potential behavioral excesses observed in children and reported by parents include: attention seeking, habits and rituals, overactivity, aggression/destructiveness, wandering away, undifferentiated displays of affection, noncompliance, and general stubbornness. Emotional difficulties such as worries, fears, and sleep difficulties are not at all uncommon in children with Down syndrome and can be added to the more general list of behavioral concerns.

The negative impact of behavior excesses and deficits can be both direct and indirect. Inappropriate behavior may lead to rejection by other children. Certain behavior problems such as running off or poor safety discrimination and problem-solving skills are likely to cause parents to restrict play outside of the home thus, limiting play contacts and activities for the child with Down syndrome (Byrne et al., 1988).

It is inappropriate to look at such problematic behavior without considering the various behavioral strengths displayed by individuals with Down syndrome. In many cases these include: general sociability and acceptance of others, sensitivity and empathy, artistry and creativity, and a strong sense of family and community. Such strengths are often overlooked in our appreciation of the individual with Down syndrome. These qualities contribute to the very positive impact that individuals with Down syndrome often have on their environment and the people in them.

Down Syndrome and Behavior: Myths and Stereotypes

Individuals with Down syndrome historically have been described as sharing a common temperamental style with clear and predictable patterns of behavior. Children with Down syndrome have been labeled as being uniformly affectionate, placid, docile, and gentle, with a good sense of fun, as well as being very self-willed and stubborn. The danger in such stereotypes is that it becomes easy to restrict oneself to looking only for these characteristics and even inadvertently reinforcing them. This can be true for behavior at home, school, or in public places. By focusing on the stereotype, it is very easy to lose track of the individual child.

A great deal of research in Down syndrome has focused on such questions as: "Is there a typical personality type in Down syndrome?" "Are these children different behaviorally from those without Down syndrome?" "Are individuals with Down syndrome at risk for significant behavioral and emotional problems by virtue of their diagnosis?"

Earlier research for the most part painted a fairly bleak picture of Down syndrome. It is important to note the inherent bias, as this research focused on lower-functioning, under-stimulated individuals in institutions who had great limitations on most aspects of their lives. More recent research has demonstrated the benefits of the stimulation and nurturance available in normal home environments, not only on the children's cognitive abilities but also on their social, emotional, and behavioral functioning.

Current research on the behavior of children with Down syndrome benefits from being more systematic, with a more sophisticated approach to measurement. Comparisons are made in this research to the behavior of siblings, to that of others with a developmental delay not associated with Down syndrome, and to children without such delays. It is common (approximately 75%) for parents of children with Down syndrome to report some behavioral difficulties at some point in their child's development. The incidence of severe behavioral difficulties, however, has been assessed to be roughly equivalent to that seen in the general population of children (8–15%) (Cunningham, 1988). This research suggests that, while there may be a higher prevalence of certain types of problems with certain children at certain ages, no clear "Down syndrome personality" emerges.

It is now clear that there is considerable individual variation in developmental progress, behavior, and general temperament across individuals with Down syndrome. The temperament of infants and very young children with Down syndrome has been demonstrated to be very similar to that of other children. Temperament refers to the basic behavioral style of individuals. In infants and young children this is characterized by their activity level; regularity in their biological functioning (hunger, sleep, bowel movements); readiness to accept new people and new situations; adaptability to changes in routine; sensitivity to noise, bright lights, and other stimuli; whether a child's mood leans towards cheerfulness or unhappiness most of the time; intensity of responses; distractibility; and degree of persistence. Based on these characteristics, different temperament types have been identified including "easy," "difficult," "slow to warm," and "intermediate" (Chess et al., 1976). The proportion of infants and children with Down syndrome falling into each of these types has been found to be roughly equivalent to that seen in samples of normal children. Huntington and Simeonsson (1987) evaluated a sample of 12–36-month-old infants with Down syndrome and found that 42% could be classified as "easy," 16% as "difficult," 13% as "slow to warm," and 29% as "intermediate." This compares well with Fullard et al.'s (1984) sample of nonhandicapped infants where 38% were classified as "easy," 12% as "difficult," 6% as "slow to warm," and 44% as "intermediate." The similarities between the groups with respect to temperamental style are important to note. In addition, the individual differences within the group of infants with Down syndrome reminds us of the heterogeneity of this population.

Influences on Behavior

Differences in personality and behavior are attributable to a variety of factors. These include environmental influences, the individual child's mental and physical abilities, inherited characteristics and genetic makeup, as well as changes associated with general development.

Environmental influences include such things as the qualitative aspects of the home and school environments as well as social opportunities and community perceptions and reactions. These environments provide opportunities for stimulation and learning through exposure and modeling as well as consequences for appropriate and inappropriate behavior. In the same way that the environment can recognize effort and the development of responsible age-appropriate behavior, attention to less desirable behaviors (even negative attention) can contribute to it recurring. Behaviors that are "cute" in a 4-year-old with Down syndrome may be very inappropriate in other situations or at a later age.

Behavior is influenced by mental and physical abilities. Limitations in problem solving, attention, and/or communication skills in children with Down syndrome can lead to less appropriate ways of dealing with conflict situations and often higher levels of frustration. There is great variability however in the levels of cognitive and physical abilities among children with Down syndrome, with relative weaknesses in some being the strengths of others. Particular physical difficulties (e.g., hearing and visual problems) can further alter the everyday experiences of the child with Down syndrome, affecting not only their mood but their ability to comply. An example would be a child who has chronic sinusitis due to a congenital nasal malformation. The resulting headaches will affect attention, mood, and motivation across all situations.

At a more basic level, behavior can be affected by genetic and inherited characteristics. Individuals with Down syndrome are as likely as any other child to inherit temperamental characteristics from their parents. Although much behavior is learned, temperamental style and general personality are more likely to be innate. Also, there are differences that are more closely associated with the chromosomal abnormalities present in Down syndrome. These affect physical attributes as well as cognitive abilities. Certain behavioral problems (i.e., toileting) can be more directly linked to the developmental delays typically associated with the chromosomal disorder.

Finally, we cannot overlook the very important changes associated with normal development and how they impact on behavior. As children with Down syndrome grow older they acquire new knowledge and experiences that further shape their behavior. Children with Down syndrome are not immune to the physical changes associated with puberty, including the hormonal changes that can affect mood and behavior. Often, however, they may be less well equipped cognitively and/or emotionally for these changes. We cannot underestimate the impact of such changes on parents who strive to cope with the various challenges associated with raising a child with different needs.

Stages of Development and Behavior

There appear to be key developmental challenges associated with different stages of development that can increase our understanding of the behavior of children with Down syndrome at different ages. Infants with Down syndrome have been described as quiet and unlikely to be difficult. On average they cry less, sleep more, and are less demanding than other newborns. Many of these babies have poor muscle tone and sleep more than other babies, making feeding more challenging. Typically, such problems are overcome with time, allowing for healthy and normal attachment relationships to occur. By three months of age, babies with Down syndrome, for the most part, resemble other babies.

Preschoolers, including those with Down syndrome, show great variability in temperament. The behavior of children with Down syndrome, however, is generally similar to that of children at a similar developmental level. That is, their actual level of cognitive, physical, and adaptive functioning may be more similar to that of a slightly younger normal child and the behavior that they display is more likely to fit this pattern as well. Although communication and individuation/separation are often the main challenges at this age, there appear to be fewer tantrums in young children with Down syndrome initially. The terrible twos do exist for these children but they may manifest themselves as the terrible three to fives. As in other children, once children with Down syndrome become more mobile and able to explore their own environment, behavioral challenges increase. At the same time, frustration at not being able to express their wants, due to difficulties with communication, can precipitate behavioral difficulties at this age (and beyond). Paying attention to the child's speech and language needs at this age and providing more effective means of communicating (e.g., some functional signs) can decrease everyone's frustration.

School-aged children with Down syndrome typically are interacting more with the outside environment. It is a time of testing their own limits and the limits of others. They still have the curiosity of much younger children without necessarily having the judgment and problem-solving skills of their chronological age group. Generally, they are slower at reacting to what is being requested of them, due to a combination of auditory processing and attentional difficulties as well as noncompliance. Wandering off, attention seeking, and noncompliance are not uncommon at this age. Children with more significant communication problems and with more numerous minor health problems (e.g., upper respiratory and ear infections) appear to be at greater risk for developing behavior problems (Sloper et al., 1988). Children with Down syndrome are as susceptible to developing the behavioral, emotional, and psychiatric difficulties that might begin to appear in other children of the same age. It has been suggested that children with Down syndrome may be more inclined to display the impulsivity, distractibility, and overactivity associated with a diagnosis of Attention Deficit Hyperactivity Disorder, although the attentional difficulties may be qualitatively different and have different etiologies. This is an emerging area of clinical and research interest that will be important to follow in the years to come (Green et al., 1989; Pueschel et al., 1991).

Although the focus of this chapter is birth to puberty, these early experiences provide the foundation for the social, emotional, and behavioral functioning of the adolescent and adult with Down syndrome. Communication and reasoning continue to improve with age, although the opportunities available to the individual with Down syndrome may not necessarily keep pace. The individual's awareness of his or her own abilities or disabilities increases as each person faces the developmentally appropriate issues of identity formation and increasing independence. The potential for emotional problems during this period is the same for the individual with Down syndrome as for others facing the challenges of day-to-day living. Children, adolescents, and adults with Down syndrome can experience problems with anxiety, depression, conduct disorder, grieving, and general coping with life.

Parent/Child Interactions and Behavior

Parents' attitudes towards the diagnosis of Down syndrome, their general style of parenting and behavior management, and the expectations that they have for their child are all key elements in the psychosocial development of their child and in the family's ability to cope with the behavioral challenges that may arise.

Parent/child interactions are truly a two-way street, with both parties bringing their own coping strengths and liabilities to the mix. Accordingly, all that is going on in the parent's life will influence how that parent interacts with the child with Down syndrome, which in turn influences the child's behavior and how that child will cope. It is important, therefore, for parents to attend to their own needs and to deal with stressors that may be unrelated to the child with Down syndrome, as these will have an impact on individual, couple, and family functioning. Parents of children with Down syndrome experience quantitatively more stress than many other parents, although the majority cope very well with this stress. When parents have more difficulty coping, as evidenced by increases in marital distress and parental depression, their families also display more behavior problems.

MANAGEMENT OF BEHAVIOR

Being a parent is a difficult job at the best of times and dealing with the behavioral difficulties of a child with a developmental delay can tax anyone's skill and patience. The majority of parents whose children with Down syndrome display behavioral difficulties have good management skills. They are good parents in a more challenging situation. The following suggestions can be viewed as ways of "fine tuning" existing parenting skills.

Maintaining a positive approach to parenting is paramount as it fosters a sense of competence in the parents, a supportive atmosphere in the home, and helps to build on strengths and to develop the child's independence and self-esteem. It is important to remember that most behavior is learned, whether it is appropriate or inappropriate. What has been learned can also be unlearned; it is often easier to promote appropriate behaviors through praise and attention, thus allowing fewer opportunities for inappropriate behavior, than to focus solely on the elimination of problem behaviors.

Parents and other caregivers should consider the child's developmental level and should not underestimate each child's potential. If there are no expectations for a child to learn adaptive behaviors, then it is unlikely that the parent will provide the opportunities for the child to develop them. Exposing the child to tasks that are age-appropriate, even if acquisition may take longer, will give the child the opportunity to develop a feeling of accomplishment and may also decrease the burden felt by parents who would otherwise do everything for the child.

It is important to be as consistent as possible in the expectations for the child and in the consequences that follow both appropriate and inappropriate behavior. The importance of consistent routines cannot be emphasized enough, as they provide the child with a consistent learning experience and decrease the need to test limits. Consistent routines should not be equated with a regimented lifestyle, as opportunities for play and self-expression are important aspects to development as well.

Consistency should extend to all those involved with the child (e.g., daycare providers, teachers, siblings, extended family) and entering each situation with a commitment to communication and collaboration will help maintain such consistency.

When fostering the development of a new behavior, or working on the elimination of a less appropriate behavior, it is important to focus attention on one behavior at a time. This decreases the load on both the parent and the child and allows all to build upon previous successes.

In spite of everyone's best efforts and intentions, behavioral difficulties are likely to arise. It is very important to pay particular attention to the nature and parameters of the problem behavior. In other words, what exactly is the behavior that is of concern, when did it start, and how often does it occur. It is equally important to consider the precipitating factors that may have triggered the behavior and the consequences that might be maintaining it. Sometimes these factors have less to do with the child directly and more to do with the family as a whole (e.g., change in family routine due to change in parent's work schedule).

The remediation of behavioral difficulties often requires creativity on the parents' part and parents should not hesitate to seek suggestions from others who have experienced similar problems. Often a change in the environment is sufficient to decrease its occurrence (e.g., child-proofing a home).

Finally, parents should not ignore their own stress, as it will interfere with their ability to deal with conflicts involving their child in an adaptive fashion. The way that parents cope provides a model for the child with Down syndrome as well for other children in the family. Coping with these issues sometimes requires parents to seek additional support. Friends and informal support networks of parents having similar experiences are important sources of ideas and encouragement. Parents should not hesitate to seek more formal supports for more chronic or severe individual coping problems or child behavior problems. It is easier to rectify a new problem than to change a chronic pattern of behavior.

SUGGESTED READINGS AND REFERENCES

Baker BL (1989): "Parent Training and Developmental Disabilities." Washington: American Association on Mental Retardation.

Baker BL, Brightman AJ (1989): "Steps to Independence: A Skills Training Guide for Parents and Teachers of Children with Special Needs" (2nd ed.). Baltimore: Brooks.

Becker WC (1971): "Parents are Teachers." Champaign: Research Press.

Byrne E, Cunningham CC, Sloper P (1988): "Families and Their Children with Down Syndrome: One Feature in Common." London: Routledge.

Chess S, Thomas A (1987): "Know Your Child." New York: Basic Books.

Chess S, Thomas A, Birch HG (1976): "Your Child is a Person." New York: Penguin Books.

Cunningham C (1988, rev. ed.): "Down's Syndrome: An Introduction for Parents." Cambridge, MA: Brookline.

Cunningham CC, Sloper P, Rangecroft A, Knussen C (1986): "The effects of early intervention on the occurrence and nature of behaviour problems in children with Down syndrome." Final report to the Department of Health and Social Services. Manchester, UK: University of Manchester.

Essa E. (1983): "A Practical Guide to Solving Preschool Behavior Problems." Albany: Delmar.

Fullard W, McDevitt SC, Carey WB (1984): Assessing temperament in one- to three-year old children. J of Pediatr Psychol 9:205–217.

Green JM, Dennis J, Bennets LA (1989): Attention disorder in a group of young Down's syndrome children. J Ment Defic Res 33:105–122.

Hanson MJ (1986): "Teaching the Infant with Down Syndrome: A Guide for Parents and Professionals." Austin, TX: Pro-Ed.

Huntington GS, Simeonsson RJ (1987): Down syndrome and toddler temperament. Child Care Health Dev 13:1–11.

Meichenbaum D (1983): "Coping with Stress." Toronto: John Wiley & Sons Canada.

Meichenbaum D, Jaremko M (1984): "Stress Prevention and Management." New York: Plenum Press.

Meyer D, Vadasy P, Fewell R (1985): "Living with a Brother or Sister with Special Needs: A Book for Sibs." Seattle: University of Washington Press.

Patterson GR (1971): "Families." Champaign: Research Press.

Powell TH, Ogle PA (1985): "Brothers and Sisters: A Special Part of Exceptional Families." Baltimore: Brooks.

Pueschel SM (ed.) (1987): "New perspectives on Down Syndrome." Baltimore: Brookes.

Pueschel SM (ed.) (1978): "Down Syndrome: Growing and Learning." Kansas City, MO: Skeed, Andrews, & McMeel.

Pueschel SM, Bernier JC, Pezzullo JC (1991): Behavioural observations in children with Down's syndrome. J Ment Defic Res 35:502–511.

Rottenberg BA, Hitchcock S, Harrison ML, Graham M (1983): "Parentmaking: A Practical Handbook for Teaching Parent Classes About Babies and Toddlers." Menlo Park, CA: The Banster Press.

Selikowitz M (1990): "Down Syndrome: The Facts." Oxford: Oxford University Press.

Sloper P, Cunningham CC, Knussen C, Turner S (1988): "A study of the process of adaptation in a cohort of children with Down syndrome and their families." Final report to DHSS.

Turnbull HR, Turnbull AP (1985): "Parents Speak Out: Then and Now" (2nd ed.).

Whelan E, Speake B (1980): "Learning to Cope."

Aspects of Behavior from Birth to Puberty

Anna Zambon Hobart

For almost twenty years in Italy, children with a disability have been included in the compulsory school system. This means all children between the ages of three and 14. Special schools and nursery schools for the disabled have all but disappeared, and self-contained classes for the disabled in public schools were finally eliminated in 1980. Legislation dating back to the 1970s limits class size to 20 children, including one child with a disability. Supplementary support teachers and therapists are provided for these classes. They include speech and language therapists, physical therapists, psychologists, and so on. The law assigns local responsibility for coordination between the schools and local public health units. The shift from special schools to inclusion also entailed changes in the objectives and methods of the entire educational system.

Today, twenty years later, people with a disability in Italy are more a part of the community than anywhere else in the world. Full inclusion has proved to be a mutually enriching experience for people with a disability and for the rest of us as well.

Our team was formed in 1977, and consists of school and clinical psychologists, doctors, social workers, and parents. In the course of these years we have seen an average of 210 families a year, and we have followed these from the Rome area for several years. It was clear from the onset that inclusion gave children with a disability a chance to express their individuality. We soon realized by observing their behavior in different contexts that except for the extra chromosome, a psychomotor delay, and particular somatic features, people with Down syndrome had nothing else in common. The time had come to set aside statistics as well as laboratory data, tests, and research done on special schools and institutions, and observe their behavior in the most natural context, which is among their normal peers.

Only 8% of children and young adolescents with Down syndrome included in the elementary and junior high schools of Rome show behavior problems, according to interviews of teachers in 1991, as compared to 12% in 1985 and about 20% in the previous years. The improvement is due to additional experience in how to cope on

37

the part of the teachers. Eight percent is a minority. Nevertheless, we will describe some elements at risk in the early years that might become problems around puberty or later.

The development of the love-object relationship of children with Down syndrome follows the same stages as that of any child and is, in a few cases, even more rapid (Zambon Hobart, 1991).

We have observed children with excellent social behavior, and some who were obstinate, aggressive, and hard to handle. I should like to say a few words about these later, because their parents most often come to us for help when they reach the age of puberty or after. I believe that these are children who had great difficulty in making a successful psychological separation from their mothers, children who find it hard to differentiate themselves from their mothers and function as autonomous individuals with a clear and separate identity.

Studies in baby and young-child observation and clinical psychoanalytic work have shown that the process of differentiation and individualization involved in a child's psychological growth consists of emerging from the symbiotic sphere that envelopes mother and baby at the beginning of life.

As Margaret Mahler says, it is a kind of symbiosis in which the baby together with the mother feels as if it were part of an omnipotent system, "a dual unit within a single boundary" (Mahler et al., 1975). There is a lack of distinction from the mother, fusion and confusion with her, and it is only gradually that a baby begins to differentiate and understand that it is a separate being. The understanding that he or she is separate is also connected with the development of motor skills. As a child grows, he or she is gradually less fused and confused with mother. When a baby is held in the mother's arms and begins to stiffen and draw back to have a better look at her, the baby starts to differentiate at an intrapsychic level as well.

The early experience of symbiosis is extremely important for children with Down syndrome. They are less physically independent because of their global delay, and this may entail greater and longer-lasting psychic dependency with aspects of fusion and omnipotence. They remain for a longer time amalgamated mentally as well as physically with the mother. The baby's sense of omnipotence comes from the mother, who is experienced as the omnipotent source of all pleasure and all discomfort. A mother feels great tenderness for a baby who smiles at her and thus reassures her that this is truly her baby. This tenderness may coexist with an altogether natural sense of rejection for this child who is so different from what was expected. This ambivalence may, in turn, foster in the baby a sense of ambivalence within the fusion. The contradictory aspects of this early phase may well survive subsequent stages of development and take the form of attacks on the mother alternating with moments of great tenderness.

These features of omnipotence and ambivalence may emerge and persist, and in some cases they may create problems in the future. Some parents encourage a child's early exploration of the surrounding world. Other parents may collude with their child's symbiotic needs and discourage any attempt at psychic separation, perpetuating the child's sense of fusion. A child's first steps are away from mother, not towards her, and this may arouse anxiety in her that the child also feels (Mahler et al., 1975). Some parents may think that their child is mentally as well as verbally mute and use their words, their hands and their intelligence as a kind of auxiliary ego for the child.

The child's reaction will also depend on his or her individual constitution. Very few children do not develop a capacity for independent action. In such cases, we have always found some preexistent difficulties in the home environment. However, the great majority of children display socially acceptable behavior, have a degree of self-sufficiency, and make distinct progress in speech when they enter a normal nursery school. But some children soon begin to behave in ways that arouse concern about their future development. These children may alternate aggressive behavior with moments of tenderness, especially with the mother. They are described by their parents as children who always want to run away. They are obstinate and provoking, but they are also extremely affectionate. It was very interesting to note that in the great majority of these cases (children from the age of two until the end of elementary school), when we asked the parents how the child behaved at school and in other people's homes, they gave us a different and much more positive image, an image also confirmed by the teachers. We are collecting interesting data on such behavior differences.

The great capacity of people with Down syndrome to adjust their behavior to different settings from an early age and into adolescence and adult life made us wonder how these defense mechanisms worked. A child who is self-sufficient in nursery school, who feeds himself and obeys the rules and then goes home to behave in an obstinate and omnipotent way, is a child who is trying with difficulty to get out of the symbiotic orbit, and to become a separate individual. For whatever reason, the child may feel suffocated by a situation that seems to block growth. It is as if he or she were saying, "you treat me like someone with Down syndrome—I'll show you!" The defense mechanism here is essentially the child's use of the disability in an omnipotent way. In extreme cases, this omnipotence may be more damaging than the primary disability.

We think that the problem of omnipotence and ambivalence arising from the long period of symbiosis in the mother's arms is connected to the need to touch that is often lying in wait. Children and young people with Down syndrome often live in a world that is extremely tolerant of inadequate behavior on their part. In the early days of inclusion, we often saw nursery school teachers holding children with Down syndrome on their laps, while the rest of the class proceeded with their normal activities. Often a child with Down syndrome would come into a classroom and be greeted with exaggerated enthusiasm, and the child's achievements celebrated more than those of the other children. Such teacher behavior is now extremely rare.

A child with Down syndrome is often given a "place of honor" at home, with family friends, and in a host of other social contexts, and has to make much less of an effort than others to be the center of attention.

We have also observed children around the age of three, who are quite sociable with their companions without disability, become unusually curious or very cautious on first meeting another child with the syndrome, as if they recognized each other's being different. What does this being different mean to a child who has the syndrome? Clearly it is not what it means to the child's parents. In the early years it may mean something that allows the child to conquer the world with far fewer obstacles than other children have. At this point he or she may not yet have understood that the difference is a disability, and may think it is something quite precious that his or her siblings ought to have too. We have seen jealous siblings create some disability for themselves to get more attention from their parents. One little four-year-old asked his parents, "when I get Down syndrome, will I be able to sleep with you?"

A survey was conducted in 1985 of 110 children with Down syndrome in elementary schools in Rome. Their teachers used the words "friendly" and "helpful" in 88% of the cases to describe the attitude of classmates towards their companion with Down syndrome. In 12% of the cases in which children with the syndrome behaved in an omnipotent way, the attitude of their classmates was described as "patient," "tolerant," or "indifferent."

One mother said that her ten-year-old son was lying on the sofa watching television instead of straightening up his room, "I can't," he said. "Why not?" she asked. "Because I am different." "Different how?" "Don't you realize I have Down syndrome?" "You have Down syndrome when it's convenient for you!" was the mother's reply. Many parents understand that their child may be using the syndrome for his or her own convenience. Other parents may consider any inadequate behavior as a function of the syndrome and fail to react (Zambon Hobart, 1991).

It is our opinion that excessive duration of infantile behavior in children with the syndrome is closely linked to the way the child experiences the problem of identity. As a child grows up and develops an individual personality, he or she begins to realize that he or she has a disability.

Much more often than one would expect, parents believe that their children don't know they have the syndrome. It is as if they think, "You don't need to know, I know it for you." And this denial only perpetuates the symbiotic fusion of infancy. These parents, wanting to protect their children, deny the truth and submerge them in a world of falsehood.

Parents who can speak of Down syndrome with their child may be very reassuring, because they make it clear that they too have accepted the reality of the situation the child has always lived with. This enhances the child's sense of identity and fosters a clearer and more serene sense of self. Sometimes this does not happen, and then the parents' denial becomes denial on the part of the child as well. Thus, there is a present and future risk of being submerged in a world of omnipotent fantasy, while having to deal with an everyday world that seems increasingly unacceptable. There may appear early signs of depression that can even take a dramatic form at some time in the future. The contrast between an omnipotent and infantile self-image—as an astronaut, for example—and a disabled self that cannot even tie his or her own shoe laces may cause psychic pain that has the same matrix of depression any of us could experience.

We have observed an extremely interesting difference between depression in a person with Down syndrome and a person with no disability. Some depressive symptoms in a young person with the syndrome seem to be closely linked to the immediate situation and hence easier to deal with. Worried parents come to us for help around the time of puberty. One of their worries is that sexuality may burst forth without sufficient control by the mind. Their concern is absolutely unfounded according to research we conducted in 1985 on 50 students included in junior high schools in Rome. Parents with this concern may try to prolong the preadolescent period and block the child's demands to be respected in his or her capability to function as a separate individual.

The reactions of adolescents with the syndrome may be more unexpected and more dramatic than those of young persons without a disability, but their inadequate behavior may be more reversible. A person with the syndrome has fewer defense choices.

He or she may suddenly stop communicating. The parents of an adolescent boy came to our office because their son had not spoken or listened to them for some months. They were afraid this was some kind of incomprehensible Down syndrome behavior. While we talked with the parents, the boy went into the next room, and a social worker asked him to help make photocopies that were needed right away. The boy had been treated as if he were a competent adult, and he responded with great efficiency. What is more, he had a long conversation with the social worker, all to the great surprise of the parents. Three years have gone by since that day, and the young man, who turned out to be very creative in the kitchen, is now writing a cook book.

On another occasion parents were terribly worried because their fourteen-year-old daughter had refused to go to school for a week. She stayed in bed all day and even ate her meals in bed. She kept the television on all the time and would not speak to her parents. They were afraid her mind was deteriorating because of the syndrome, and they felt helpless. In the course of our conversation, however, it emerged that for some time the girl had wanted to be allowed to go to school by herself. It was a twenty-minute walk, and all her classmates went to school on their own. But the mother insisted on accompanying her. The daughter reacted in a way that we have seen in many cases. It was as if she were saying to her parents, "if you treat me like a little child, then I'll act like a baby." The next day the girl went to school by herself.

A boy memorized the shopping list his mother wrote for him so he would not look like a child who has to show the grocer the shopping list. This boy, like many of his contemporaries, is forced to make a great effort in order to be treated with the respect due his chronological age. The dramatic intensity of an adolescent's defenses (stopping communication, refusing to leave the house, tearing up clothing, refusing to eat, etc.), may be connected to his or her difficulty in expressing suffering in another way. Therefore, this may not necessarily represent an irreversible psychiatric problem or a problem connected with Down syndrome. Further research is needed in this direction.

In conclusion, the great majority of our children and young adolescents with Down syndrome do not have behavioral problems. When problems do arise, they may be worked out by using a clinical approach similar to what we would use for such problems in "normal" children or adolescents. However, there are some potential risks in all cases. There is the risk of prolonged symbiotic fusion with the mother, and its concomitant features of omnipotence and ambivalence. In their early years, children may make an intelligent use of their disability as a secondary gain. In later years they may use their disability to "punish" their parents if they feel their needs for independent growth are not being respected. From adolescence on, an important source of psychiatric problems may be confusion about identity, when a person with a divided self-image is forced to deal with an unsatisfactory quality of life.

REFERENCES

Ferri R (Ed.) (1987): "Il Bambino Down a Scuola. Seminario di Studi. Roma, Ottobre 1985." Bergamo: Juvinilia.

Ferri R, Spagnolo A (Ed.) (1989): "La Sindrome di Down." Roma: Il Pensiero Scentifico.

Mahler M et al. (1975): "The Pyschological Birth of the Human Infant. Symbiosis and Individuation" New York: Basic Books.

Regione Lazio—ABD (1991): "Analisi dei Bisogni e Rispondenza dei Servizi Territoriali." SDN #1.

Zambon Hobart A (1991): "Sviluppo Sessuale. Il Problema dell'Identità" Roma: Quaderno ABD #14.

Social Life, Dating, and Marriage

Roy I. Brown

INTRODUCTION

This chapter begins with some commentary on interviews with people who have Down syndrome and are married. They are in their 30s and 40s. In each instance the other partner does not have Down syndrome but has some disability, e.g., cerebral palsy.

Vignettes on Marriage and Partnership

Pat and Jim. Yes, I got married a long time ago. '73 I think. Got engaged a long time ago. Married 14th February, don't remember—19th, Valentine's Day. Met at rehab center. Date I got engaged decided I wanted to get married—a long time in-between. Went out on picnics and go places in the city. He asked me to become engaged. I said yes. To get married. I said yes. *[Why did you say yes?]* Oh, I liked to be married. Do things together to do other things. Before married lived in a group home. *[What do you like about marriage?]* Happy, nice, do things, do stuff, listen to music. *[Was it different from before marriage?]* Oh yes! *[How?]* I don't know. I like to be with him most of the time. Feels better, just part of life. *[What do you mean?]* Well it's up to the woman or man. Can't put this in words. Feels good to marry if date someone. *[What's it like?]* Go out in the evening, get groceries *[Are there rows?]* No. *[Do you get cross with each other?]* No, once he scratched me but it was an accident. He's good to me. Jim buys me everything. He chooses clothes. I choose clothes. Get groceries together. Both do cooking. *[Thought of having children?]* No, I can't have any. I had operation. Good idea. *[Would you want a child?]* No. *[Does Jim want one?]* No. Jim was married before. *[Tell me what it was like to get married.]* Lots of gifts—beautiful. Wanted to get married like my sister. I'm an auntie and that is all right. Minister marry me. Cousin was bridesmaid. Great grandmother was there. Mum stayed in Texas. Jim's mum had passed away. Brothers and sisters didn't come. Had a white dress—I still have it. Have an engagement and wedding ring but I can't get it off. Jim was sick and I had to look after him and see he eats right and everything. Now's he's better and a big stomach already.

Jane and John. They live in a basement apartment in a pleasant city area. They

43

have someone in to clean and the owners of the house are professionally involved in the field of disability and provide some voluntary support. They say Jane and John are the happiest married couple they know.

Jane says: I cook the meals and bring it to him. Get $810 per month from government. *[Is it enough money?]* Oh, it's plenty. Having a living room, bathroom, bedroom, and kitchen. *[Do you love each other?]* Of course, have to love—in the heart. Everybody loves who's married. *[If he is not there?]* Then, I hurt. We hug. *[Is it good to hug?]* Yes. *[Why?]* I feel better. We get angry, have cross words sometimes. I vacuum—he does the dishes. My money goes to mother. She thinks I'd spend it all. I would! When I got married I got more friends. When we go out he walks ten paces ahead of me. He's the timekeeper!

Gretchen and Joe. They live in a basement apartment.

He took me out for coffee and to a fun park. He asked me to marry him. I said yes. We got married in his church—lots of brothers and sisters came. I wore white. He had a blue suit. It was exciting cutting the cake *[they were married about 4 years ago].* We had a woman preacher. We have someone in to clean. We both cook. We go to a local bar together. We get pizza.

[The wedding photos came out and each of two volumes were fully described. He works in a bottle depot and gets $32 to $37 a week, supplemented by government funds. They have their own bank account. Each statement she made she checked with him. She often put her arm around him or touched him. She knelt beside him while he sat on the seat. The house was full of cards and drawings strung across the living room. The bedroom was full of female pinups, which I was proudly shown. This interview was set up by a mum who belongs to the Ups and Downs Group, and has a very young son with Down syndrome. She was excited to see this home and the relationship. She said it showed her what was possible!]

After the wedding we went on a honeymoon to Disney World. We both had cameras. We had a pet cat called Tiger. Joe decorated the Christmas tree. *[We were shown the photograph.]* Joe took me out for my birthday. *[Although Gretchen did most of the talking, she kept on saying "ask Joe." Joe could not talk very well but by the continual reference to Joe he became included in the conversation and took the lead in showing us the apartment.]*

There are other stories. One of an initially happy marriage where the wife had Down syndrome and the husband a minor handicap and a job. They had two children, one of whom has cerebral palsy. The couple have just separated.

Donna was married and is very competent. She has a job and volunteers for a Down syndrome group. She felt her husband was abusive and made sexual demands she did not appreciate. She decided to leave the marriage and is presently doing very well and has little further interest in partnership.

ADULT DEVELOPMENT

The change in our expectations for people with Down syndrome has changed enormously over the past 30 years. In the early 1900s, the average life expectation for people with Down syndrome was only 9 years. By the 1950s, most people with this condition were reaching their 50s, and today 1 in 10 may be expected to live to 70 years of age (Selikowitch, 1992). Medical intervention, the move towards a more normal lifestyle within the community rather than institutionalization, and the availability of a range of behavioral and social interventions have probably all combined to produce this greater longevity. But this brings new challenges. First, greater longevity for people with Down syndrome means the majority of parents will be outlived by their child. Parents therefore are faced with either arranging for additional support through a group home or other residential arrangement, and are likely to seek guardianship and trusteeship to look after their son or daughter after they have died. There is another way of looking at this challenge. Given a normal life expectancy approaching that of the general population, the person with Down syndrome should be provided with a normal lifestyle and be prepared for this. This includes the prospects of dating, partnership, and marriage (Edwards, 1988).

The aim of this chapter is to underline issues relating to such development. Social learning over the lifespan becomes critical, and there is now sufficient evidence to indicate how this might be put into effect, and that marriage and partnership can be rewarding and successful for people with Down syndrome.

LIFESPAN AND QUALITY OF LIFE

It is important to take a lifespan approach built within a quality of life model where consideration is given to all aspects of living—school and education, social skills, home living, employment, and leisure and recreation. It is critical to recognize that such an approach is not made up of sudden events and interventions but thousands of small issues, concerns, and interventions. It requires attention to a wide range of minor experiences that need to occur on a regular and "experimental" basis. We know that adolescents who are disabled are more dependent on parents, for example, in setting bedtime, providing wake-up calls, agreeing to use of the telephone, controlling friendships, selecting school attendance and activities, than adolescents of similar age who are not disabled. The range of opportunities and the practical experience of choice are critically limited for those with Down syndrome (Brown & Timmons, 1993).

Human growth is based on accumulation of knowledge, including experience, and the transfer of that knowledge to every area in which the individual functions. Many of the challenges confronted in the field of Down syndrome arise from specific skill training given in artificial environments that restrict opportunities for broad-ranging experiences and diminish opportunities for transfer of skills. This problem of transfer has been noted in the literature for many years (Ward, 1990). The individual with Down syndrome should, from birth, be provided with as natural an environment as possible in which a wide range of stimuli are experienced. Thus, schooling should be in regular classrooms with opportunities to learn and practice in the home and local community. For these reasons, segregation in special schools and classes or adult training workshops is likely to inhibit social and recreational development. Obviously, only some of these areas can be discussed in this chapter. The particular examples are taken from 1) the field of self-image, 2) leisure and recreation, and 3) friendship, social network, and relationships.

THE DEVELOPMENT OF SELF-IMAGE

Brown, Bayer, and Brown (1992) found that many adults with developmental disabilities, including people with Down syndrome, developed poor self-images over the years. Such individuals found it difficult to make friendships, probably because they were inhibited in terms of exploring their environments and making relationships in an appropriate fashion. In this study individuals showed decreased self-image in perception of their skill attainment in 18 areas of functioning (such as reading, budgeting, and making friends). The same individuals were then given opportunities to take part in much more normal relationships in the community through a quality of life choice model, where the individuals selected the activity in which they wished to be involved, the environment in which they wished this learning to take place (often this was the home of the individual, either living with their parents or other people with disabilities) and the person who would work with them (they were able to choose their partner, intervener, or teacher from a reasonably wide range of personnel available). These interventions, which took place over several weeks to several months, resulted in considerable development. Not only did individuals perceive themselves as improving in objective terms, it was possible to measure the amount of improvement correlating with their perception. Perhaps even more startling was the improvement in activities where intervention was not taking place. The conclusion was that when intervention took place within natural situations with choice, individuals started to learn more effectively, with a parallel improvement in their self image. The latter then positively affected a wide range of other activities. This is a cost effective way in which to carry out rehabilitation (Bayer, Brown & Brown, 1988). Such intervention must, by its very nature, be coordinated with the family. Reasonable risk-taking and collaboration are essential.

LEISURE AND RECREATION

One area of interest was that of leisure and recreation. Persons with Down syndrome tend to spend a large proportion of time in spectator activities with relatively little involvement in physical, social, and self-actualized activity, where individuals make their own choices and plans. The relative lack of these activities probably has major effects on adult development. For example, data in the Brown et al. study suggest that individuals with Down syndrome probably started reducing their frequency and breadth of activity in recreation during their twenties. The factors causing this decrease, however, probably commenced in earlier years, because individuals did not function in natural environments, and in some cases it was possible to observe the encouragement to carry out only sedentary or spectator activities (e.g., "this keeps them quiet"). It is essential that a stimulating environment with broad-ranging activities in leisure be increased over the years. This could also play a role in terms of improving health, expanding motivation and also improving self-image for individuals who would then function in empowering environments.

RELATIONSHIPS

Parents and professionals recognize that the lack of developing friendships represents a major stumbling block to full integration in the community. Attempts have been made to promote friendships, often to no effect. Parents, in desperation, have sometimes paid people to perform as friends. Yet in the Brown et al. (1992) study once relations started to develop, other positive experiences followed. For example, individuals would invite another person with a disability to go for lunch or dinner with them. Individuals indicated that they recognized that others did not have the same opportunities as themselves. In one instance the individual said "I took her out because Joan is handicapped like I used to be."

The quality of life model put forward suggests that the development of self-image, including natural environments and natural choices, provides an atmosphere that enables friendship, dating, and partnership to take place. There have also been a number of studies that suggest ways in which this can be further encouraged. Friendship is more likely to develop if it is first recognized that young people with Down syndrome have the same needs, interests, and concerns as other adolescents. Among those with Down syndrome there is great variability as with any group of young people. For example Bibby and Posterski (cited in Denholm, 1993) showed that among normal teenagers "friendship, music, mother, girlfriend or boyfriend, stereo, father, dating, television, sports, and reading" were ranked in this order for the top ten sources of greatest enjoyment. In terms of valued goals, friendship was at the top of the list, and this was closely followed by "being loved," along with "success in what the individual does" and "having freedom." Although goals were noted, the above stress the importance of natural relationships, the importance of high self-image, and the requirements of family life and choice. Some activities and environments are more suitable than others in promoting friendships. Firth and Rapley (1991) list political action, singing, acting, social dancing, special-interest clubs, and church. There are also activities and encounters that do not promote relationships. These include going out for coffee or a meal, mall walking or shopping, spectator sports, and bowling. Many of these "poor opportunities" for friendship development are common activities for people with Down syndrome.

There need to be changes towards more social and mobile situations where relationships can more easily develop. In such empowering environments a positive self-image can develop, and such activities enhance other attributes, including effective language and social skills. The development of relationships, however, implies not just successes but also the learned ability to accept failure or rejection. As one mother noted (Lawrence et al., 1993), by being in a normal environment with normal opportunities, her son had learned how to accept rejection. The thrust is towards the development of normal and spontaneous relationships and this is unlikely to occur by providing paid "friends" as companions or by relying on professional staff.

Many people with Down syndrome refer to professional staff as their friends, probably because these are the relationships that they find most acceptable and commonplace in special services. Again, Firth and Rapley (1991) and Brown et al. (1992) recommend and practice the development of social opportunity in natural environments guided, as needed, through skilled professional field-workers who understand that the goal is towards normal relationships. Therefore, activities where people with and without disabilities can meet in a nonformal social setting are to be encouraged. Some structure is required. For example, Litchy and Johnson (1992) describe how it is possible to set up dinner meetings where people come together to discuss their experiences and their aims for the future, thus promoting a discussion of experience while encouraging future orientation and forward planning.

In the development of relationships, long-term associations may follow. That these can be successful is shown by the vignettes described earlier. What is important about these relationships, as in all normal relationships, is that they provide a means of supporting individuals in a friendly and loving environment with the opportunity to capitalize on each other's assets rather than isolating each person to survive on their deficits. In the vignettes, examples of this material support can be seen. Individuals turned to each other, partnered each other in activities, and shared or partitioned responsibilities between them. The development is only likely to occur if there are regular opportunities for giving, sharing, and experiencing. Individuals need to learn how to deal with the negatives of relationships as well as the positive, not only as receivers of behavior, but also as presenters of behavior. For example, to be able to forgive is seen by normal adolescents as a very important characteristic. To not embarrass other people is also seen as highly relevant. Such learning does not take place by regarding people with Down syndrome as different, but rather recognizing that, though infinitely variable among themselves, they have more in common with other people than differences. It is in the normal development of family life with support and help that development can take place.

PLANNING

The above represent some of the specific ideas about and examples of the development of relationships, but the challenges facing each individual and family are different. Because of this, Lawrence et al. (1993) suggest a format for planning that requires bringing together a few friends and professional supporters to help the family, and particularly the individual, make a detailed plan for social, friendship, and partnership issues. It is important that the young adults have representatives of their choice with whom the parents also feel comfortable. Commitment to the agreed plan is essential. The planning or support group will need to help the individual resolve issues or revise plans as issues arise. Such a model provides a network, helps the individual to make decisions, extends responsibility to the young adult, and relieves parents of some of the pressures of continuous parenting. Some of the references included in this chapter provide further ideas and resources for this type of action and problem solving. The aim is not to force choice on the individual, but to encourage individuals to provide their own choices while the group provides the processes through which the goals may be achieved.

ACKNOWLEDGMENTS

I am grateful to Ms. Laurel Griffen, who provided some of her experiences and suggestions. She had Down syndrome. I also recognize with thanks the input of the marriage partners who provided the commentary on Down syndrome and marriage.

REFERENCES

Bayer MB, Brown RI & Brown PM (1988): Costs and benefits of alternative rehabilitation models. *Aus. & NZ J Dev Dis* 14(3/4):277–281.

Brown RI, Bayer MB & Brown PM (1992): "Empowerment and Developmental Handicaps: Choices and Quality of Life." Toronto: Captus Press; London: Chapman and Hall.

Brown RI & Timmons V (1993): Quality of Life—Adults and Adolescents with Disabilities. *Exceptionality Education Canada* (in press).

Denholm CJ (1993): Developmental needs of adolescents: Application to adolescents with Down syndrome. In Brown RI (Ed.): "Building our Future. The 1992 National Conference of the Canadian Down Syndrome Society." Calgary: Canadian Down Syndrome Society and Rehabilitation Studies, the University of Calgary.

Edwards J (1988): Sexuality, Marriage and Parenting for Persons with Down Syndrome in Pueschel SM (Ed.): "The Young Person with Down Syndrome: Transition from Adolescence to Adulthood." Toronto: Brookes.

Firth H & Rapley M (1990): "From Acquaintance to Friendship: Issues for People with Learning Disabilities." Kidderminster: BIMH Publications.

Lawrence PL, Brown RI, Mills J & Estay I (1993): "Adults with Down Syndrome: Together We Can Do It! A Manual for Parents." Ontario: Captus Press and Vancouver: The Canadian Down Syndrome Society.

Selikowitch M (1992): Down syndrome: The facts. In Brown RI (Ed.): "The 1992 National Conference of the Canadian Down Syndrome Society," pp. 3–25. Calgary: Canadian Down Syndrome Society and Rehabilitation Studies, the University of Calgary.

Ward J (1988): Obtaining generalization outcome in developmentally delayed persons: a review of the current methodologies. In Brown RI & Chazan M (Eds.): "Learning Difficulties and Emotional Problems." Calgary: Detselig.

The Myth and Realities of Depression and Down Syndrome

Louis Rowitz and Elaine Jurkowski

A major myth in the area of disability is that people with Down syndrome are always happy. Accompanying the myth is a stereotype of a happy child with Down syndrome. The stereotype does not look beyond childhood, nor does it consider the complex quality of life issues that concern people with disabilities and their families throughout life. This myth homogenizes a whole group of people with Down syndrome and argues against the diversity that is possible when the lives of people with disability are viewed more comprehensively. This chapter makes certain assumptions that immediately call the myth into question. First, people with Down syndrome live long and often productive lives. Thus, Down syndrome is not only a problem of childhood. Second, people with Down syndrome have different life experiences; they are not all alike. Third, and perhaps the most controversial assumption, not all people with Down syndrome are happy all the time. People with Down syndrome have mood swings like all people without Down syndrome. The realities of life bring with them all the emotional turmoil that day-to-day community living engenders. All people experience emotional highs as well as emotional lows. This means that all people are depressed at times. Thus, the critical dimension of any discussion of these mood changes relates to the extremes of the mood changes.

Depression is not an uncommon problem. It has been estimated that 50% of the general population will experience depression during their lifetime (Canadian Mental Health Association, 1992). While this incidence rate may seem high, the prevalence of disorders that exist but are never treated is also significantly high, as has been documented in a number of classic epidemiologic studies (Hollingshead & Redlich, 1958; Srole et al., 1962; Bland et al., 1990). While these studies have been used to project the actual prevalence of depression within the general population, epidemiologic studies relative to individuals with mental disabilities, and more specifically Down syndrome, are limited.

The increasing lifespan of people with Down syndrome allows them to experience more of life's realities for longer periods of time. Poverty, unemployment, frustration over a lack of social relationships, social isolation, family conflict, and other life experiences must be faced and reactions to these events inevitably will occur. In this chapter we will explore the lives of some people with Down syndrome. First, a review of the literature will demonstrate the state of our present knowledge about the occurrence of depression in adolescents and young adults with Down syndrome. Second, we will present data from an exploratory survey of parents with older offspring with Down syndrome concerned with incidents of depression.

REVIEW OF LITERATURE

In 1992, Burt et al. argued that clinical and subclinical depression were common in adults with Down syndrome and with other forms of mental retardation. They also found that there was an association between depression and dementia that did not seem to appear in people without Down syndrome. The researchers also found that the people with Down syndrome who had more severe forms of depression also tended to have lower performance ratings on specific measures of mental age, memory, and adaptive skills.

In an earlier paper, Reiss et al. (1982) pointed out that people with mental retardation showed a full range of emotional and personality disturbance. They also found that people with mental disabilities had poor coping skills related to stress. Moreover, there were few mental health professionals trained to work with people with both mental retardation and mental illness. Reiss and his colleagues presented the concept of "diagnostic overshadowing" to demonstrate how symptoms of mental illness were often ignored in the presence of another disorder, such as mental retardation, which took precedence in the diagnostic process.

In an interesting book chapter, Harris (1988) reported on the dearth of information on depression and Down syndrome. Information was generally limited to a number of case studies. Harris believed that part of the reason for this lack of information was that it was very difficult to undertake research on the depression and Down syndrome connection because of the level of cognitive development in these individuals and a lack of agreement on diagnostic criteria for the recognition of depression in people with Down syndrome.

In a survey of psychopathology in 497 persons with Down syndrome, Meyers and Peuschel (1991) found an overall prevalence of psychiatric disorder of 22%, which they argued was a lower prevalence figure than in people with other forms of mental retardation. They also pointed out that adults with Down syndrome living in the community showed evidence of major depressive disorders in about 6% of the sample over 20 years of age.

A study done in Great Britain viewed 378 adults with Down syndrome (Cooper & Collacott, 1993). Forty-two of these adults (approximately 11%) had a past history of at least one depressive episode. In addition, they found that the younger the age at first episode, the poorer the adaptive behavior scores when compared with a matched control at follow-up. The researchers concluded that being older serves as a protection factor in maintaining adaptive functioning following a depression episode. In another paper, Collacott et al. (1992) noted that those individuals with Down syndrome showed a different spectrum of mental disorders than those without the syndrome. People with Down syndrome seem to be less vulnerable to mental disorder than others with mental retardation. However, the individuals with Down syndrome did show a greater percentage of cases with depressive disorders and Alzheimer dementia than other individuals with other forms of mental aberration.

METHODS

Subject–Group Selection

The sampling frame utilized in this study was comprised of a convenience sample of parents of adult children with Down syndrome in three different geographic areas. The National Down Syndrome Society provided contacts for two regional associations, which included families in the Los Angeles area (n = 75 families) and a New York group (n = 12). The sampling frame consisted of membership lists of the group's roster of families with an adolescent or adult child with Down syndrome. A further sample of parents was drawn from the Adjustment Training Center (ATC) in the northeastern corner of South Dakota, under the assumption that this sample would serve as a contrast to the two samples from the coastal urban areas. For the South Dakota sample, surveys were submitted to all parents or caregivers of this center's Down syndrome population (n = 38).

Because of the unique characteristics of the three study populations and the potential bias in convenience studies, the present study is considered to be an exploratory survey in search of some preliminary information on the relationship between Down syndrome and depression.

Instrumentation

The survey instrument used in the parents' component of the study was developed through a combination of research tools and scales. The initial section on demographics (items 1–7) was adapted from a previous instrument entitled "Consumer Perception Survey" (Jurkowski & Voloschin, 1992). This was followed with the Center for Epidemiologic Studies Depression Scale (CES-D) (Radloff, 1971) with twenty items. Five additional items were added to validate these items using additional criteria of situational and chronic depression given in DSM III-R. These items related to the longevity of specific symptomatology. Four items were added and adapted from the Chadsey-Rusch Loneliness Inventory (Chadsey-Rusch et al., 1992) and Telleen's Social Support Inventory (Telleen, 1988). An open-ended question was added to give some qualitative information to the survey.

DEMOGRAPHIC CHARACTERISTICS

The parents' samples led to an overall response rate of 60% (75 respondents). The respondents were either married (42.5%) or paid caregivers (52.1%). About 16% of the parent sample were separated or widowed. The majority of the respondents were mothers of the offspring with Down syndrome or were female caregivers. Sixty-four percent of the people with Down syndrome in the study were less than 29 years of age. The educational level represented in the samples showed at least a college education for both parents in 76.7% of the cases. The mothers who responded were homebound in 21.1% of the cases or working within professional or management jobs (26%). The great majority of the sample were white (92%). An interesting finding related to the fact that 47.7% of the respondents identified themselves as retired or not otherwise fitting into the occupational groups presented.

The sample people with Down syndrome primarily lived at home (47.8%). Some (25.7%) lived in group settings of six or more people, supported living settings (15.4%), or independent living (11.3%). Relative to where the people with Down syndrome lived, about 40% lived in South Dakota, 18.3% in New York and 42.3% in California. With regard to the vocational settings in which the people with Down syndrome resided, 30.6% were in workshop settings, 15.3% were in supported employment programs, 15.3% in community employment, 11.1% in some form of mainstream program, 9.7% in day activity programs, and the remainder of the samples in other diverse programs.

RESULTS

Within the reported findings of the CES-D, and verified by the additional questions developed from DSM III-R, the respondents indicated that the incidence rate of multiple symptoms related to depression was 47.9% of the total sample. An interesting inconsistency occurred in that a number of respondents identified their offspring with Down syndrome as "happy and well adjusted" and also reported symptoms of depression as measured on the study instrument scales. Part of the explanation for this apparent inconsistency related to the possibility that respondents were not always aware that certain behaviors may in fact be linked to the incidence of depression.

Within the study population, the incidence of depression was highest among those with no reported leisure activities (75%). In contrast, the incidence was lowest in cases with greater than seven reported specific leisure activities (9.59%). Respondents reported specific types of leisure activities including bowling, sports-related activities, arts and theater, crafts, community recreational activities, and peer support groups. Within the sample of people with Down syndrome, about 11% reported no leisure activities at all, 30.1% reported up to three specific activities, 41.1% reported between four and six activities, and more than seven types of activities were reported by 17.3% of the sample.

The data indicated that the individuals who lived at home were not more depressed than individuals living in other settings. The data did indicate that there was a dramatic increase in incidence among individuals residing within congregate living quarters of six or more individuals. In fact, the incidence rate was highest within this group in contrast to those reported to be living at home, within supported living settings or in independent living settings.

There was a dramatic difference between type of vocational setting and the incidence rate of depression. Individuals involved in supported work, competitive employment, or in community colleges showed the lowest incidence of depression, while those in mainstreamed or segregated settings represented the highest rates of individuals with depression. Thus, the present study, although exploratory in nature, did demonstrate that individuals integrated within community-based settings were at less risk for depression and/or maladaptive behavior. There was some evidence that mainstreamed settings may also be somewhat artificial in nature and not representative of the real world.

A number of researchers have argued that various types of formal and informal social supports might diminish the effects of depression over the long run. The present study explored the issue of social support. The evidence in this study pointed out that there is a lack of awareness about the effects of depression on people with Down syndrome. In fact, it appeared that health providers were not aware of the possibilities of depression in individuals with Down syndrome. The result of this lack of information explains the lack of specific treatment interventions for this population. Parents and other caregivers have noticed the changes in behavior in their offspring or charges, but have not associated these behavioral changes with depression. It is also striking to note that mental health therapists were sought out for support by 35.8% of the respondents but only 18% of those with depressive symptomatology used mental health therapists (see Table 1). In addition, there was a difference when supports would be sought or utilized. Specifically, it was found that in those situations where an individual displayed behavior related to depression there was a tendency not to seek help from other siblings, grandparents, aunts, or neighbors. Clergy tended to be sought for support by individuals with a demonstrated incidence of depressive symptomatology.

There was an interesting relationship between parental education and the in-

Table 1. Social Supports and Patterns of Utilization for Social Support

Source of Social Support	Seeks support often, sometimes, and most of the time	Seeks support most of the time	Tendency (nondepressed versus depressed)
Family	74.08%	55.56%	54.55 vs. 87.5%
Spouse of respondent	70.1%	32.84%	32.8 vs. 37.32%
Other children	34.3%	22.39%	19.41 vs. 17.9%
Grandparents	44.78%	13.43%	17.9 vs. 26.87%
Aunts	32.2%	4.41%	10.2 vs. 22.05%
Neighbors	35.8%	4.48%	8.57 vs. 0%
Teachers	34.8%	6.06%	13.64 vs. 21.22%
Specialists	42.43%	13.64%	18.1 vs. 29.41%
Vocational instructors	42.43%	18.18%	12.1 vs. 6.06%
Mental health agency personnel	45.5%	22%	13.2 vs. 8.82%
Therapists	35.8%	13.43%	4.48 vs. 17.9%
Supervisors	33%	13.64%	16.77 vs. 25.7%
Coworkers	42.43%	10.61%	4.55 vs. 6.06%
Clergy	56.72%	11.94%	4.5 vs. 7.46%
Peers	49.2%	15.38%	18.5 vs. 30.7%

cidence of depression in individuals with Down syndrome. The incidence rate was lowest for caregivers with graduate degrees and parents with a college degree. In addition, parents who were in professional jobs, which may or may not require a college education, showed offspring with the highest incidence of depressive symptomatology, in contrast to families in which the mother was at home, where the incidence rate was very low.

Finally, parents identified needs for several types of services that could promote the mental health of their offspring with Down syndrome. The most significant recommendations included the following:

- The development of activities through park and recreation programs
- Physical activities to include aerobics
- Support groups and counseling groups
- Community education related to mainstreaming persons with Down syndrome
- Transportation services
- Singles activities
- Supported-living options

It is interesting that specialized mental health services were not listed as a critical need. Parents tended to pick services that would enhance the quality of life of their offspring rather than increase the therapeutic services that their offspring might need.

CONCLUSIONS AND SUMMARY

This study calls into question the myth that people with Down syndrome are always happy. Parents and caregivers report significant evidence for depression in almost 50% of the study sample of adolescents and young adults with Down syndrome. However, generalization of the results to other Down syndrome populations must be made with extreme caution because of the biased nature of the present sample. Another important finding from the present study relates to the lack of knowledge about depression on the part of the parent and caretaker respondents. Some supporting information from other data on service providers collected by the authors showed a similar lack of knowledge of the incidence of depression in people with Down syndrome as well as strategies for treating the disorder in this population.

Although the present study was exploratory in nature, a number of interesting themes emerged to guide other research. First, research needs to go beyond small clinical studies to look at the epidemiologic aspects of the problem of depression in special populations. Aggregated information is necessary for appropriate causal information to be determined and also for new interventions to be developed. Second, the importance of exploring symptomatology from a parent/caregiver perspective are important. If parents and caregivers are to be responsive to the needs of individuals with depression and Down syndrome, they need to know what to look for in terms of behavioral manifestations of the mental disorder. Central in the process is the need for parent education. On the other side, mental health professionals need to be trained to look for the symptoms of depression in special populations. They need to learn how to develop treatment interventions appropriate for people with Down syndrome.

Third, there was a great amount of confusion in the literature about the connection between Down syndrome, Alzheimer disease, and depression. This was an issue in the present study of the parent/caregivers in that these respondents' perceptions were that mental health providers and health providers do not know the present state of knowledge about these problems. Moreover, the problems associated with diagnostic overshadowing need to be avoided. Thus, it is important to once again stress the need for education on a variety of fronts including education and training for service providers, mental health providers, educators, families, and, ultimately, the community at large. It is anticipated that such education will begin to address the confusion between Down syndrome, depression, and Alzheimer disease. This education and training should create sensitivity to the critical issues necessary to build coping and adaptation skills for those people with Down syndrome as they adjust to adulthood within a community setting. In addition, it is necessary to develop more support groups and opportunities for people with Down syndrome to develop problem-solving skills and meaningful social and recreational outlets with their peers.

Fourth, parent/caregivers gave important information related to the types of services needed. They seemed to believe that the reason for many of the behavioral aberrations that were noted may be due to a lack of social activities for the person with Down syndrome. If quality of life can be improved, then the implication is that some of the behavioral problems may diminish or vanish. Parent/caregivers are also disenchanted with the service providers that they use. They believe that they often know more than these providers do.

In summary, there is only limited information available on the relationship between Down syndrome and depression. This exploratory study has attempted to document some of the risk factors associated with this symptomatology as well as to document the fact that depression may be more prevalent than we realize. More data are needed to explore these issues in more detail in diverse populations in multiple settings.

REFERENCES

Bland R, Newman S, Orn H (1990): Health care utilization for emotional problems: Results from a community survey. Can J Psychiatry 35, June:397–400.

Burt D, Loveland K, Lewis K (1992): Depression and the onset of dementia in adults with mental retardation. Am J Ment Retard 96, 5:502–511.

Canadian Mental Health Association (1992): Mental Health Network. July.

Chadsey-Rusch J, DeStefano L, O'Reilly M, Gonzalez P, Collet-Klinenberg L (1992): Assessing the loneliness of workers with mental retardation. Ment Retard 50, 2:85–92.

Cooper D, Collacott R (1993): Prognosis of depression in Down's syndrome. J Nervous & Ment Dis 181, 3:204–205.

Collacott R, Cooper S, McGrother C (1992): Differential rates of psychiatric disorders in adults with Down's syndrome compared to other mentally handicapped people. Brit J Psychiatry, 161:671–674.

Harris J (1988): Psychological adaptation and psychiatric disorders in adolescents and young adults with Down syndrome. In Puesdel S (Ed.): "The Young Person with Down Syndrome, Transition from Adolescence to Adulthood." Baltimore: Brookes.

Hollingshead AB, Redlich FC (1958): "Social Class and Mental Illness in a Community Study." New York: Wiley.

Jurkowski E, Voloschin (1992): "Consumer Perception Survey." Unpublished manuscript. The University of Illinois at Chicago.

Meyers B, Peuschel S (1991): Psychiatric disorders in persons with Down syndrome. J Nerv & Ment Dis 179, 10:609–613.

Radloff LS (1977): The CES-D scale: A self-report depression scale for research in the general population. Appl Psych Meas 1:385–401.

Reiss S, Levitan G, Szyszko J (1982): Emotional disturbance and mental retardation: Diagnostic overshadowing. Am J Ment Defic 6:567–574.

Srole L, Langner TS, Michael ST et al. (1962): "Mental Health in the Metropolis: the Midtown Manhattan Study," Vol. 1. New York: McGraw-Hill.

Telleen S (1988): "Parenting Social Support, Reliability and Validity." Unpublished manuscript. The University of Illinois at Chicago.

Alzheimer Disease: A Health Risk of Growing Older with Down Syndrome

Arthur J. Dalton

INTRODUCTION

Everyone has to face the prospects of a number of health risks with increasing age. Changes in vision, hearing and sensitivity to touch, temperature and pain can all occur with age. Older individuals are also familiar with decreased flexibility and efficiency in physical activity, increased likelihood of heart attacks, cancer, and several other conditions. Not surprisingly, therefore, persons with Down syndrome also must consider the fact that they will have to face health risks as they grow older. However, many of the health risks that occur with increasing age are different for persons with Down syndrome. For example, they are less likely to suffer from high blood pressure, heart disease, heart attacks, emphysema, chronic lung disease, heart attacks, emphysema, chronic lung disease, and bone fractures (Haveman et al., 1989). The development of auditory and visual problems as well as a higher incidence of epilepsy are well-known problems. Less well known is that they may have a higher risk for the development of thyroid abnormalities (Percy et al., 1990a), arthrosis (a form of arthritis of the joints), and osteoporosis (Haveman et al., 1989), superoxide dismutase abnormalities (Percy et al., 1990b), immune system changes (Mehta et al., 1993), and Alzheimer disease. This report focuses on Alzheimer disease because it represents the most significant health risk faced by aging individuals with Down syndrome who live beyond the age of 40 years.

CASE HISTORY: DAVID

Mr. and Mrs. Davis of Indianapolis, Indiana, have recently described a lifetime of affectionate caring and support for David, their 46-year-old son with Down syndrome, who is now suffering from some of the signs of Alzheimer disease (Davis, 1992). David showed the first signs when he was about 33 years of age. He was slowing down and unable to perform in the workshop program the way he used to. He developed difficulties in bowling, one of his favorite leisure activities. He then developed seizures which, at first, were poorly controlled by medication that caused unexpectedly serious side effects. He now needs more or less continuous care, is disoriented, and no longer seems to enjoy watching television. His mood changes suddenly and his vision is becoming poor. He has hearing difficulties that make it hard to communicate with him. He now has dental, digestive, and elimination problems.

For his parents, David has become more than they can cope with. They feel the agonizing impact of their own diminishing stamina at this stage in their lives.

This story is gradually becoming more common as individuals with Down syndrome live longer and healthier lives under the care of their family or service providers and, consequently, face an increased risk of Alzheimer disease. Unfortunately, our understanding of the causes, diagnosis, treatment and prevention of Alzheimer disease and its relationships with Down syndrome are very limited at the present time.

ALZHEIMER DISEASE: WHAT IS IT?

Alzheimer disease is a fatal, progressive, degenerative disease of the brain that affects about 11% of all individuals over the age of 60 years (Terry, 1976). There are distinctive changes in the brain of affected individuals, including the loss of millions of nerve cells and the widespread appearance of senile plaques and neurofibrillary tangles, which have been described by many investigators (for example, Wolstenholme and O'Connor, 1970; Katzman et al., 1978). Over a period of years, these physical changes in the brain cause significant deterioration of its intellectual and communication capabilities and the skills of daily life, and, ultimately, all of its other functions. The most evident symptoms of Alzheimer disease may appear as barely subtle changes in memory followed by increasing difficulties in language and orientation and decline in mobility. These signs may then be followed by changes in personality and a gradual deterioration in many other functions over a period lasting from as little as a year to longer than 20 years. However, each person affected with Alzheimer disease will show only some of the signs, these will be different from person to person and they will not necessarily appear in the same sequence as the disease progresses.

SUSCEPTIBILITY OF PERSONS WITH DOWN SYNDROME
TO ALZHEIMER DISEASE

Individuals with Down syndrome are uniquely susceptible to Alzheimer disease. It has been known for more than 60 years that the brains of nearly all individuals with Down syndrome who die after the age of 40 years show clear-cut evidence of Alzheimer disease (Struwe, 1929). However, there are a few exceptions. Whalley (1982) reported the absence of any pathology in the brain of a 49-year-old woman with Down syndrome and a similar report has been made by Janota (in an article by Sylvester, 1984) from examination of the brain of a 4-year-old person with Down syndrome.

There is a large gap in our knowledge about the characteristics of the clinical manifestations and course of Alzheimer disease in persons with Down syndrome (Dalton, 1992). The clinical signs and symptoms of Alzheimer disease in persons with Down syndrome were first described in English by Jervis (1948), and reviews of the current status of knowledge are numerous (see, for example, Lott, 1982; Sinex and Merril, 1982; Dalton and Crapper-McLachlan, 1986; Dalton and Wisniewski, 1990; Schupf et al., 1990; Dalton et al., 1993). The symptoms, though difficult to observe for many reasons, seem to be similar in persons with Down syndrome when compared to those from the general population who develop Alzheimer disease. The chief difference seems to be the age of onset. Persons with Down syndrome develop symptoms 20–25 years earlier. While it is generally assumed that the brains of most (if not all) individuals with Down syndrome will have the characteristic brain lesions of Alzheimer disease, it is equally apparent that not all of them will develop the clinical manifestations of dementia. Explanations for this situations have been numerous and many speculations have been offered (see reviews by Rabe et al., 1990; Oliver and Holland, 1986; Wisniewski and Rabe, 1986). To complicate matters further, it has not been conclusively shown that the brain pathology and the possible factors that produce it are identical in persons with Down syndrome and those with Alzheimer disease without Down syndrome.

CAUSES OF ALZHEIMER DISEASE: UNKNOWN

The loss of millions of brain cells is the most dramatic physical evidence of the disease. The process whereby these nerve cells die in such numbers and the significance of the selective losses in particular regions (such as the nucleus basalis) and the death of specific types of nerve cells are not known. The search for infectious or transmissible agents, genetic or inherited abnormalities, and environmental toxins have yielded a large and important body of knowledge but no specific cause(s) for Alzheimer disease has been established. No infectious or viral agent has yet been identified and there have been no reported instances of one affected person transmitting the disease to any other. The neurofibrillary tangles and the senile plaques which are found in widespread regions of the brains of affected individuals have been the subject of intense research over many years (see recent reviews by Iqbal et al., 1993; Wisniewski and Wisniewski, 1992) and data from such studies hold promise for the development of potential bio-markers useful in diagnosis and rational approaches to drug therapies. Unfortunately, it is not clear whether the neurofibrillary tangles and/or the senile plaques are causes of Alzheimer disease or whether they simply represent the debris or consequences of some as yet undetermined process of unidentified causative event. The possibility of a genetic basis for Alzheimer disease has received a significant boost since the discovery of a location on chromosome 21 for the genetic blueprint for an important protein associated with deposits of beta-amyloid in senile plaques and blood vessels of the brain (Robakis et al., 1987). While this gene may lead to the overproduction of beta-amyloid, there is no proof that it causes Alzheimer disease either. Understanding the molecular events involved in the production, breakdown, modification, and regulation of beta-amyloid may yield important new treatment strategies.

DIAGNOSIS OF ALZHEIMER DISEASE

There is no test or procedure that can identify the presence of Alzheimer disease before the onset of clinical manifestations. Furthermore, there is no test that adequately monitors the total range of deficits induced by Alzheimer disease and no single test is useful throughout the entire course of the disease (Dalton et al., 1993). Of particular significance, diagnosis of individuals with Down syndrome must rely on procedures that have been developed for individuals who do not have Down syndrome. Some of these procedures can be expected to yield incorrect information because many diagnosticians do not have sufficient experience with individuals with Down syndrome. Therefore, follow-up evaluations conducted at appropriate intervals may be particularly important to help improve the accuracy of diagnosis. Because there is no specific test for Alzheimer disease, evaluation must be sufficiently extensive to rule out every other possible explanation. A "tentative" diagnosis of Alzheimer disease can then be given on the basis of exclusion. These procedures rely heavily on the report of behavioral, psychological, and other changes reported by family members or care and service providers who have constant association with the affected individual. The diagnostic procedures may involve several stages spread over several weeks or months and include a visit to a neurologist specializing in the functions and disorders of the brain. Laboratory studies of blood specimens will be required to rule out a long list of possibilities. An electrocardiogram to assess heart function, an electroencephalogram to assess abnormal electrical brain activity, imaging studies using a computerized brain scan (CTT) or magnetic resonance image (MRI) to assess the possibility of brain tumors or other physical abnormality in the brain, and neuropsychological evaluations to assess learning, memory, intellectual, and other aspects of psychological function may also be included in the evaluation. An accurate diagnosis is very important because the prognosis for Alzheimer disease is so poor and there are many conditions that resemble Alzheimer disease but could be effectively treated if detected and correctly identified. Some of these problems have been addressed recently in a review of the clinical aspects of the association between Alzheimer disease and Down syndrome (Dalton et al., 1993). Diagnosis of Alzheimer disease among persons with Down syndrome is difficult to make. Many treatable conditions, such as thyroid abnormality, vitamin deficiency, or depression, can be confused with Alzheimer disease. Moreover, some conditions occur more often not because the individual is growing older but because of the extra chromosome 21 present in each cell. Examples of such conditions include sleep apnea, cataracts, susceptibility to influenza and other infections, as well as epilepsy. Increased aggressiveness and acting-out behaviors may not be related to Alzheimer disease.

While all individuals with Down syndrome are at risk, some are known to have lived as long as 82 years of age and retained all of the functional competencies they possessed throughout their lifetime. The Office of Mental Retardation of the State of New York has information on more than 230 living persons with Down syndrome living in New York State who are 60 years of age or older and, of these, more than 50 persons are over 70 years of age at the present time. Unfortunately, the current health status of these individuals, including the incidence and prevalence of Alzheimer disease, is not known. Preliminary data bearing on this issue has been described in a recent survey conducted in New York State. In a recent survey in New York State 244 (1.6%) out of 6840 individuals with Down syndrome over 40 years of age who are receiving services from New York State institutions and not-for-profit service providers have been diagnosed or suspected of having Alzheimer disease (Janicki and Dalton, 1993). Half of those suspected or diagnosed with Alzheimer disease were individuals with Down syndrome, indicating that this diagnosis is four to five times more common among individuals with Down syndrome than other developmentally handicapped individuals of comparable age, level of function, health, and lifestyle factors.

DISCUSSION

This report has focused on Alzheimer disease because it is one of the most important health problems of growing older with Down syndrome. Unfortunately, the existing knowledge on the subject has been almost entirely published in technical journals, which are easily accessible only to those who can find their way through the complexities of information retrieval systems of university libraries. Public awareness has heightened to such an extent in the past 15 years that Alzheimer disease has become a household word and a term that may be incorrectly assigned to an older person with Down syndrome who is showing any change in conduct or behavior. Our incomplete understanding of Alzheimer disease and its connection with Down syndrome has a major impact on everyone affected as well as their families and care providers. Accurate diagnosis is particularly crucial because of the complex interplay of the life-long impact of the trisomy condition, with its more familiar age-related changes in sensory, motor, language, communication, and intellectual abilities, with the subtle, insidious alterations in functions caused by Alzheimer disease. Proper recognition, sensitivity, and greater attention to the individual's needs are essential elements in maintenance of quality of life at this time in the life of the aging person with Down syndrome as well as lessening the impact on family members and caring service providers. Inaccurate diagnosis also hampers research studies that seek to establish the incidence and prevalence of Alzheimer disease, to identify as yet unknown risk factors, and to establish patterns of disease frequency and severity among family members and relatives.

ACKNOWLEDGMENTS

This report was supported in part by NIA grant 5RO1-AGO8849 and a grant from the Velleman Foundation.

REFERENCES

Dalton AJ (1992): Dementia in Down syndrome: methods of evaluation. In Nadel L, Epstein CJ (Eds.): "Alzheimer Disease and Down Syndrome," pp. 51–76. New York: Wiley-Liss.

Dalton AJ, Crapper-McLachlan DR (1986): Clinical expression of Alzheimer's disease in Down's syndrome. Psychiatric Clinics N Am 9:659–670.

Dalton AJ, Selzter GB, Adlin MS, Wisniewski HM (1993): Association between Alzheimer's disease and Down's syndrome. In Berg JM, Holland AT, Karlinsky H (Eds.): "Alzheimer's Disease and Down Syndrome: Their Relationships." London: Oxford University Press.

Dalton AJ, Wisniewski HM (1990): Down syndrome and the dementia of Alzheimer disease. Intern Rev Psychiatr 2:43–52.

Davis D (1992): David. Down Syndrome News, November:121–123.

Haveman N, Maaskant MA, Sturmans F (1989): Older Dutch residents of institutions with and without Down syndrome: comparisons of mortality and morbidity trends and motor/social functioning. Aus NZ J Devel Disabil 15:241–255.

Iqbal K, Alonso A, Gong CX, Khatoon S, Kudo T, Singh T, Grundke-Iqbal I (1993): Molecular pathology of Alzheimer neurofibrillary degeneration. Acta Neurobiol Exper 53:325–335.

Janicki MP, Dalton AJ (1993): Alzheimer disease in a select population of older adults with mental retardation. Irish J Psychol 14:38–47.

Jervis GA (1948): Early senile dementia in mongoloid idiocy. Am J Psychiatr 105:102–106.

Katzman R, Terry RD, Bick KL (1978): "Alzheimer's Disease: Senile Dementia and Related Disorders." New York: Raven Press.

Klatzo I, Wisniewski HM, Streicher E (1965): Experimental production of neurofibrillary degeneration. J Neuropath Exp Neurol 24:187–199.

Lott IT (1982): Down syndrome, aging and Alzheimer's disease: a clinical review. Ann NY Acad Sci 396:15–27.

Mehta PD, Dalton AJ, Mehta SP, Percy ME, Wisniewski HM (1993): Increased beta2-microglobulin (beta2-M) and interleukin-6 (IL-6) in sera from older persons with Down syndrome. Adv Neurosci 87:95–96.

Oliver C, Holland J (1986): Down's syndrome and Alzheimer disease: A review. Psycholog Med 16:307–322.

Percy ME, Dalton AJ, Markovic VD, Crapper-McLachlan DR, Gera E, Hummel JT, Rusk ACM, Somerville MJ, Andrews DF, Walfish PG (1990a): Autoimmune thyroiditis associated with mild "subclinical" hypothyroidism in adults with Down syndrome: a comparison of patients with and without manifestations of Alzheimer disease. Am J Med Genet 36:148–154.

Percy ME, Dalton AJ, Markovic VD, Crapper-McLachlan DR, Hummel JT, Rusk ACM, Andrews DF (1990b): Red cell superoxide dismutase, glutathione peroxidase and catalase in Down syndrome patients with and without manifestations of Alzheimer disease. Am J Med Genet 35:459–467.

Rabe A, Wisniewski KE, Schupf N, Wisniewski HM (1990): The relationship of Down syndrome to Alzheimer disease. In Deutsch SI, Weizman A, Weizman R (Eds.): "Application of Basic Neuroscience to Child Psychiatry." New York: Plenum.

Radetsky P (1992): Alzheimer's stepchild. Discover 13, September:84–90.

Robakis NK, Wisniewski HM, Jenkins EC, Devine-Gage EA, Houck GE, Yao X-L, et al. (1987): Chromosome 21 locus for gene for beta-amyloid protein. Lancet i:384–385.

Schupf N, Zigman WB, Silverman WP, Rabe A, Wisniewski HM (1990): Genetic epidemiology of Alzheimer's disease. In Battistin L (Ed.): "Aging Brain and Dementia: New Trends in Diagnosis and Therapy," pp. 57–78. New York: Liss.

Sinex FM, Myers RH (1982): Alzheimer's disease, Down's syndrome and aging: The genetic approach. Ann NY Acad Sci 396:3–13.

Struwe F (1929): Histopathologische Untersuchungen uber Entsehung und Wesen der senilen Plaques. Z Neurol Psychiatr 122:291–307.

Sylvester PE (1984): Aging in the mentally retarded. In Dobbing J, Clarke ADB, Corbett JA (Eds.): "Scientific Studies in Mental Retardation," pp. 262–282. London: the Royal Society of Medicine and MacMillan Press.

Terry RD (1976): Dementia, a brief and selective review. Archiv Neurol 33:1–4.

Whalley LJ (1982): The dementia of Down's syndrome and its relevance to etiological studies of Alzheimer's disease. Ann NY Acad Sci 396:39–53.

Wisniewski HM, Rabe A (1986): Discrepancy between Alzheimer-type neuropathology and dementia in persons with Down's syndrome. In Wisniewski HM, Snider A (Eds.): "Mental Retardation: Research, Education and Technology Transfer." Ann NY Acad Sci 447:247–260.

Wisniewski TM, Wisniewski HM (1992): Alzheimer's disease and the cerebral amyloidoses. In Kostovic I, Knezevic S, Wisniewski HM, Spilich G (Eds.): "Neurodevelopment, Aging and Cognition," pp. 157–172. Boston: Birkhauser.

Wolstenholme GEW, O'Connor M (1970): "Alzheimer's Disease and Related Conditions." Ciba Foundation Symposium. London: Churchill.

Woollard DC, Pybus J, Woollard GA (1990): Aluminum concentration in infant formulae. Food Chem 37:81–94.

III. Role of the Family

Perspective

John Taylor

I will be 27 years old on the 22nd of September. I live with my mother and am the youngest of 4 children. My oldest sister Laurie is a writer, actress and film maker. She and her husband Murph won two ACE awards for the documentary they made about me called "Yours To Keep." My sister Mary is a singer and song writer and has recently returned to college to become an occupational therapist. My sister Bridget is finishing her doctorate in psychology at Rutgers University, and works with autistic children. When I was born, and the doctors told my mother I had Down syndrome, they told her I would never be able to do much of anything. Well let me tell you a little bit of what I have done.

After I finished school, I had to get a job. I had to learn about going on job interviews, about being able to take responsibility, and getting along with others. The problem was, where could we find someone who would be willing to hire a person who has a handicap? My family and I talked about it. And we decided my sister Laurie would write letters to different places. I went on some interviews and got a job as an animal assistant. I like the animals, and I like the people. But after several weeks, I got laid off. Actually, I got fired. That was no fun. So my mother decided I should get some experience working with a counsellor. So I got a job through the ARC working in a candy factory. I wrapped candy in plastic and I liked my work and my counsellor. But the horrible thing about the job was that I only got $17 a week. That made me angry and frustrated because I worked very hard. Lucky for me, I was asked to audition for a movie called "The Seventh Sign." I went to New York and read for the part. They liked me and I went out to Hollywood, California for five weeks.

The director was Carl Schultz. I had to learn my lines and wait around a lot and put in long hours just like everyone else. They didn't treat me like a retarded actor, they treated me like all the other actors. I especially liked that. I made a lot of money from the movie, and I still get residuals. After I finished the film, I decided I didn't want to go back to the candy factory. I took the summer off and went upstate to my aunt's house to think about my life and to have a vacation. At the end of the summer, my brother-in-law Murph wrote a letter to Sam Goody Record Store and told them about me. He told them I loved music and asked them if they could give me a job. They said I could come for an interview. That was in October of 1987. I got the job and have been working as a retail sales associate at Sam Goody ever since. I wait on customers, alphabetize the cassettes, and sometimes I set up the displays. I recently learned how to do special orders and my boss is teaching me how to use the register. My boss gets many compliments on my work from the customers. In April of 1988, I was Employee of the Month, and I just received an award for my excellent customer service.

I still want to do more acting. I have a manager named Brian Glass, and he sends me on auditions for movies and Off-Broadway plays. He sometimes sends me for roles that are not specifically written for people with Down syndrome.

In the past few years, I have gone to Washington DC with the National Down Syndrome Society to testify before Congress. I told Senator Daniel Inouye and Senator Tom Harkin how important it is to get money for research on the cause of Down syndrome, and money to help people with Down syndrome to get jobs.

I have a girlfriend named Adria. I have known her since we were five years old. We have been going out for 5 years, and in December of 1988 I gave her a diamond. She is very pretty and very smart. She also has a job and someday we would like to get married. I hope that in the future, doctors will tell parents of children who have Down syndrome to give them a chance, to encourage them to be whatever they can be. Thank you.

Sisters and Brothers of Persons with Down Syndrome: An Intimate Look at Their Experiences

Judy S. Itzkowitz

THE SIBLING RELATIONSHIP

The sibling relationship is an especially powerful and potent relationship (Dunn and Kendrick, 1982). According to Bank and Kahn (1982), the relationship between brothers and sisters is usually the longest relationship in a human being's lifetime; in most cases, it is longer in duration than the relationships human beings have with parents and with a spouse. Furthermore, the genetic and biological make-up of a person is most similar to his or her sibling. As communities and society have changed, these changes have influenced the nature of the sibling bond. For example, Bank and Kahn (1982) indicate that the following variables have influenced the sibling relationship: smaller family size, longer human life span, divorce and remarriage, geographic mobility of families and family members, maternal employment, the various alternatives to child care, competitive pressure, and family stress. As Lobato (1990) indicates, the sibling relationship has numerous functions, including teaching cognitive language, social, motor, and moral skills, providing children with emotional experiences and opportunities for expressing love, affection, intimacy, etc., developing identity and personality, as well as providing children with important social opportunities whereby development and learning are enhanced. A wide range of emotions and experiences have been associated with the sibling relationship. This has been confirmed through scientific research and the retrospective responses of siblings themselves. Furman and Buhrmester (1985) queried siblings aged 11 and 13 to learn about how they described their relationships. At least 65% of the siblings reported positive qualities such as companionship, admiration, prosocial behavior, and affection. The negative characteristics of antagonism and quarreling were reported by 91% and 79% of the respondents respectively. It is not unusual to hear the following words used to describe the sibling relationship: fun, jealousy, learning, competition, fighting, loving, and challenging. The research on sibling relationships is replete with studies examining numerous variables and their impact on the relationship: age spacing between siblings, gender, birth order, disability condition, family character-istics, and parent characteristics (Stoneman and Brody, 1993). A more detailed review of this literature can be found in Itzkowitz (1989), Powell and Gallagher (1993), and Stoneman and Brody (1993).

THE SIBLING RELATIONSHIP WHEN A BROTHER OR SISTER HAS SPECIAL NEEDS

The experiences associated with the sibling relationship when a brother or sister has Down syndrome will be discussed based upon the research and anecdotal ac-counts of siblings of individuals with disabilities. There has been little specific research looking solely at the experiences of siblings of persons with Down syn-drome. Therefore, the experiences commonly shared by siblings of persons with disabilities will be highlighted. It is important to remember that the relationship among siblings is first and foremost the sibling relationship; the relationships shared between brothers and sisters where neither child has a disability are quite similar to relationships where a brother or sister happens to have special needs. Although the sibling relationship changes over time, the experiences that will be discussed are part of the human condition; at some point in our lives, each one of us had to cope with challenges and may have had to experience these feelings. These experiences may pose more challenges to siblings of persons with disabilities. Yet, many siblings indicate that they have learned a tremendous amount from their brother or sister with special needs and acknowledge the contributions that their sibling has made and continues to make to their life.

Brothers and sisters of persons with special needs share some common exper-iences. Many siblings are concerned about their brother or sister who has special needs. They are interested in helping their sibling, yet many are unsure what they can do to help. For some children, this may lead to frustration; having a goal of wanting to help, yet being unsure about what they can specifically do. Many brothers and sisters are interested in learning about the disability or special needs; they are curious about Down syndrome and the professionals who work with their brother or sister with special needs; they may have many other questions, too.

It is not unusual that young children may have some misperceptions about the disability. For example, some children may think that they caused the disability. A child of five years of age informed me that she thought that because she had tickled her mother during the pregnancy this caused her brother to be born with Down syndrome. Another child thought that the Down syndrome was catching. These misconceptions should be dealt with in an up-front honest manner so that the child receives accurate information at an age-appropriate level.

Sometimes brothers and sisters may feel anger, sadness, guilt, or disappointment about their sibling's disability. As adults, it is important to assist children in seeing the value of these feelings. For example, anger is related to a standard that has been violated in some way. Guilt may be related to the beliefs possessed about how people should be. Children need reassurance that all of their feelings are valid along with opportunities to express their feelings in appropriate ways. Sometimes, young people may feel separate, alone, or different. It is important to support siblings in recognizing that they are not alone; that there are other people who are going through similar kinds of experiences in life. Providing children with opportunities to get together with other siblings of the disabled might assist them in recognizing that they are not alone and enable children to share their experiences in a safe milieu (Itzkowitz et al., 1985). Other feelings that may arise include feeling embarrassed about the brother or sister with special needs, experiencing jealousy because the sibling with special needs receives considerable attention, or feeling left out because a parent is spending more time with the child with Down syndrome. Many siblings see themselves in the role of "the other mother," or "the surrogate parent." It is important that brothers and sisters are given choices about the amount of responsibility and the roles they assume with their disabled sibling. They are young people first, and brothers or sisters of siblings with special needs second. Powell and Gallagher (1993) indicate that siblings may express concerns focusing on the child with disability (e.g., the cause of the disability, the child's feelings and prognosis, what services are needed, how to help, where the child lives and goes to school, and the future); their parents (e.g., dealing with parents' feelings and expectations, communicating with and helping parents, participating in child-rearing activities, and dealing with how parents spend time); themselves (e.g., their feelings, their own health, their relationship with their sibling, finding out that their brother or sister has Down syndrome); their friends (e.g., talking with friends about their sibling, dealing with teasing, interacting with friends, coping with their friends' reactions to their brother or sister with Down syndrome, dating); the community (e.g., going to school with their brother or sister with special needs, dealing with parental efforts to achieve an inclusive education for the youngster with Down syndrome, coping with community awareness and acceptance); and adulthood (e.g., decisions about guardianship, their own current and future relationship with their sibling with Down syndrome, their role when their parents are unable to support the young adult with Down syndrome).

Even with these concerns, siblings learn to cope with the challenges and feelings that may arise. Although siblings may experience any of the feelings and concerns just described, the relationships of brothers and sisters with their disabled siblings are also filled with many benefits, including feeling pride at their brother's or sister's accomplishments, appreciating individual differences, the gifts of life, "the little things in life," their family life, feeling enthusiasm, having a heightened sensitivity to others, acquiring compassion, empathy, and an appreciation for individual differences and diversity, experiencing enhanced communication within their family, learning to deal with and accept challenges as valued lessons in life, acquiring the ability to be flexible and deal with change, and wanting to make a contribution in life. Certainly, many siblings feel an intense love for their brother or sister with Down syndrome and for their entire family as a whole. Summers, Behrs, and Turnbull (1989) listed these positive contributions to the family when a child happens to have a disability: increased happiness, greater love, strengthened family ties, strengthened religious faith, greater pride and accomplishment, greater knowledge about disability and diversity, learning not to take things for granted, learning to be patient, expanding career development, personal growth, and living life more slowly. Families who are able to communicate openly and honestly about their experiences as well as see their experiences as opportunities to learn are able to cope more effectively with any of the challenges that may arise through living with a young person with Down syndrome. As I have written, "My experience with my retarded [sic] sister has been one of the most important in my life. It has at times been stressful and emotional, but ultimately a very positive influence. It has definitely shaped my life and channeled my interests in ways I would otherwise have not pursued" (Itzkowitz, 1990, p. 188).

STRATEGIES TO FOSTER SUPPORTIVE RELATIONSHIPS AMONG SIBLINGS

It is essential that we listen to and learn from brothers, sisters, and families themselves. The strategies listed below can serve as a vehicle to support parents, professionals, and siblings themselves as they consider how to strengthen relationships among siblings.

1. Each child is a unique individual with unique strengths, needs, experiences, and contributions to make to the family and society. Each young person should share his or her unique gift with others. Each person in the family is an individual and should be treated like an individual.
2. Remember that brothers and sisters are people first, children first.
3. All children have the need to be accepted and respected for who they are, recognizing that all people have similar needs and may experience some challenges within the course of their lives.
4. Listening to children is very important. Learn from them and through their experiences. Encourage children to express themselves fully; respect what you hear. Their feelings are real and valid for them. Acknowledge the feelings that your son or daughter has as well as their experiences. Reflect upon their feelings. Assist them in learning the value of their feelings and how to act upon those feelings in effective ways. Assist children in expressing the full range of their feelings.
5. Encourage open and honest communication among all family members. Make your family a place where brave questions and brave answers are natural.
6. Provide each child with the opportunity to have their strengths, gifts, capacities, and talents—their contribution to your family and the world—recognized.
7. Encourage children to be as independent and competent as possible. Each child is capable of learning, growth, and change, just as we are as adults. Utilize the natural opportunities in life to teach life's lessons. For example, discussions about fairness and equity are important. It is important for children to learn that while life may not be fair, that does not mean that life is not good. Although it is natural for parents to want to protect their children, it is essential that children learn about the realities of life from people who genuinely care about them and love them.

8. Haim Ginott indicates that we must treat our children, not as they are, but as the people we hope they will become. Have high expectations. Dream. Give yourself permission to dream, to have dreams for yourself, your children, your spouse, and your family as a whole. Talk about those dreams, and how you can bring them to life. Create a vision of the future.

9. Ask for what you want. Encourage your children to express their needs. It is okay to ask for help and assistance from others.

10. Each of us changes from one moment to the next. Change is a vital part of any family system. Issues arise; your reaction to those issues changes across time. Be flexible. Explore different resources and solutions. Have an adventure.

11. Create situations in which everyone wins.

12. Remember that your children look to you. You are a model.

13. Provide children with information and support that is based upon their age, strengths, needs, and interests. It is important that siblings hear from you, the parent, that their brother or sister has special needs. They need to learn about Down syndrome from you first; it is critical that they see that their brother or sister with Down syndrome is valued for who he or she is—a whole person who happens to have Down syndrome.

14. Laughter is a healing mechanism. Laugh a lot and love often.

15. Use everything that happens in your life as an opportunity to learn, for your advancement. Each instance, experience, and challenge in life provides us with opportunities to learn and to grow.

16. Make sure that you take care of yourself; that way, you can take good care of others.

In closing, my hope is that the experiences within your family will make you strong; that in working together, you will create strength and harmony within your family.

REFERENCES

Bank SP, Kahn MD (1982): "The Sibling Bond." New York: Basic Books.

Dunn J, Kendrick C (1982): "Siblings: Love, Envy, and Understanding." Cambridge: Harvard University Press.

Furman W. Buhrmester D (1985): Children's perceptions of the qualities of sibling relationships. Child Devel 56:448–461.

Itzkowitz JS (1990): "The Needs and Concerns of Brothers and Sisters of Individuals with Disabilities." (Doctoral dissertation, University of Connecticut, 1989). Dissertation Abstracts International 50:2453A.

Itzkowitz, JS et al. (1985): Sibling day: A workshop for brothers and sisters of children with handicaps. Sibling Information Network Newsletter 5:2–3.

Lobato D (1990): "Brothers, Sisters, and Special Needs. Information and Activities for Helping Young Siblings of Children with Chronic Illnesses and Developmental Disabilities." Baltimore: Brookes.

Powell TH, Gallagher PA (1993): "Brothers and Sisters: A Special Part of Exceptional Families" (2nd ed.). Baltimore: Brookes.

Stoneman Z, Brody G (1993): Sibling relations in the family context. In Stoneman Z, Berman

PW (Eds.): "The Effects of Mental Retardation, Disability, and Illness on Sibling Relationships. Research Issues and Challenges," pp. 3–30. Baltimore: Brookes.

Summers JA, Behr SK, Turnbull AP (1989): Positive adaptation and coping strength of families who have children with disabilities. In Singer GHS, Irvin LK (Eds.): "Support for Caregiving Families: Enabling Positive Adaptations to Disabilities," pp. 27–40. Baltimore: Brookes.

Project Child

Barbara Moore

Over the years a major concern of families of children with Down syndrome has been the need for self-reliance and independence for those children. Persons with Down syndrome now live longer; therefore it is imperative that they master at an early age social skills essential for employment and independent living.

Parents have a tendency to be very protective, and this hinders the child's ability to separate from his or her parents at a time when such independence is expected. As a result, children do not develop confidence in their independence and their social skills can be critically inadequate.

Children with disabilities must be allowed to venture from the protectiveness of their own family environment, to adapt to new and varied people, surroundings, and situations. Time and again, parents have expressed a desire for alternative programs. They would like some respite in order to relax and spend quality time with their spouse and other children. At the same time, they want their child with Down syndrome to be exposed to circumstances that will help develop skills necessary for maturation.

Project Child was developed by the National Down Syndrome Society. This program provides respite for the family and exposure to the community for the child. The participants of Project Child are children aged 5–12 with Down syndrome. The children are carefully matched with a volunteer host family and the exchanges begin. The Association for Retarded Citizens–San Diego is happy to have the privilege of offering Project Child.

The idea of having a vacation for their son or daughter is very inviting to families. The exchange occurs one weekend every six weeks for one year, resulting in about 8 mini-vacations. Before an exchange can occur, each child is painstakingly matched with a volunteer host family. Once the match is made, the exchanges may begin. The first visit lasts approximately 4 hours. This is an introductory visit, preceding the regular visits.

The child who enters the program is now exposed to new games and toys. He or she may find that the rules of their host home are different from their own. At this time, a new realm of independence and self-esteem begins to be cultivated.

The volunteer host family is, for the first time, exposed to a child with Down syndrome. The family may find that besides the need for a little extra time to accomplish tasks, this child is not so unlike their own children. The host family's children learn from this experience as well. It is our hope that if they have experience with a person with a disability, in the future they will realize that it is only another of many differences between themselves and others.

In addition to the vacation for their son or daughter, the child's family now has a regularly scheduled respite time once every six weeks. Some parents decide to do some catching up with their other sons or daughters. Other reported experiences include a romantic evening along with soft music, wine, and cheese, a romantic walk along the beach at night, and one mother even decided to paint her son's room.

After a short while, it becomes apparent that it is necessary for the families to come together as a group periodically. These outings provide the families opportunities to share ideas and enjoy one another's company. They also provide safe environments for the children of both families to be exposed to many community affairs.

The children's "cultural" minds have been enriched by visits to the theater. They have attended plays at the outdoor Starlight Bowl, the Civic Theater, and the Old Globe Theater. They have heard a concert of chamber music and viewed the Nutcracker at Christmas time. Attending sports events has been a completely new experience for the children. They were able to see baseball, hockey, basketball, and football games. Many of the children are interested in cars and motorcycles, so attending Monster Truck shows and Super Motor Cross races has been a special thrill. They have also attended Stars on Ice and Disney on Ice shows, to name only a few events.

How does Project Child provide magic to the children? The answer is very simple—David Copperfield. We were able to view one of Mr. Copperfield's magic acts at the Civic Theater.

These experiences through Project Child are more than just entertainment. For all participants, they are lessons in diversity and citizenship. The children as well as the adults get a bigger view of the world in which they live. For the children for whom Project Child was developed, it may be the catalyst to a life full of activity and exploration, a life to which they may not otherwise have been introduced.

The goals of Project Child are as follows:

- To enable children with Down syndrome and other developmental disabilities to develop the social skills they require for independent living and employment in adulthood.
- To provide an integrated environment, thereby creating unique learning and recreational opportunities.
- To provide a regular, planned respite service for the child's family.
- To develop community awareness and understanding of Down syndrome.

Project Child has met all of these goals and more. It is hoped that, from their experiences, these children have been able to develop goals of their own.

Support for Families of Children with Developmental Disabilities: A Revolution in Expectations

Valerie J. Bradley

OVERVIEW OF PUBLIC POLICY IN FAMILY SUPPORT

The first and primary natural environment for members of any society is the family. To say that children belong in families and that those family connections are of lifelong and primary importance states the obvious. However, only in recent years have we begun to recognize that persons with mental retardation and other developmental disabilities are also entitled to be part of a family. This represents a clear break with the past, when families were strongly encouraged by medical and social service professionals to seek institutional placements for children born with severe disabilities (McKaig, 1986).

During their childhood years, over 90% of persons with mental retardation and other developmental disabilities now live with their families (Ashbaugh et al., 1985). However, changes in the American family—increased numbers of working mothers, more single-parent families, smaller family size, and lack of available extended family—suggest that families have diminished resources at their disposal to provide the care required by their family member with a disability (Agosta and Bradley, 1985; Schorr, 1988). Additionally, children with severe multiple disabilities and complicated medical conditions are surviving past infancy and living at home. The presence of such children is in part the result of improved neonatal intervention that has reduced mortality among increasingly smaller and more premature infants as well as the availability of a variety of home-based technologies that in the past would only have been seen in hospitals (e.g., respirators, heart monitors, etc.).

The development of family support policy has proceeded in three phases. In the first period, the era of institutionalization and segregation (roughly ending in the late 1960s), the governing norms were primarily medical and the impetus was to separate people who were "sick" and vulnerable. During this period, families who had children with disabilities had only two alternatives—to maintain the child at home 24 hours a day or to place the child in an institution. The initiation of two major federal programs toward the end of this era Medicaid (1966) and Supplemental Security Income (1974), at least made it possible for income-eligible families to secure needed therapies, equipment, and other basic supports for their children.

This period was followed by the era of deinstitutionalization and community development (1970s to the mid 1980s). The impetus for this shift was based on the growing acceptance of the developmental model and its presumption that the provision of specialized training and therapeutic services could assist people with mental retardation and other developmental disabilities to grow and learn. For families, this era of "active treatment" led to increased services directed at the child with a disability, though not necessarily at the family as a whole. The Individualized Education Plan, mandated by the Education for All Handicapped Children Act (PL 94-142), became the organizing vehicle for the prescription of developmental services such as speech therapy, physical therapy and behavioral intervention.

The third and current period, the era of community membership, is marked by an emphasis on functional supports to enhance community integration, quality of life, and individualization. The concept of functional supports offers an alternative to a continuum of specialized services by focusing on the creation of a network of formal and informal supports that people with disabilities need to meet day-to-day demands in their homes and communities (Ferguson and Olson, 1989). With respect to children and families, functional supports are viewed as interventions for the family as a whole as well as the child. The assumption is that the presence of a child with a disability affects the functioning of the entire family and that failure to nurture family functioning places the child at risk for out-of-home placement.

A more "wholistic" approach to the provision of services and supports to families of children with disabilities places new demands on service providers. A major challenge is how to provide supports that maximize natural as well as specialized services.

GROWTH OF THE FAMILY SUPPORT MOVEMENT

Frustrated by the lack of opportunities and services, parents have historically initiated programs for their sons and daughters with mental retardation and other developmental disabilities. Most recently, parents are concentrating their advocacy efforts on the creation of family support programs defined by individual family needs. This movement is fueled by changed expectations among families, an evolution in values in the disability field, and concurrent shifts in program approaches. When conceptualized in this family centered fashion, family support offers flexible service, focuses on the entire family, changes as family needs change, encourages families to use natural community supports, and provides convenient access to coordinated services and resources.

An increasing number of states, with guidance and/or pressure from parents, have begun to recognize their responsibilities to families and are increasing the support and services they provide (Knoll et al., 1990). In 1972, Pennsylvania became the first state to initiate a family support project. Currently, all but a handful of states provide some form of support to families who have children with mental retardation or other disabilities. While respite care is by far the most prevalent support that states provide for families, an increasing number of states offer a range of services including home and vehicle modification, training, case management, counseling, nursing, and home health care.

It is to the credit of grass roots lobbying efforts by families that the concept of family support is beginning to be accepted at both state and national levels (Smith et al., 1987). Parents who have testified before Congress, their state legislatures, and the boards of regional and local service agencies have been successful in initiating or expanding the support and services available to families caring for children with mental retardation or other disabilities.

Parents base their call for family support on the fact that it is the most cost-effective service the state can provide. By supporting families and aiding the integration of children with disabilities in their home communities and neighborhood schools, the state will shape the future demand for adult services in a manner that places much greater reliance on the resources that already exist in our communities rather than on more expensive specialized settings. They further argue that families should increasingly be included in the design, implementation, and monitoring of family support programs.

In a study completed in 1990, the Human Services Research Institute determined that family support services make up only about 1.5% of the total budget of services for people with developmental disabilities (Knoll et al., 1990). Further, though about 46 states had some form of family support, it was by and large limited to respite services and, in 15 states, less than 100 families were served in family support programs. Though each new fiscal year brings substantial growth in family support programs around the country, there are also reports that some programs no longer exist because they were pilot projects that did not become permanent (e.g., in Arkansas). Further, many family support initiatives are not firmly established by legislative mandate and therefore are susceptible to the vicissitudes of the state budgetary process. These factors underscore the often tentative and embryonic nature of family support services in the United States.

While support for families may take a variety of forms (see Table 1), the major goals of state family support programs are to: 1) deter unnecessary out-of-home placements, 2) return persons living in institutions back to families, and 3) enhance the care-giving capacity of families (Agosta and Bradley, 1985). The Wisconsin Department of Health and Social Services (1985) gives the following explanation of their Family Support Program:

> The program is intended to ensure that ordinary families faced with the
> extra-ordinary circumstances that comes with having a child with severe
> disabilities will get the help they need without having to give up parental
> responsibility and control.

To enhance the practice of family support and to promote sharing of information across states, the Administration on Developmental Disabilities sponsored a conference in Washington, D.C. in 1990 that brought together parent representatives and

Table 1. Taxonomy of Family Support

Services
　Core services:
　　Respite & child care:
　　　Respite
　　　Child care
　　　Sitter service
　　Recreation:
　　　Recreation
　　　Camp
　　Supportive:
　　　Extra-ordinary/ordinary
　Needs:
　　Family counseling
　　Family support groups
　　Siblings groups
　　Transportation
　　Special diet
　　Special clothing
　　Utilities
　　Health insurance
　　Home repairs
　　Rent assistance

　　Traditional developmental services:
　　　Behavior management
　　　Speech therapy
　　　Occupational therapy
　　　Physical therapy
　　　Individual counseling
　　　Medical/dental
　　　Skill training
　　　Evaluation/assessment
　　　Nursing
　Case management/service coordination
　Financial assistance:
　　Discretionary cash subsidy
　　Allowances
　　Vouchers
　　Reimbursement
　　Line of credit

　Environmental adaptations:
　　Adaptive equipment
　　Home modification
　　Vehicle modification
　Systemic assistance
　　Information & referral
　　Advocacy

　Training
　　Parent training
　In-home assistance:
　　Homemaker
　　Attendant care
　　Home health care
　　Chores

staff of Developmental Disabilities Planning Councils in 12 states. At the conclusion of the two-day meeting, the group affirmed the following principles:

Children, regardless of the severity of their disability, need families and enduring relationships with adults in a nurturing home environment. As with all children, children with developmental disabilities need families and family relationships to develop to their fullest potential. Adults with developmental disabilities should be afforded the opportunity to make decisions for themselves and to live in typical homes and communities where they can exercise their full rights and responsibilities as citizens.

Family support should be readily available and should not require the family to fight for it.

Families should be involved in planning, designing, and evaluating family support at all levels of the system including federal, state, and local.

Family support services should be community centered, family centered, integrated, and coordinated.

Family support should be designed to be sensitive to cultural, economic, social, and spiritual differences.

Family support should include interagency coordination and collaboration.

Family support should be directed at the whole family and should be aimed at keeping families together.

Family supports should be flexible.

This direct and committed call to affirm the family, all families, is, despite its apparent simplicity, at the heart of a national re-examination of how human services should be designed and provided. The impetus for developing a family policy is not limited to the field of mental retardation and developmental disabilities, but is also being echoed across the human services community. The 1991 report by the National Commission on Children provides a generic and comprehensive analysis of the needs of families nationwide and advances several family support principles. The National Conference on State Legislatures (Wright and King, 1991) has also highlighted the importance of family support policy in a recent monograph on developmental disabilities. All of these policy initiatives and refinements point to a growing national consensus regarding the relationship of healthy family functioning to the well-being of all children regardless of their disabilities or vulnerabilities.

CONCLUSIONS

Research suggests some important lessons for those who are designing family support systems. Specifically, the role of the service coordinator or family facilitator emerges as central to the ability of the family to secure resources and to make connections in the community. Families rate this facet of their family support program very highly. There are many obvious reasons why this is the case, not the least of which has to do with the difficulties families face in gaining access to complex service systems. The role played by the family facilitators in these programs is also different from that of a conventional case manager since it involves more of a partnership or collaboration between the paid staff person and the family member. Finally, families report that just having a sympathetic person at the other end of the line who is willing to give advice, come over to help cope with a crisis, or simply listen is a significant support for them and their families.

The change in the role of case managers raises an additional design issue—the importance of training and retraining to ensure that staff in family support programs have a firm grounding in the programmatic assumptions that underlie the program. Such training is crucial given the ways in which family support programs depart from more conventional services. For staff, this means developing more collaborative approaches and vesting more of the decision making and determination of needs with the family. These approaches are not necessarily part of current training for case managers and other staff, and without an aggressive campaign to reorient existing personnel, standard operating procedures will persist.

Studies suggest the importance of some form of flexible funding within family support programs in order to meet the idiosyncratic needs of families of children with disabilities. Given the extreme variability in the types of things that families say they need, it is virtually impossible to design a family support program that can anticipate all of these needs and provide for them. The only way to ensure that family support programs are capable of responding in a flexible fashion is by including a cash component. While the family subsidy program in Michigan offers the most flexibility by providing families with "no strings attached" monthly stipends, there are many other ways of making cash available to families for specific purchases (e.g., through vouchers, cash reimbursement, etc.).

Interviews with families around the country graphically point out the difficulty that families face in attempting to gain access to services and the extent to which they are made to feel that they must "beg" for services and/or are demeaned for asking for help. This attitude not only is disempowering of families but it may dissuade some people from seeking needed services. This tendency to treat potential clients as supplicants rather than equals can be rectified by a strong affirmation of the principles of empowerment and family commitment as part of the design of any family support program. Such principles should not only be part of the specific mission of discrete family support agencies but should also be present in statute and regulation (see state family support laws in Colorado, New Hampshire, and Oregon).

A major way of ensuring that these principles are in fact reflected in program implementation is to create oversight mechanisms that involve families in a direct monitoring role. It follows that if family support programs are "family focused," then families should be involved at various levels to ensure that programs continue to live up to the expectations that were initially vested in them. For instance, New Hampshire and Louisiana have included family support councils as a key ingredient in their family support programs. These councils are vested with the responsibility of evaluating the conduct of family support providers. The inclusion of families in these capacities should provide an early warning system regarding any compromise of the original governing principles.

The needs of families are not only idiosyncratic but span a number of agencies (e.g., health, social services, Social Security Administration, education, etc.). Services are currently organized in a way that puts the onus on the family to seek out and apply for services from each agency in turn. The result is an onerous burden for families who already face more than their share of time-consuming tasks associated with caregiving. In order to relieve families of some of this responsibility, designers of family support programs should build in an interagency component. This can be accomplished in several ways including joint agency sponsorship, interagency councils, integrated agencies at the local level, and so forth.

One of the biggest challenges for those who design family support programs is to address the very real isolation and stigma faced by families of children with mental retardation and other disabilities. Such isolation can be seen in the strong need expressed by families to find recreational and leisure time activities for their families and in their anecdotal reports of shrinking social contacts resulting from the pressures of caregiving as well as the withdrawal of some friends and relatives from the family. One of the aims of a family support program, therefore, should be to assist families to make connections in their communities and to take advantage of natural support systems in their own neighborhoods. This assistance should also be directed at helping families to identify integrated recreational programs and to ascertain the types of supports that might be required to successfully gain access to such community services.

The family support movement is being touted as a critical element in the emerging community system. Given this increased interest in family support, it is important to explore some of the limitations of the program as well as some realistic cautions. First, it is important to keep in mind that family support programs cannot be a substitute for basic foundation supports, including health care, income assistance, parental leave opportunities, and day care. Family support programs should not, therefore, be sold to policy makers as the sole or sufficient intervention on behalf of families with children with disabilities but rather as "whatever it takes" over and above these basic safeguards to maintain a child in the home.

It should also be recognized that even the best family support programs will not, in every case, prevent the placement of a child out of the home, either temporarily or permanently. Not all families will be able to meet the challenges of a family member with a disability and some families will seek placement in order to preserve the integrity and functioning of the remainder of the family. In these instances, public policy must assure that other resources are available and that such alternatives are also family based (e.g., adoptive families, specialized foster families, etc.). Family support policy that stresses the maintenance of children within natural families should also not be used as a sword to diminish or attack those families forced to make a placement.

Further, there is also a danger that family support programs will be promoted as a way of reducing the demand for services and reducing waiting lists. Family support should not be seen as a substitute for the provision of services to adults who, like their brothers and sisters, deserve to be given the opportunity to pursue their lives as independent adults. If family support becomes a thinly disguised means of shifting the responsibility for people with disabilities back onto the family, the basic principles underlying the movement will be betrayed and the trust of families in the service system will be further eroded.

In line with this issue is the need to address how adult children will be treated within family support programs. Clearly, many adults—both those with disabilities and those without—continue to live with their parents after they reach the age of majority. Recent economic contractions coupled with inflated housing prices have made this phenomenon more prevalent in the past decade. Thus, it would seem arbitrary to design eligibility requirements that cut off entry to those families with a family member over 21 years. However, there should also be a sensitivity to the emerging adult and the importance of ensuring that his or her choices regarding where to live are respected. In other words, family support for families with adult family members should be provided when it is determined with certainty that the wishes of the person with a disability as well as the family are taken into account.

It will also be important as family support gains legitimacy in disability policy to ensure that it is not simply a white, middle class program. This fear is supported by the fact that the political movement for family support has been led primarily by middle class and upper-middle class families. If family support programs are also to reflect the needs of minority families and families living in poverty, policy makers and program administrators will have to include these constituencies in the design of programs and will have to assess the most efficacious ways of reaching out to these communities.

The need for family support should also be seen as an important issue for women, who are the primary caregivers for children with disabilities in the overwhelming number of cases. Many women have had to put their lives on hold (e.g., professionally, educationally, etc.) to take on the responsibility of caring for their child. It is also often incumbent on women in the home to make the necessary connections with the community, to develop supports in the neighborhood and to negotiate the maze of services including the educational system. The implications of this frequent division of labor suggest that the push for family support should also be linked to other women's issues such as parental leave, child support, and day care. Additionally, those who espouse the values of family support should be cautioned not to overly romanticize the role of mother as caregiver in order to free her to pursue those personal goals that many other women are now able to pursue.

The critique that is being brought to bear on public welfare programs in general and the resulting concern for the perpetuation of dependence suggests a final issue for the future of family support programs—the incorporation of ways for families to make contributions back to the program and to other families. Many families are uncomfortable with the one-way character of publicly subsidized supports and report positive feelings about programs that offer them the opportunity to give back something. This can be accomplished in a variety of ways including bartering arrangements in which families can contribute their talents to others in the community, self-help groups where families can share their experiences and expertise, and the use of families as service brokers, coordinators, and/or advocates for other families.

This chapter is an initial effort to flesh out the outlines of an emerging service paradigm. Since the program is still somewhat formative, the analyses and findings should be treated in a similar fashion. One thing does appear certain, however. The family support movement has gained substantial momentum and acceptance and its premises are attractive to those who espouse a leaner, more consumer-focused, and locally based human services system. The challenge is to ensure that the excitement and innovation that accompany these initial efforts can be sustained in the face of budget constrictions and the tendency in human services toward inertia and routinization.

REFERENCES

Agosta JM, Bradley VJ (Eds.) (1985): Family care for persons with developmental disabilities: A growing commitment. Cambridge, MA: Human Services Research Institute.

Ashbaugh J, Spence R, Lubin R, Houlihan J, Langer M (1985): Summary of data on handicapped children and youth. Cambridge, MA: Human Services Research Institute.

Ferguson PM, Olson D (Eds.) (1989): Supported community life: Connecting policy to practice in disability research. Eugene, OR: University of Oregon, Center on Human Development.

Knoll J, Covert S, Osuch R, O'Connor S, Agosta J, Blaney B (1990): Family supports services: an end of decade status report. Cambridge, MA: Human Services Research Institute.

McKaig K (1986): Beyond the threshold: Families caring for their children who have significant developmental disabilities. New York: Institute for Social Welfare Research, Community Service Society of New York.

Schorr LB (1988): "Within our Reach: Breaking the Cycle of Disadvantage." New York: Doubleday.

Smith M, Card F, McKaig K (1987): Caring for the developmentally disabled child at home: The experience of low income families. New York: Community Service Society of New York.

Wright B, King M (1991): Americans with developmental disabilities: Policy directions for the states. Denver, CO: National Conference on State Legislatures.

Linking Parents with Parents: The Family Connection Casebook of Best Practices in Family Support*

Barbara Gibbs Levitz and Allen A. Schwartz

During the last two decades, the number of parent support groups for families of children with Down syndrome has grown in number from a handful nationally to over a thousand internationally. The one commonality of all such groups is the goal of offering parent-to-parent support. In most instances, this objective was the initial reason for the establishment of the Down syndrome parent support groups. Many also perform multiple functions such as information and referral, advocacy, promoting public awareness, parent and professional education and training, and others.

However, there may be limited access to the parent-to-parent model of support because many parent groups are informal and do not have well-defined systems for receiving and acting upon referrals from health, education, and human service agencies. This model will focus on a replicable systematic approach in providing one-to-one supports to families of children with Down syndrome and other developmental disabilities.

Family support services include a variety of ways to assist families in "whatever it takes" to strengthen their ability to care for a family member with a developmental disability at home and improve their quality of life. In New York State, these supports have been administered primarily through a wide range of provider agencies and organizations, and are typically organized as "formal" programs. This report focuses on one method of encouraging the development of informal supports through a parent-to-parent network.

THE FAMILY CONNECTION

The Family Connection of the Lower Hudson Region, exemplifies what its director believes is one of the most effective means of providing support to care givers:

*A version of this article was previously published as a report entitled *Linking Parents With Parents*, developed as part of the Family Support Services Best Practices Project of the New York State Office of Mental Retardation and Developmental Disabilities, Albany, NY.

families helping other families. It does this by systematically linking a family or care giver of a child with a developmental disability to a family that has had similar experiences or needs. The network that has evolved through The Family Connection is composed of families living in Westchester, Rockland, and Putnam Counties of New York with children of all ages and many disabling conditions. The staff who coordinate the program are parents of children with developmental disabilities.

The Family Connection was established in 1992 following earlier recommendations of a collaborative community based initiative focusing on family support issues for early intervention. The program has offered one-to-one support to approximately 60 families and more than 50 additional families have requested information on organizations, programs, and services offering family support and advocacy. Professionals working in the field of developmental disabilities also ask for information about resources for families.

> We spoke to doctors, nurses, a geneticist, a pediatrician, but nothing compared to the support and understanding from actually meeting another family. And, although these professionals were supportive and knowledgeable, we still felt a sense of doubt. How could we actually believe them; they didn't have children with disabilities. They could not experience the feelings of confusion, loneliness, anxiety, and, above all, the uncertainty that overcame us when our daughter was born with a disability.—Margarita, mother of a four-year-old daughter with Down syndrome (all names are fictitious)

> Prospective parents can buy dozens of books in preparation for "The Big Day," but no one is prepared for the day they become the parent of a child with a disability. We walked out of the hospital having to deal with two government agencies, three nonprofit groups, two companies trying to make a profit, seven doctors, conflicting professional opinions, a mountain of bills, a lifetime of uncertainties ahead of us, and feelings that ran from joy and hope to actual grief at the loss of our "normal" child.— Timothy, father of a three-year-old daughter who is medically fragile and technology dependent.

The Family Connection is a key part of The Family Resource Center at the Westchester Institute for Human Development, a university affiliated program that is part of the Westchester County Medical Center and New York Medical College. The Family Resource Center has three primary goals:

1. To encourage and enlist family participation.
2. To provide a family and consumer perspective in training professionals.
3. To promote policy development and systems change through family and consumer education and training.

The Family Resource Center is in the process of developing a family resource library for families. Also available from the Institute are a regional technology center, foster families program, and other clinical and support services for individuals with developmental disabilities. A children's center is scheduled to open where children will receive general and specialty pediatric services. The regional medical genetics center will also be relocating to the Institute.

WHY IS PARENT-TO-PARENT SUPPORT SO VALUABLE?

Families linked to other families who share similar life situations can offer encouragement, emotional support and practical information on an informal basis. Volunteer support parents are available for telephone conversations and for visits at home or in the hospital. Support from volunteer parents is neither intrusive nor threatening because it has been either asked for or offered as an option. The purpose is to provide one-to-one support and friendship at a time it is most needed and to assist families in accessing information and resources.

This kind of help is especially meaningful because families caring for a family member with a developmental disability often share a commonality of feelings and worries. Mutual concerns are authentic and deeply felt. As a result, families often form a special bond with other families facing similar challenges. The support provided usually includes several contacts. Sometimes, the initial support may develop into a long-term relationship in which knowledge and encouragement are shared. This includes exchanging ideas and strategies on everything from dealing with daily life situations to advocating for programs and services. Such enduring friendships may spill over to other family members, especially siblings and grandparents.

> I remember meeting a family, a family whose memory will never fade. A family with knowledge, unbiased feelings, and, above all, a family that had gone through what we were going through. At last! . . . a family who could share some of our feelings. How reassured we felt knowing this family and later learning that there were more families like us.—Margarita

> I'll never forget the first time another parent gave me a call. It was like someone threw me a life preserver! She had a child who was nine; she had "been there before," and I could call her anytime.—Timothy

In addition to one-to-one support, families may also wish to join existing mutual-support groups. Referral information for this resource is provided by The Family Connection. And in cases when such support groups are not available, families who have been linked through parent-to-parent contacts sometimes form their own support groups to meet their specific needs.

Families helping families represents an invaluable untapped and underutilized resource that offers commitment, empathy, immediacy and personalized support in meeting individual needs. The approach may also provide the constancy and continuity of enduring relationships. It offers flexibility as to when, where, and how support is provided, is often available seven days a week on a 24-hour-a-day basis, and may offer a method for response to crisis situations.

HOW IS THE PROGRAM DESIGNED?

The Family Connection was designed along the lines of the parent-to-parent model program. Parent-to-parent is a way of providing support to parents of children with special needs. The support comes from parents who have experienced similar life situations and confronted similar problems. New or "referred" parents, who are either beginning to meet the challenges of having a person with disability in their family or are dealing with the stresses of a transitional period, are systematically matched with "veteran" parents. The connection that occurs through the program can lead to either one-to-one support or involvement in a parent support group. There is no fee for this service.

Support parents are volunteers. They complete an informational questionnaire and are offered training (some parents come to the program with strong interpersonal and communication skills from prior education or work experiences). They are also provided with a support parent training manual that offers guidance and information about how to be a sympathetic listener and effective supporter. Some support parents are bilingual, so parents who speak a variety of languages can be assisted.

Parent coordinators of The Family Connection match parents who have recently learned that their child has special needs with support parents. Matches are made based on the child's disability and special health care needs along with secondary factors such as family characteristics, language spoken, and geographic proximity. The parent coordinators are paid staff members of the program and are always parents of children with special needs. They follow standard procedures that include collecting and recording information, suggesting resources, coordinating linkages, and following up with both the referred family and the individual making the referral.

The three parent coordinators bring special skills and experience to this program. Their backgrounds include both leading and participating in councils and task forces, presenting at parent and professional training sessions, and coordinating parent-to-parent initiatives for organizations on Down syndrome and spina bifida. Their major areas of experience include early intervention, special education, transition from school to adult life, special health care needs and multiple disabilities, service coordination and entitlement programs, and outreach to Hispanic families. Staff members also have experience in office management, data processing, project design, and administration.

A 24 hour parent network hotline telephone number is available for after office hours, in addition to a message tape at the Family Resource Center in English and Spanish.

HOW DOES THE PROGRAM WORK?

In addition to parents of newborns or newly diagnosed children, other parents contact The Family Connection when they are faced with difficult transitions as the child is entering or exiting school, beginning an inclusive school or community program, or accessing a new service. Referrals can also come from health care professionals involved with the family, or friends and relatives of the family. Six steps are followed in engaging new families and matching them with a support family.

1. A parent coordinator at The Family Connection receives a referral by phone or personal contact from either a parent or from a professional, friend, or another family member providing the name of a parent who wants to be contacted.

2. A parent coordinator speaks with the family by telephone or during a personal visit at the hospital, home, or the Family Resource Center office and, from information gathered, identifies a support parent and/or a support group and other additional resources as requested, and informs the referral source that the family was contacted. All information that is recorded is used for matching purposes and is considered to be confidential.

3. The family contacts the support parent and/or support group themselves or the parent coordinator notifies the support parent who contacts the family within 48 hours. If a referral is made to a support group, then their own procedures go into effect.

4. Additional telephone conversations or visits at home or in the hospital may be arranged between the family and the support parent and/or support group.

5. For short-term follow up, the parent coordinator contacts the family one week after the initial referral and again one month later. The family is encouraged to call or visit the Family Resource Center anytime they have questions, need information, or if they would like another support connection.

6. Long-term follow up may include recruitment for family participation in other activities such as becoming a support parent, parent education and training, to be a speaker, to join an advisory council, etc.

The support we received from that family gave us a feeling of hope. The feeling that I felt was that, someday, I too would be able to give hope to other families. And today, as I now in return support and offer hope to other families, I can only say that, had we not met this family, our lives would have taken a different turn.—Margarita

Today, the tables have turned and now I am the veteran that new parents can call. It is only because I have gone through my pains that I can help others go through theirs and it enables me to listen and support in a way that a professional never could. As volunteer jobs go this is a rather tough one to become qualified for, but the rewards almost make it worth it.—Timothy

Currently there are 100 support parents who are a part of The Family Connection network, including parents of children with a variety of disabilities including:

- mental retardation
- medically fragile and technology dependent
- pervasive developmental delay and autism
- attention-deficit disorder
- cerebral palsy and related orthopedic conditions
- genetic disorders (e.g., fragile X, Down syndrome)
- spina bifida and hydrocephalus

- speech and language delay
- visual and auditory problems
- muscular dystrophy
- craniofacial disorders
- traumatic brain injury
- seizure disorders and other neurological conditions
- prematurity and low birth weight
- fetal alcohol syndrome

LESSONS LEARNED

Parent-to-parent supports are vitally important for families of children with disabilities. Developing a centralized systematic support network has had the positive outcome of parents feeling less isolated and alone. With the help and support of other families who have "been there," parents are in a better position to make informed decisions.

The cornerstone of this program is finding a good parent-to-parent match, and helping families access resources, supports and services. The success of this program can best be measured by strengthening families and seeing many grow and become support parents for the other families.

Public awareness activities are extremely important in establishing a networking project of this nature. By sharing information and publicizing the program through radio, cable television, training programs and conferences, listings in directories, personal meetings, and brochure distribution, The Family Connection has established referral sources that include a variety of health, education and human service agencies. The program has also come to be widely known by professionals, community leaders, family members, and friends of people with disabilities.

In addition, the Family Resource Center established a regional Advisory Board composed of approximately 30 parents and professionals, who meet quarterly and are involved with ongoing outreach, referral, quality assurance, and consultant services. The board provides an avenue for families to voice their suggestions, and is an important source of feedback to the program to the program staff.

CONCLUSION

The Family Connection is designed as a parent-to-parent model program. This model is one example of the kind of community bridge building that can make a big difference in people's lives—make them feel included in a natural support network and closer to the community in which they live. It is a relatively inexpensive resource to develop in a community or region.

The program's design and materials have been shared for replication in other locations in New York State. Materials include a packet of procedural and information recording forms, recruitment letters, a brochure, and the support-parent training manual. The program is developing information packets appropriate for referred families. In addition, the parent coordinators are available for technical assistance in helping to develop similar programs.

FOR ADDITIONAL READING

Singer HS, Powers E (1993): "Families, Disability and Empowerment: Active Coping Skills and Strategies for Family Intervention." Baltimore: Brookes.

Trainer M (1991): "Differences in Common: Straight Talk on Mental Retardation, Down Syndrome, and Life." Rockville, MD: Woodbine House.

Smith, PM (1992): "You Are Not Alone: For Parents When They Learn That Their Child Has A Disability." National Parent Network on Disabilities, 1600 Prince Street #115, Alexandria, VA 22314.

Assessment and Planning and Systems Development Guides. National Center on Parent Directed Family Resource Centers, Parents Helping Parents. 535 Race Street, Suite 220, San Jose, CA 95126.

Parent To Parent National Survey Project. Beach Center on Families and Disability, The University of Kansas, 3111 Haworth Hall, Lawrence, KS 66045.

The Exceptional Parent 1994 Resource Guide: Directories of National Organizations, Associations, Products & Services. Exceptional Parent 24, 1, 1994.

Long-Term Caring: Family Experiences over the Life Course

Marty Wyngaarten Krauss and Marsha Mailick Seltzer

> The hardest part is at night, when he's laying there peacefully and you're thinking the 100,000 thoughts of what could have been and all the reasons why this happened. You think that from day one, and I think you ask that all your life. And it goes on 24 hours. It does not end—A 72-year-old mother of a 49-year-old son with mental retardation

A single event can transform not just one life, but many lives. It can change not just one stage of life, but an entire lifetime. Some events are considered "normative events" for they are expected, predictable, and occur at about the same time for most people. Examples include getting a driver's license, graduation from school, establishing one's own home, etc. Other events, however, are nonnormative, in that they do not occur in the lives of most people, are unplanned and unanticipated, and usually are not wanted or desired (Baltes et al., 1980; Brim and Ryff, 1980). Examples include temporary unemployment, divorce, traumatic injury or illness, and chronic disability. Both normative and nonnormative events have the potential to transform lives; however, nonnormative events do so in less predictable ways.

In our research, we are studying parenting a child with mental retardation as an example of a nonnormative event with lifelong consequences (Seltzer and Ryff, 1994). It is now recognized that the vast majority of persons with mental retardation live with or under the supervision of their families throughout their lives (Seltzer and Krauss, 1994). While parents are the primary careproviders, it is often assumed implicitly or explicitly that, upon their death or infirmity, one of their children will adopt the parental role (Krauss, 1990). The marked increase in the life expectancy of persons with mental retardation means that it is now, and will continue to be, the norm for adults with mental retardation to survive their parents and to enjoy sibling relationships in adulthood (Janicki and Wisniewski, 1985). Increasingly, many adults with retardation may subsequently rely on their siblings for support and possibly for direct care during their mutual old age.

This chapter reviews the basic questions that drive our research on families of adults with retardation and presents qualitative and quantitative information about aging mothers and their many decades of caregiving.

STUDY METHODOLOGY

This longitudinal study focuses on 462 families who provide in-home care for an adult child with retardation. When the study began in 1988, families met two criteria in order to participate: 1) the mother was age 55 or older, and 2) the son or daughter with mental retardation lived at home with her. Half of the families live in Massachusetts (n = 227) and half in Wisconsin (n = 235). The first phase of the study included four visits with each family in our sample, each visit occurring 18 months after the preceding one. (See Seltzer and Krauss, 1989; Seltzer et al., 1993 for more complete details regarding the study's methodology.)

At the time of study enrollment, the mothers ranged in age from 55 to 85 (mean = 64.8 years). Their sons and daughters with retardation ranged in age from 15 to 66 (mean = 33.5 years). About three-fourths had either mild or moderate retardation, and more than one-third had Down syndrome. Most (80%) have always lived at home with their parent(s). Thus, these families have provided a lifetime of care for their member with retardation.

Basic Questions Addressed

Clearly, one of the most compelling questions is *why* these mothers have elected to continue to have their son or daughter with retardation live at home with them. This is a particularly riveting question, given that the oldest mother in our sample is 85 years old and she has a daughter who is 66 years old who has never lived anywhere else.

The most common answer to this question is that they never considered any other option—either initially when their child was born or over all these years of parenting. One central theme that emerged in our interviews with mothers was their deep commitment to providing the most normal, loving, and caring environment possible. The mothers felt they were uniquely qualified to give their child the best care and that their children would not have been happy elsewhere. As one mother said,

> She was my child and I feel responsible for her. We've loved her and
> wanted the best for her. We've handled problems at home with love and
> understanding. My daughter always said she wanted to stay home.

Another common theme suggests the mutual benefits that accrue from a lifetime of caring. At this stage in their lives, many mothers derive companionship, household assistance, and a sense of stability and continuity from their continued caregiving. For example, one mother said, "She provides almost as much care for me as I do for her. She's kind and sees what I need. We both provide company for each other."

A third reason for continued parenting is a distrust of the alternatives. About one-fifth of the families in our study had at one time placed their child with retardation in another setting—usually an institutional setting when the child was much younger. Others have either heard about or observed problems in community residences. For many parents, the prospect of having nonfamily members provide the day-to-day supervision and care for their child with retardation provokes a great deal of anxiety and, indeed, fuels their resolve to continue as the primary careprovider. One mother commented that "I made the decision when she was younger— I never really had any questions about it. I think there are a lot of bugs to be worked out in group homes. They give them too much freedom. They don't use common sense. There's no continuity in staff."

These themes reveal the logic and passion of the intensely felt reasons why families continue to have their adult sons and daughters live at home with them. For most, this arrangement simply suits their family values, fulfills their sensibilities about the importance of family life, and attests to the durability and impressive strength of the emotional bonds that sustain most family systems. These families should inspire strong respect from policy makers and service providers, and not necessarily provoke images of enmeshed, overprotective family units. These are not families who are eager to change their lifetime commitment and efforts on behalf of their member with retardation.

We have also investigated how the mothers feel about their caregiving—a particularly important question given their age and the fact that most reared their children in an era when there were few services available and in which the social acceptance of their children was abysmally low. Most of the mothers are eminently proud of the care they have provided their children with retardation. They describe in quiet terms their efforts to provide the most nurturing care possible and give plenty of applause to the inspiration and actions of other parents of their generation who helped forge pathways towards dignity and humane opportunities. As one mother said,

> The first two years (1943–45) were bleak, with institutional placement the recommendation of professionals. How did we cope? Well, first we founded a parents' group. Then we helped to establish a special kindergarten class and turned it over to the school board. Also, we worked to develop our local sheltered workshop and most recently, we promoted the infant stimulation program for young families. The best way to cope is to join with other parents early on, learn together, and then you can help to provide the best possible future for all retarded children.

We conducted additional analyses to assess the current well-being among mothers in our study (Seltzer and Krauss, 1989). We used a multidimensional perspective on well-being, which we defined as physical health, life satisfaction, perceived burden of care, and parenting stress. We found considerable evidence that the mothers in our sample had at least as high a level of well-being as several relevant comparison groups. Specifically, mothers in our sample reported better physical health in comparison to other women their age with and without significant caregiving responsibilities, reported greater life satisfaction in comparison to other women who provided daily care to an elderly relative, and reported no greater burden or stress associated with parenting a child with retardation in comparison to younger mothers of children with mental retardation or women providing care to an elderly relative (Krauss and Seltzer, 1993).

These positive outcomes, at first glance, were puzzling to us. The mothers in our study averaged 66 years of age, with the oldest mother 85 years old. Most of their sons and daughters with retardation had lived at home their entire lives and had received minimal educational or other support services when they were children. Their mothers reported considerable difficulty getting competent professional help and experienced many instances of the social insensitivity and discrimination that was particularly prevalent in the 1940s through the 1970s. Most mothers also had poignant accounts of the often heroic efforts they had expended to raise their child with retardation along with their other children. The "objective" facts of their histories, diverse and unique as each one was, conveyed a common theme—the arduous task of parenting a child with retardation in an era in which little public and often spotty private support was available. Their "subjective" perspectives on their histories also conveyed a common theme—these women felt like pioneers. Their experiences opened up new opportunities for their children; they used their situations to forge a "career" as a parent; and they now gamely recounted the successes they achieved. It was clear that, at this stage in their lives, they had developed a frame for their experiences, a set of beliefs about what had happened to them, and a personal view of what this nonnormative event had taught them about themselves, their families, and about people with disabilities.

Why is it the case that our sample of caregiving mothers—whom we expected would be at *greater* risk for poor physical health, poor morale, more burden, and more stress—appear to be just the opposite? At least three factors come into play here. First, there is a self-selection process regarding which families decide to rear their son or daughter with mental retardation at home, even after the child has reached adulthood. While this self-selection factor is an important one, it must be remembered that most persons with retardation live at home in childhood and adulthood. Thus, in this respect, the families we are studying are not atypical.

A second explanation for the unexpectedly positive well-being of the mothers we are studying is that after so many years of caregiving, these parents have adjusted to their situation and accommodated to their responsibilities as a long-term family caregiver. Many parents noted that earlier in life they experienced more burden and distress associated with having a child with retardation. However, with the passage of time, many have accepted their child's limitations and developed an appreciation of his or her strengths. One mother reflected,

> Twenty-seven years ago, when Anne was born, they told me she'd only live for six years. The services were appalling back then and we had very little support. It's been a long haul, but full of love that nobody unless they've been through it can understand. She's taught me compassion and understanding. She's taught me to treat people properly.

Another mother in her 70s told us,

> It wasn't positive when he was young, but we've enjoyed seeing him progress. These are the golden years of caregiving.

A third explanation for the favorable well-being of our sample relative to comparison groups is that the mother may be deriving benefit from the adult child with retardation. Some receive direct support from their son or daughter. For example, many of the adults with retardation in our sample did chores around the house. In some situations in which the parent was becoming physically frail, the able-bodied son or daughter was essential for the maintenance of the household. One mother told us that her son

> . . . is a joy to have around. He gives me support and helps me with his father, who has Alzheimer's. As long as I am able, I'll keep both of them at home.

In addition, many mothers—widows in particular—described the importance of the companionship provided by their son or daughter and the strong emotional bonds of affection that exist between them. One widow told us,

> We are good for one another. She is my friend. Although there have been difficult times, I can't imagine life without her. She would not be happy . . . and neither would I. She keeps me young.

It also appears that some parents have maintained their health and emotional fortitude *because of* the caregiving role, which gave them a continued sense of purpose in life. These mothers appeared to have responded to the challenge of rearing a child with retardation by developing new adaptive capacities, reaching into previously untapped personal reserves, and envisioning new opportunities for growth and development. As one mother told us,

> This child has taught me an appreciation for the little things in life that we all take for granted. My other children learned about love and caring for others from Cindy. I don't ask, "Why me?" I ask, "Why not me?"

For any one or a combination of these reasons, the mothers in our sample currently are, on balance, a well-functioning group of aging women. While few deny that they have experienced grief, frustrations, and many disappointments, most of the mothers in our sample now report more gratification than frustration.

However, we know that there will be profound changes in all of these families during the next few years, because the aging of the family unit will pose challenges more difficult than any they have faced in the past. All of these families will face a "caregiving gap," which will emerge after the mother is no longer able to function as the primary caregiver. While there is a great deal to be learned about what the future has in store for the mother and for the other family members, in many families a sibling of the adult with retardation will bridge the caregiving gap.

We have also studied the long-term care plans described by mothers in our study. Four basic patterns of long-term care plans emerged from our analyses (see Fig. 1). These patterns are based on the mothers' anticipation of the durability of family care and on mothers' anticipation of out-of-family placement.

The first dimension, durability of family based care, was determined by whether there was someone else in the family who would take over if the mother could no

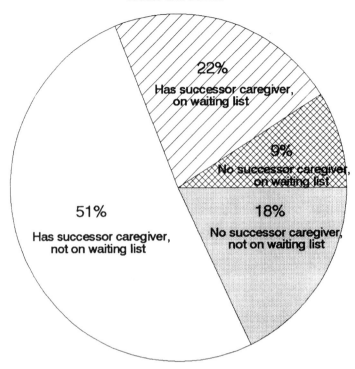

Fig. 1. Long-term care plans as reported by mothers.

longer provide care. We designated this person as the "successor caregiver." The second dimension, willingness to consider out-of-family placement, was determined by whether the parent had added the son or daughter's name to a waiting list for residential services. These are separate dimensions; the relationship between them was not statistically significant.

Half (51%) of the mothers anticipate continued family based responsibility: they could identify a successor caregiver and did not have their child's name on a waiting list for residential services. In contrast, only 9% anticipate relinquishing the responsibility solely to the public residential system: these mothers could not identify a successor caregiver and had placed their child's name on a residential waiting list. Almost a quarter (23%) anticipate a mix: they had named a successor caregiver *and* had their child's name on a waiting list. For these mothers, it is assumed that they will, in fact seek residential placement, but will also rely on continued family involvement to supervise the care of their adult member with retardation. Alarmingly, we point out that 18% of the mothers had no provisions in place for their child: there was no successor caregiver and their child's name was not on a waiting list.

Our analyses have yielded three basic conclusions. First, most of the older parents in our study feel very positively about their caretaking decisions. They interpret the decision to raise their child at home as consistent with their sense of family responsibility and parental duty. Despite the difficulties they enumerate around specific issues, the "bottom line" of their decision is seen as being in the credit rather than the debit column.

Second, even at this stage of life, active attempts to place children are the exception rather than the rule. While a third of the families have their child's name on a waiting list, the waiting list is often used simply to provide a sense of security for the parents.

Third, while most families indicate another family member will in fact assume responsibility for the overall well-being of the adult with retardation, few expect this transfer of authority to include residential placement with the relative.

These findings attest to the durability of family ties across the life span, but also suggest that even among parents in their 60s, 70s, and 80s, planning for the inevitable residential relocation of their adult child with retardation is met frequently with avoidance and denial. This is clearly a significant issue for service providers, as well as the siblings of adults with retardation, who will inherit a tremendous responsibility.

There is a serious fragility in the long-term care plans among these families— plans that involve siblings may be implicit rather than explicit. New and creative strategies need to be developed to incorporate siblings into the care planning for their brothers and sisters. This fragility will not disappear until there is a more reasonable supply of community residential programs, a more equitable and predictable array of services for families, and a greater social, political, and fiscal appreciation for the complexity of families who shoulder the responsibility for millions of persons with developmental disabilities. We cannot continue to ignore this durable social force, which has demonstrated for centuries that retardation requires and receives a lifetime of commitment. This is a critical agenda for the remainder of this century and into the next. We have seen how families "practice" their caregiving roles. It is time to develop and implement the policy to support their efforts.

ACKNOWLEDGMENTS

This research is supported by a grant from the National Institute on Aging (R01 AG08768) and from the Joseph P. Kennedy, Jr. Foundation. Support is also provided by the Starr Center for Mental Retardation at Brandeis University and the Waisman Center for Human Development at the University of Wisconsin–Madison.

REFERENCES

Baltes PB, Reese HW, Lipsett LP (1980): Life-span developmental psychology. Ann Rev Psych 31:65–110.
Brim OG Jr, Ryff C (1980): On the properties of life-span events. In Baltes PB, Brim OG, Jr (Eds.): "Life-span Development and Behavior," vol. 3. New York: Academic.
Janiciki MP & Wisniewski HM (Eds.) (1985): "Aging and Developmental Disabilities: Issues and Approaches." Baltimore: Brookes.
Krauss MW (1990): Later life placements: Precipitating factors and family profiles. Paper

presented at the 114th Annual Meeting of the American Association on Mental Retardation, Atlanta, GA.

Krauss MW, Seltzer MM (1993): Current well-being and future plans of older caregiving mothers. Irish J Psych 14:47–64.

Seltzer MM, Krauss MW (1989): Aging parents with adult mentally retarded children: Family risk factors and sources of support. Am J Ment Retard 94:303–312.

Seltzer MM, Krauss MW (1994): Aging parents with co-resident adult children: The impact of lifelong caregiving. In Seltzer MM, Krauss MW, Janicki MP (Eds.): "Life Course Perspectives on Adulthood and Old Age." Washington, DC: American Association on Mental Retardation.

Seltzer MM, Krauss MW, Tsunematsu N (1993): Adults with Down syndrome and their aging families: Diagnostic group differences. Am J Ment Retard 97:496–508.

Seltzer MM, Ryff C (1994): Parenting across the lifespan: The normative and nonnormative cases. In Featherman DL, Lerner RM, & Perlmutter M (Eds.): "Life-span Development and Behavior," vol. 12. Hillsdale, NJ: Erlbaum.

Aging and Down Syndrome

Janet S. Brown

Advances being made in scientific research, health care, educational methods, training, and employment opportunities on behalf of persons with Down syndrome have created helping resources that were scarce or nonexistent earlier in this century.

Changing attitudes and growing awareness about Down syndrome among parents, educators, the health and social service professions, the legal community, and legislators hold the potential for making lifetime planning more readily accepted and easier than it is today for the families of the thousands of older adults with Down syndrome.

Rapid advances in clinical treatment during this century have been responsible for the increase in the life span of men and women with Down syndrome. Ninety years ago children survived to a mean age of nine. Today, as many as 80% of adults with Down syndrome live to age 55, and some beyond that. Most of the other adults have lived with their families their entire lives. Others, institutionalized in early life, returned home when deinstitutionaliztion became an almost general public policy approximately 20 years ago. Although mandated, community services that were established were either insufficient, inadequate, or nonexistent, and did not enable those discharged to grow to the maximum of their potential.

Medical observations have confirmed that physical maturation occurs earlier in persons with Down syndrome than in the general population. There is also a higher than normal incidence of some diseases. Individuals with the syndrome who live beyond the age of 35 will develop the pathological signs of Alzheimer disease, but not all will develop the dementia that accompanies it. It is currently believed that the incidence of Alzheimer disease in this population is overrated. Only an estimated 20% of the Down syndrome population can be said to have it. The incidence in the general population is 30% of those over the age of 80. Other causes of noticeable behavior changes are being actively investigated.

The aging parents of the growing number of older adults with Down syndrome, and their concern about the well-being of their adult children when they are no longer able to care for them, has brought the situation to a critical point. In 1987 a survey determined that in the United States there were 63,000 persons waiting for residential services. It is estimated that one third to one quarter of that number had Down syndrome. In 1988 another survey showed nearly 76,000 were waiting for day

99

programs. It can be assumed that the same proportion of persons with Down syndrome is represented in these figures as well. In New York State there are 14,000 developmentally disabled persons on the waiting list for alternative living arrangements, with the possibility of settling 1,300 a year. The wait in New Jersey is estimated at ten years for a list of 4,000; in Connecticut it is about the same.

There are social, legal, and financial aspects to consider in planning for continuing care, all with an overlay of understandable anxiety and deep emotion. Where a person will live, for example, when a parent can no longer care for him or her due to illness, death, or inability to cope with challenging behavior is important, but is only a part of what needs to be considered. It would be an understatement to say that for the older adult with Down syndrome for whom no advance plans have been made there are more questions than answers.

Many specialists have done substantial research on the many aspects and implications of a family's challenges in providing continuing care. Throughout the studies three major concerns appear: first for the person with Down syndrome, second for the rest of the family, and third for the service-delivery system.

Lack of many elderly parents' willingness to explore the steps to be taken to achieve the maximum independence and potential possible for their child is a generally recognized problem. Differences in cultural background influencing the attitudes toward care and treatment of children, men, and women are an influence not fully understood in the United States. Many cultures consider developmental disabilities supernatural illnesses for which there is no cure—illnesses that are stigmas and punishment for families.

Recognition of the changing demographics in the United States has resulted in the establishment of a federal Office of Alternative Medicine. In New York City, for example, funds have recently been given to Haitian, Russian, Dominican, Asian, and Hispanic organizations to make health services culturally relevant. For these groups, developmental disabilities and mental illness have been low on the priority list for treatment.

Lack of access to information or misinformation regarding legal and financial matters have led elderly parents to make inappropriate decisions resulting in situations totally contrary to their best intentions. Lack of advance planning inevitably leads to crisis planning.

Assuming that the optimum situation exists and parents (more likely to be the mother alone at advanced ages) are willing to make short-term and long-term plans, have openly discussed the matter with siblings, or, in the instance of only children, with other potential supporters, and included the person concerned to the limit of his or her ability to participate, there are actions that can be taken. In the United States individual states vary in their regulations, just as resources vary in number, location, and capacity to serve.

Each family has unique requirements; therefore, consideration needs to be given to the combination of actions that will best protect the interests of the relative with Down syndrome. Whatever the starting point of planning, periodic reviews are essential to insure that safeguards for person and property are consonant with changing conditions and needs of the individual and family. Planning needs to be regarded as an ongoing process and the best interests of the person with Down syndrome weighed as changes occur. There is a growing body of literature useful for guidance (see Suggested Reading).

For parents and involved family members making a decision about ongoing care the following questions must be answered:

1. Has a parent written a letter of intent? A letter of intent is the first step in organizing a life plan. It is, in essence, a set of instructions describing what the parent wishes future caregivers to know. The letter of intent gives essential information about medical history and care, educational background, employment training experiences, insurance coverage, benefits, social activities, religious affiliations, behavior management, preference for living arrangements, final arrangements, designated advocate or guardian, trustees, and other pertinent information about family members that will be of help to another caregiver. The location of all records such as social security information and birth certificates, for example, are important to include in a letter of intent. The existence of the letter should be known to the family or other potential caregivers. Preparing a letter is a valuable way of starting lifetime planning. No legal help is needed. The letter should be reviewed yearly and modified whenever new situations occur and information added.

2. Does the older adult need an advocate or a guardian? Effective implementation of a letter of intent depends on the people selected to follow its instructions. Even if a group or independent living arrangement is part of the picture, an advocate—a family member, friend, or agency representative—is essential to look after the person's best interest. A recent innovation in the mental health field is to teach self-advocacy skills to adults with disabilities.

An alternative to an advocate is a guardian, a person who is appointed by a court to look out for the child's interests. The law assumes that an individual over the age of 18 is competent to manage his or her affairs. This means that no matter how severe the disability, in the eyes of the court the person who has reached majority has the right to make decisions about the future. Parents are no longer considered the legal guardians. Guardianship proceedings vary from state to state, but there are general categories from which to choose, depending on the level of competence and other factors, such as guardian of the person, guardian of the estate, limited guardianship, or plenary guardianship. Plenary guardianship gives broad powers.

Initiating the guardianship proceeding requires filing a petition with a court. There are a growing number of lawyers who are knowledgeable about laws relating to developmental disabilities. Workshops are being offered nationwide by Down syndrome parent support groups and local and state organizations. Guidelines, readily available from many sources, enable families to do much of the preliminary information gathering themselves. The guardianship proceeding can be expensive. It also requires a finding of "legal incompetence" of the older adult with Down syndrome. Sometimes guardianship arrangements are started by parents having themselves appointed guardians after the child's 18th birthday and naming successor guardians in a will. Although this discussion is concerned with older adults, ideally parents should think about lifetime planning when the child is born.

3. Have financial plans been made to insure quality of life? Families with children who have disabilities require financial planning. In most cases, such children cannot be expected to earn enough, if employable, to meet their financial needs. Government benefits play an essential role, as lifetime care is costly. In the instance of the older adult with Down syndrome, the potential of increased incidence of physical ailments can mean higher medical costs.

Rules and regulations covering government benefits are complex. Some programs are federally run, others are directed by states, and still others are jointly financed by state and federal agencies under federally mandated guidelines. It is necessary, however, to make sure that whatever benefits to which the person is entitled are in place: Social Security, Supplemental Security Income, Medicare, and Medicaid.

Trusts can be established to supplement government benefits, but should be done in consultation with an attorney or trust department of a financial institution. Wills need to be written so as not to jeopardize government benefits. Even a small inheritance may cancel entitlements and be exhausted in a relatively short time.

In light of the currently limited opportunities for the older adult to find living arrangements other than at home—a group home, community residence, supported living apartment, or adult foster care—Developmental Services/Home and Community-Based Services, now commonly known as the Medicaid Waiver, should be sought. The Waiver represents a "user friendly" way of thinking about developmental disabilities. It was approved federally in December 1992 and became operational July 1, 1993. Some states have had a plan in place for several years; 49 out of 50 states have now adopted plans to comply with the waiver. About 15 emphasize services at home, the rest community residences.

The passage of the Americans With Disabilities Act is proof that public views regarding disabilities have changed. It is now recognized that a person with a disability has the same basic needs as anyone else, and services that addressed only therapies emphasizing the disability have been broadened to include basic needs. A patient or client is now more respectfully considered a customer or consumer. In Florida, for example, a new kind of service provider—an Independent Support Coordinator (ISC)—serves the whole person, not just one specific need. ISCs implement and monitor services under the waiver amendment; they work independently of case managers and government or nonprofit agencies providing other services; they serve a manageable number of individuals and their families, and are available at all times.

Whatever the state's approach, it is required to follow the design to integrate fragmented services into holistic systems. Individuals and families can have more control in deciding their own needs; costs of services are expected to be dramatically reduced.

Families with assets will want to develop estate plans for themselves to avoid probate and also to be particular about drawing a will. In the even of death, if there is no will with a trust for beneficiaries with disabilities, the state will write a will and distribute property according to its own probate laws. The laws were originally written for the general public and did not take into account families with special needs. A recent case in point in upper New York State concerned an older adult with Down syndrome who inherited a sizeable amount of cash and income-producing real estate from elderly parents who died within a few months of each other, plus cash from a deceased aunt. The man is unable to manage money; government benefits have been cancelled; two sisters are sustaining considerable expense to have the will probated. It's an example of good intentions gone awry. Whether resources are large or small, each sibling needs to have a will taking the same special considerations into account.

4. Have families thought about the living will and the durable power of attorney? Medical technology and medical ethics have not run a parallel course. The living will and durable power of attorney have been developed to give people some control over what happens in case of catastrophic illness or injury. The power of attorney for health care is more flexible than the living will as it permits a trusted person to act on the patient's behalf and enables that same period to oversee medical care.

The power of attorney for property is designed to give someone power to manage property when the parent is no longer able to do so. The power of attorney for property is an alternative to guardianship and protects financial interests for parent and child without the need of a guardianship proceeding.

5. Have parents had open communication with other children or trusted relatives about their plans? Unspoken assumptions about care of the older adult with Down syndrome can cause apprehension, anxiety, and anger. Sibling support groups now being established in many communities (the Association for Help of Retarded Children group in New York City has been meeting monthly for 12 years) have highlighted the need and desire for siblings to be involved in lifetime care and planning. Ability or willingness to accept responsibility changes over time, and open discussion, though painful or difficult for some, can be the key that opens the door to appropriate action. The end of a lifetime of care may be the hardest step of all for aging parents to accept, even though experience has shown that older adults, once adjusted in a stimulating, less-sheltered environment, do grow socially and can achieve increased measures of independence.

6. How can aging, protective parents be reached? This is a difficult question. Professionals in the field and siblings may need to recognize that there will be instances in which resolution of lifetime plans for older adults with Down syndrome will only be done on a crisis basis. Until patterns change, service systems and courts will need to be prepared for the contingency.

Siblings who are concerned can look for the network that will support them in efforts to put plans into effect for the time when they may be responsible for care or decision-making when parents are no longer living or are no longer able to carry out their daily responsibilities. This support may help them convince parents that planning is protection not abandonment. It is good to note that young siblings are being recognized as having a special role in the family, and groups have been organized for them. They will be better prepared for the future.

More opportunities need to be created for older adults with Down syndrome to participate in day programs when living away from home is not acceptable to the parent. Eliminating the age barrier to involvement in senior citizen centers that now exists in many states can provide socialization and ease the way to eventual transition. Awareness of the need for planning must be stimulated in the helping professions so that encouragement can be integrated with their services.

Plans for retirement should be considered as part of the employment picture if the person with Down syndrome goes to work. Physical conditions will probably reduce ability to work until 65, but a person who has the structure of a job will want and need ongoing stimulation and satisfaction.

The use of respite services in and out of the home should be encouraged to help with eventual transitions for parent and adult child. Respite services can demonstrate to parents that others can and do care for their child.

Options for services under the Medicaid Waiver should be explored as a way to provide the most useful kinds of help for the whole family. It has to be recognized that during the waiver shake-down phase, it takes time, effort, and patience to negotiate a new system. If successful, it can be hoped that the provision of new services will engender trust and provide the impetus for making future plans.

With a distance yet to go, society has come a long way in its attitudes toward Down syndrome. With today's involved and aware parents there is hope that the next generation of older adults with Down syndrome, and their families, will have had the benefit of thoughtful planning for their future.

SUGGESTED READING

Moss S (1992): "Aging and Developmental Disabilities: Perspectives from Nine Countries. The International Exchange of Experts and Information in Rehabilitation." University of New Hampshire (The Institute on Disability, a University Affiliated Program).

Russell LM, Joseph S, Grant A, Fee RW (1993): "Planning for the Future." Evanston, IL: American Publishing.

"Questions and Answers About Down Syndrome" (1992). New York: National Down Syndrome Society.

IV. Cognitive Development and Language Acquisition

Perspective

Paloma Garcia Cecilia

I am from Majorca, Spain, and before I start about my own life, I want to mention something very important for me because I heard Andy Trias say what he felt when they told him he had Down syndrome and he didn't know (see Section V). The same thing happened to me, but in a different way. I knew it in a way by the activities program I attended, and then I understood more or less what my parents felt when they had me. I wished that my parents had told me I had Down syndrome early on.

Although I am a person with Down syndrome, I went to a normal school, to the British Council School, where I stayed about 25 years. There I won the first certificate in English, and the most wonderful thing that happened to me was that it was the first time that I went to the United Kingdom, and not only this, but also because it was a step, a very important step for me. I learned another language that was not mine, and I was capable of going over to the United Kingdom, to hear people speak in English, and understand them.

During my studies, I ran an English magazine. I was on the editorial staff, and there I wrote several critiques of plays, films, poetry, stories and other things.

The reason why I went over to Majorca to live was because I felt that it was a time to be a bit independent by myself and support myself in life. Also because I felt various strong ties with my parents and my brother (my only brother) and five sisters that I have. There, in Majorca, I studied for our Spanish graduation, and after this graduation, I was awarded by the Ministry of Education and Science a certificate.

I enjoy reading very much, classical and modern authors, and also some poetry. I do quite well in swimming. I love classical music and opera, the theater, cinema, and also I like famous painters like Velasquez, Van Gogh, and Michelangelo. I went to Rome. That's why I like Michelangelo.

I believe that parents, professionals, and scientists must continue giving their support, their courage, their own experiences and knowledge, to give to all of us who suffer from Down syndrome something that is so human and important. I believe that we must leave behind those clichés that some people use about us. Because we are also people and we can know how to defend ourselves if we are able to have your support and your ability to show us, in a way, how to do it.

But the thing that is not always very clear for us people with Down syndrome is to know how to use our independence, and I think that is our goal. And why not give us more opportunity to grow. Let that superprotection that some parents have for their children, let that word be ripped completely out of the dictionary.

Finally, I want to express my gratitude in being with all of you and hope we will be able to come back here and share, once again, another Down syndrome conference. Thanks.

Neural and Cognitive Development in Down Syndrome

Lynn Nadel

Understanding brain and cognitive development in individuals with Down syndrome is an essential part of any plan to effectively intervene in the lives of these individuals in ways that will allow each to achieve their fullest potential. We have a long way to go before reaching this point. This chapter presents a brief overview of current knowledge in this area.

NEURAL DEVELOPMENT

It is generally assumed that there are a range of problems with brain development in individuals with Down syndrome. What is not at all clear is when in development these problems emerge, and how general they are. The best evidence at this time suggests that for most measures brain development is within normal range through the first 2 months of life, after which differences begin to emerge. A variety of neurochemical systems seem largely normal at birth (Brooksbank et al., 1989), as does the formation of myelin (Wisniewski and Schmidt-Sidor, 1989), a fatty substance that covers many nerves and helps them to function normally. Although there are some differences at birth, they are relatively minor. While we cannot exclude the possibility that serious problems, or forerunners to such problems, exist prenatally and just after birth, the general picture is one of measurable differences only emerging later in life.

Just how general are the problems that do emerge? Until recently, this question would have been answered with an assertion that neural deficits are probably observed in all systems, in line with the assumption that mental retardation is also seen across-the-board. However, the best evidence now suggests that defects in brain development are quite selective. Only some systems are affected, while others are apparently nearly normal. If there is any principle that seems to apply here, it is that the later developing parts of the brain are particularly likely to be affected (see Nadel, 1986). This is consistent with indications that noticeable defects only show up late in development, typically after birth. Should it turn out to be the case, this would have important implications for understanding the selective nature of the defect in brain development, as well as opening up potential avenues for structural intervention. The brain structures that, in particular, seem to be important in this regard include the cerebellum and the hippocampus, as well as specific cell layers of the neocortex (Nadel, 1986). All these structures share the feature of including granule cells, which have a unique proliferative profile that leads to delayed maturation.

BEHAVIORAL AND COGNITIVE DEVELOPMENT

Once again, we do not know enough about behavioral and cognitive development to make clear statements about the situation for individuals with Down syndrome. There is evidence that specific difficulties exist with certain fundamental sensory and motor capacities. One particular issue worth noting is the prevalence of hearing difficulties, which can account for at least some of the observed difficulties with language.

With regard to cognitive functions, it is important to raise the same questions as those raised with regard to the brain; that is, when are problems first observed, and how general are they?

The evidence suggests that problems in the area of cognitive function only emerge some time after infancy. Although it is quite difficult to assess cognitive function in really young infants, when this is done, infants with Down syndrome seem normal. Thus, infants with Down syndrome show normal classical conditioning (Ohr and Fagen, 1991), and normal acquisition of simple concepts of number and counting (Caycho et al., 1991). As suggested by our examination of brain development, real problems with cognitive development only begin to emerge after some months or years.

Concerning the issue of the generality of deficits in cognitive development, the evidence is again consistent with what is observed in terms of brain development; that is, deficits appear to be selective rather than across-the-board. One example comes from work on the emergence of various forms of spatial learning. Peter Mangan, in my laboratory, tested children with Down syndrome on three spatial-learning tasks, which differed in terms of the kind of information the children had to use in order to perform well (Mangan and Nadel, 1992). The basic task (see Fig. 1) involves remembering the location of a toy hidden under a pie plate. The experiment was performed in a room containing a large circular platform with 12 holes, each covered by a plate. In the first version of the task, the children had to remember to choose the pie plate on the right, or on the left, or straight ahead, in order to find the toy. We call this the Response Task. In another version of the experiment, the toy was hidden under a plate that had a specific, unique, color. All the children had to remember to find the toy in what we called the Cue Task was to search under the colored plate. In the third version of the experiment, the toy was always hidden under the same plate, in the same location. In this Place Task version all of the plates were of the same color, and the children had to remember where the correct plate was located in order to find the toy. In this case the children started from a different spot on each trial, so that simply going left, right, or straight ahead would not lead to consistent success (in contrast to the Response Task).

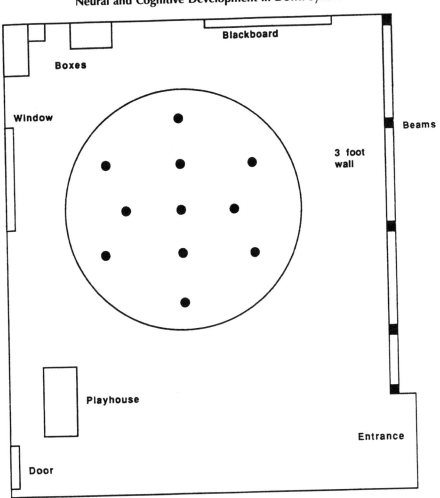

Fig. 1. The test environment, showing the spatial arrangement of the holes in the platform and the location of cues visible from the platform.

When the correct plate was identifiable by left–right turns, or by color, children with Down syndrome were relatively normal in their ability to find the toy (Figs. 2 and 3). When the correct plate was identifiable only by its location, children with Down syndrome were deficient (Fig. 4). The real difference emerged on the "memory probe" part of the experiment. Here, children were shown the location of the toy under a plate, and then were removed from the experimental apparatus for a delay interval. After the delay, children were returned to the platform and allowed to search for the toy. Figure 5 shows that the children with Down syndrome made twice as many errors as did normally developing children in this memory task. This highly

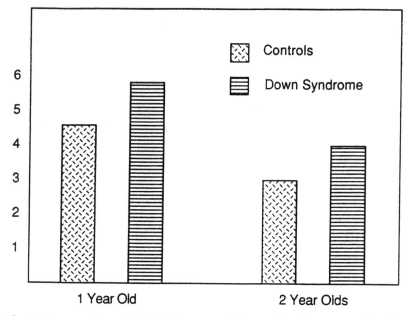

Fig. 2. Mean number of trials during successful test session for response learning.

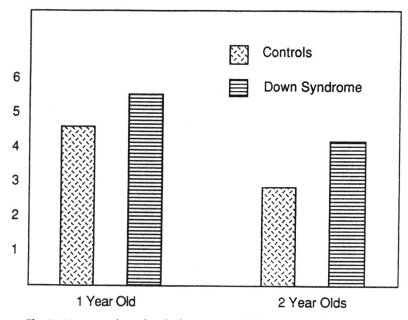

Fig. 3. Mean number of trials during successful test session for cue learning.

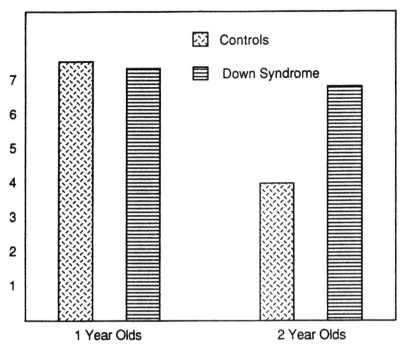

Fig. 4. Mean number of trials during successful test session for place learning.

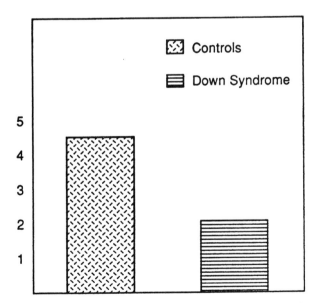

Fig. 5. Mean score on memory probe in place learning task.

selective result suggests that the brain areas responsible for learning about locations might be selectively compromised in Down syndrome. This is particularly interesting in that this kind of location learning is known to depend upon the hippocampus. Recall that we already noted the hippocampus as a late-developing brain structure that might be selectively deficient in terms of development. It is also worth pointing out that this brain structure is one of the first to show deterioration in Alzheimer disease. It is now well known that all individuals with Down syndrome show the neuropathological signs of Alzheimer disease by the age of 35–40 (see Dalton, this volume; Lott, this volume). Taken together these facts point to improper development of the hippocampus as a likely contributor to the cognitive difficulties observed in children with Down syndrome.

LANGUAGE

In the study of language development one is concerned again with exactly how to characterize the difficulties observed in individuals with Down syndrome. Are these problems generally observed in all aspects of language or are they selective, affecting only certain aspects of language?

Language function encompasses many separate abilities, including hearing, understanding the sounds that make up words (phonology), understanding the meanings of the constituents of words (morphology) and words themselves (semantics), understanding the meaning that derives from the order in which words are put together (grammar or syntax), being able to articulate and in other ways produce meaningful utterances, understanding the pragmatics of language use, and more.

Down syndrome seems to affect some of these abilities more than others. There is evidence that one of the earliest aspects of language learning, the "babbling" that infants engage in during the first year of life, is relatively normal in infants with Down syndrome (Dodd, 1972). There is also evidence that word learning is within normal range (Chapman et al., 1990). What appears to be most affected is the acquisition of syntax, or grammar. There is also evidence that particular problems exist in the phonological component of language, which involves the perception and production of speech sounds, as well as how these sounds are "represented" in our memory systems. Some of this work is discussed in greater detail in Fowler (this volume).

PROSPECTS FOR IMPROVEMENT

In thinking about how to approach intervention, and to help each individual with Down syndrome achieve his or her maximum potential, the facts outlined above suggest some interesting possibilities. The fact that serious problems only emerge after birth is important in thinking about the timing of intervention. Notwithstanding the fact that Down syndrome is a genetic disorder that takes effect from the very start of prenatal development, some currently unknown factors mitigate the impact of this disorder until after birth. Unless there are subtle, undetectable differences earlier on, this seems to allow for intervention at an early enough stage of development to have a considerable impact.

Another important factor to bear in mind concerns the enormous variability in outcomes from individual to individual. Again, given the identical underlying genetic cause, this variability suggests a great deal of latitude in how the Down syndrome phenotype unfolds. This variability means that there are certain conditions, still unknown, that can lead to very high functioning at least in some individuals with Down syndrome (see Rondal, this volume). We must find out what these conditions are, and to replicate them as widely as possible.

Yet another fact of critical importance is the selective nature of the observed defects. This opens up the possibility of concentrating on those particular abilities and capacities in each individual that are relatively preserved, in contrast to those that are less preserved. This is really no different than what one does with all children—figuring out what they are good at and what they are not so good at, and letting this guide one's approach to their early intellectual development.

Another important point is that there seems to be a particular problem in individuals with Down syndrome with the stability of learning. There are now several indications that learning in individuals with Down syndrome has a particularly unstable character. One might say that it rapidly "decays," or is forgotten. In normally developing children, learning episodes build on one another over time, creating the progressive accumulation of knowledge and skills that we are familiar with. In individuals with Down syndrome there is serious instability, of unknown origin, that hinders this accumulation of learning in some way. This fact suggests that special attention should be paid to ensuring that learning is strongly consolidated and perhaps repetitively drummed in. A related point is that progress is often observed in individuals with Down syndrome well into the second decade of life, in areas where learning is normally completed at an earlier age. This suggests that educational efforts should not be abandoned after the early years, even when progress is not always what one would hope for.

We know even less about prospects for improvement at the neurological level. The brain is a good deal more plastic than we once thought, but whether or not the neuromaturational problems seen in Down syndrome can be reversed remains completely unclear. There is some recent evidence that improper development of the hippocampal system (as a function of hypothyroidism) can reverse under some conditions allowing the hippocampus to reach normal values over time (Farahvar and Meisami, 1993), but whether this can apply to other cases of improper brain development, such as in Down syndrome, is completely unknown.

WHAT WE NEED TO KNOW

We desperately need more and clearer information about neural and cognitive development. Although we know a good deal now, there is still a great deal more to learn. In particular, much of what we learned until recently was gained from studies of individuals with Down syndrome who were not given the benefit of the very positive interventions and other strategies provided in recent years. It is no accident that the apparent potential of children with Down syndrome has risen dramatically in the past decade; this clearly reflects the fact that many, if not most, of these children have been provided opportunities and living situations that were not available to earlier generations. These enhanced conditions have helped us understand that the potential of individuals with Down syndrome is greater than what we had previously thought. In turn, we must now carefully study the progress of this newer, advantaged, generation to get a clearer picture of the exact nature of brain and cognitive development in Down syndrome.

It is also critical to have better knowledge about these early stimulation programs, and the various ways in which the potential of each child can be fully and optimally realized. While recent research and much observation and anecdotal evidence indicates that early stimulation programs can lead to real benefits, little is known about which programs work and, most importantly, why they work. Only when we know the answer to this question will we be able to design optimal strategies and promote the fullest life for each child with Down syndrome.

REFERENCES

Brooksbank BWL, Walker D, Balázs R, Jøorgensen OS (1989): Neuronal maturation in the foetal brain in Down's syndrome. Early Human Devel 18:237–246.

Caycho L, Gunn P, Siegal M (1991): Counting by children with Down syndrome. Am J Ment Retard 95:575–583.

Chapman RS, Kay Raining-Bird E, Schwartz SE (1990): Fast mapping of words in event contexts by children with Down syndrome. J Speech Hearing Disorders 55:761–770.

Dodd BJ (1972): Comparison of babbling patterns in normal and Down syndrome infants. J Ment Defic Res 66:35–40.

Farahvar A, Meisami E (1993): Recovery of rat hippocampal regions from early hypothyroid retardation: A study of volume, surface area, cell number and cytochrome oxidase staining. Soc Neurosci 23:1313.

Mangan P, Nadel L (1992): Spatial memory development and development of the hippocampal formation in Down syndrome. Paper presented at the 25th International Congress of Psychology, Brussels, Belgium.

Nadel L (1986): Down syndrome in neurobiological perspective. In Epstein CJ (Ed.) "The Neurobiology of Down Syndrome." New York: Raven Press.

Ohr PS, Fagen JW (1991): Conditioning and long-term memory in three-month-old infants with Down syndrome. Am J Ment Retard 96:151–162.

Wisniewski KE, Schmidt-Sidor B (1989): Postnatal delay of myelin formation in brains from Down syndrome infants and children. Clin Neuropath 8:55–62.

The Development of Early Language Skills in Children with Down Syndrome

Jon F. Miller, Mark Leddy, Giuliana Miolo, and Allison Sedey

This chapter will present a brief summary of recent findings from our research on early language learning in children with Down syndrome. While some of this work has been published or presented at national research meetings, the focus here will be on major findings and their implications for research and clinical practice. Four areas will be addressed: 1) a new measure of early language learning, 2) the unique language-learning profiles of children with Down syndrome, 3) anatomical differences that may be associated with speech intelligibility, and 4) using augmentative communication systems.

MEASURING EARLY LANGUAGE LEARNING: THE VALIDITY OF PARENT REPORT MEASURES

One of the most dramatic findings of our recent work has been documenting the validity of parent measures of vocabulary acquisition in children with Down syndrome. It has always been assumed that the families of children with handicapping conditions would be unreliable in reporting their children's progress. Our data suggest that this is not the case; in fact, the parents of children with Down syndrome are just as reliable in reporting vocabulary production as the parents of typically developing children. Families of children with Down syndrome report their children's vocabulary progress with accuracy equal to parents of typically developing children. These results have been confirmed in a longitudinal study of vocabulary development (Miller et al., in preparation). These results suggest that parent-report measures like the MacArthur Child Development Inventories (Fenson et al., 1993) will provide us with a very powerful clinical methodology that is cost effective and can provide uniquely productive language data. Issues relevant for using parent-report measures for monitoring language performance are:

1. Parent-report measures of language performance can provide accurate information on the language performance of children with Down syndrome up to 30 months of mental age.

2. Parent-report measures can be repeated frequently without fear of "learning" affects on performance, making these measures ideal for monitoring intervention progress.
3. Parent-report measures access children's total vocabularies rather than vocabulary subsets derived from language samples.
4. Parent-report measures access all of the parents knowledge of their children's performance.
5. Parent-report measures can be used to record gesture and signed communication as well as oral language production.

UNIQUE LANGUAGE LEARNING PROFILES

Children with Down syndrome demonstrate a unique profile of language development. The results of our studies, and those of other researchers, document deficits in language-production skills relative to language comprehension and cognitive skills in these children. Our data document several unique features of these language-production problems. First, delays in language production are evident in only 50% of the subject sample up to 24 months of mental-age development. By 36 months of mental age almost all children with Down syndrome exhibit productive language deficits relative to mental-age progress. Second, deficits in language production are more pronounced in syntactic skills compared with vocabulary development. While 50% of the children exhibit deficits in vocabulary development, the remainder appear to be developing vocabulary consistent with their cognitive progress. All subjects exhibit deficits in acquiring syntactic skills. The specific causal mechanisms responsible for these deficits have not been identified to date. We are pursuing this issue in research sponsored by the National Institutes of Health.

We have learned from earlier research that productive language deficits do not appear to be accounted for by differences in parental language input, hearing status, general health status, or structural differences in the speech-production mechanism (Miller, 1992a; Miller 1992b; Miller et al., 1989a; Miller et al., 1989b; Miller et al., 1992a; Miolo et al., 1992; Sedey et al., 1992).

Issues relevant for monitoring language production are:

1. Expect language production to be delayed relative to language comprehension and general nonverbal cognitive skills. Language production skills are not a good predictor of language comprehension skills.
2. Delays in acquiring the syntax of English will be more pronounced than the acquisition of vocabulary skills.
3. Only 50% of children with Down syndrome seem to evidence deficits in vocabulary skills, while almost 100% of our subjects exhibited deficits in syntax by 36 months of mental age.
4. The rate of progress in acquiring language-production skills gets slower with advancing chronological age, though language learning continues through adolescence.

ANATOMICAL DIFFERENCES THAT MAY BE ASSOCIATED WITH SPEECH INTELLIGIBILITY

Persons with Down syndrome are biologically distinct as the result of an extra copy of the 21st chromosome. Almost every organ system of the body is affected (Lott and McCoy, 1992). The impact of these differences on speech production has been documented in a detailed review of the literature on the anatomy and physiology of persons with Down syndrome (Leddy and Miller, in preparation; Miller et al., 1992b). The latter review documented several differences that may be associated with the continued problems children with Down syndrome experience with speech intelligibility. We believe that the numerous central nervous system anomalies, along with differences in speech structures, such as the vocal cords, the oral cavity, and facial muscles, may restrict speech production in some persons with Down syndrome.

Central Nervous System (CNS)

Researchers examining the CNS of persons with Down syndrome have found smaller structures, including reduced cerebral hemispheres, fewer and smaller cerebral sulci and gyri, and a smaller cerebellum. At the cellular level, persons with Down syndrome have fewer cortical neurons, decreased neuronal density, abnormal dendrite structures, altered cellular membranes, and delayed neural myelination. These anatomical irregularities in the CNS are likely to reduce the accuracy, speed, and consistency of neural activity, indirectly disrupting the precision, sequencing, and timing of speech movements.

Vocal Cords. Current research (Leddy, in progress) on the vocal cord structure of persons with Down syndrome has found swollen vocal cords, with areas of redness and irritation. This suggests that the vocal cords are stiffer and vibration is interrupted, resulting in the hoarse voice frequently associated with Down syndrome.

Oral Cavity. Evaluation of the mandible, maxilla, and nasal bones reveals a smaller mandible, poorly developed maxilla, and absent nasal bones. The result is a smaller oral cavity, leaving less room for the tongue, which may "appear" to be too big for the mouth, to move during speech.

Facial Muscles. The facial muscles that attach to the upper lip of typically developing persons are distinctly separate, but the same muscles are fused together in individuals with Down syndrome. There is also an extra muscle in individuals with Down syndrome going from the corner of the mouth to the back of the head (Bersu, 1980). These muscular deviations have the affect of limiting lip movement for speech production.

These findings suggest that numerous anatomical and structural differences in persons with Down syndrome may be related to their disrupted speech production. The implication of this work suggests correcting structural deviations where possible, e.g., correcting dental overbite with braces, and to provide early motor–sensory stimulation to optimize oral function for speech.

USING AUGMENTATIVE COMMUNICATION SYSTEMS

We have evaluated the communication systems of our sample of children with Down syndrome in several studies to determine the extent augmentative communication systems have been employed by families and schools to improve overall communication. Overall we found that 75% of our children had been exposed to manual signing systems at some time during their development. Most of these systems were introduced when the children were between two and four years of age, though some children had sign introduced after the age of five. The usual reason given for introducing sign was to improve initial communication when early verbal attempts at communication were unintelligible. More than 20% of our families refused to have sign systems introduced with their children, believing signed communication would interfere with the acquisition of intelligible speech. Our data show that children acquire signed vocabulary, which expands their total (oral and signed) vocabularies. This suggests that signed vocabulary adds additional communication power to the child's functional communication system. Parents report that early signed communication reduces the child's frustration and provides the child with a clear method for referencing objects, actions, wants, needs, and people in the child's environment. Parents also report that as the child is more successful in communicating orally; i.e., speech is more intelligible and, the use of signs diminishes. The introduction of sign communication systems, if done properly, does not inhibit in any way the development of oral language skills (Miller et al., 1991; Sedey et al., 1991).

Issues in implementing signed communication systems are:

1. Sign systems should be introduced when children become intentional, acting on their environment communicatively, using gestures, vocalizations, or both.
2. Sign-system content should initially represent words that are relevant for the child in important communicative contexts, such as home, play activities, meals, pets, family members school activities, computers, lunch, snacks, etc.
3. Sign vocabularies should be focused on basic wants and needs to augment communication; sign should not be taught as a second language.
4. Families should learn to use the signs introduced to the child. Languages are learned through practice.
5. Sign should be taught and used as an extension of the child's natural gestures, a regularization of the gesture system. This will promote spontaneous communicative use of the sign system.
6. Remember, sign systems are introduced to facilitate communication when speech is unintelligible. As speech becomes more intelligible, the use of signs becomes unnecessary and children will spontaneously stop using them.

There is a great need for a standardized methodology for developing early sign systems for children with Down syndrome that can be used by families and schools. At present, children are introduced to a variety of sign systems, each developed independently by professionals working with the child and family. The focus of any sign system must be on communication, not method.

ACKNOWLEDGMENTS

This work was supported in part by research grant No. RO1-22393, NIH, NICHD, Jon Miller, Principle investigator and Behavior and Social Science Research Grant No. 12-197 from the National March of Dimes, Jon Miller and Lewis Leavitt, Principle Investigators.

REFERENCES

Bersu E (1980): Anatomical analysis of the developmental effects of aneuploidy in man: The Down syndrome. Am J Med Genetics 5:399–420.

Fenson L, Dale P, Reznick S, Thal D, Bates E, Hartung J, Pethick S, Reilly J (1993): "The MacArthur Communicative Development Inventories." San Diego: Singular Publishing Group.

Leddy M (in progress): The relationship among select vocal function characteristics of non-institutionalized adult males with Down syndrome. Department of Communicative Disorders, University of Wisconsin—Madison.

Leddy M, Miller J (in preparation): Anatomical bases for speech production deficits in individuals with Down syndrome. Waisman Center, University of Wisconsin—Madison.

Lott I, McCoy E (Eds.) (1992): "Down Syndrome: Advances in Medical Care." New York: Wiley-Liss.

Miller J (1992a): The development of speech and language in children with Down syndrome. In Lott I, McCoy E (Eds.): "Down Syndrome: Advances in Medical Care." New York: Wiley-Liss.

Miller J (1992b): Lexical acquisition in children with Down syndrome. In Chapman RS (Ed.) "Child Talk: Advances in Language Acquisition." Chicago: Year Book Medical.

Miller J, Miolo G, Sedey A (in preparation): The validity of parent report measures of early language for children with Down syndrome. Waisman Center, University of Wisconsin—Madison.

Miller J, Miolo G, Sedey A, Pierce K, Rosin M (1989a): Predicting lexical growth in children with Down syndrome. Paper presented at the annual convention of the American Speech-Language-Hearing Association, St. Louis, MO.

Miller J, Rosin M, Pierce K, Miolo G, Sedey A (1989b): Language profile stability in children with Down syndrome. Paper presented at the annual convention of the American Speech-Language-Hearing Association, St. Louis, MO.

Miller J, Sedey A, Miolo G, Rosin M, Murray-Branch J (1991): Spoken and signed vocabulary acquisition in children with Down syndrome. Poster presented at the annual convention of the American Speech-Language-Hearing Association, Atlanta, GA.

Miller J, Sedey A, Miolo G, Murray-Branch J, Rosin M (1992a): Longitudinal investigation of vocabulary acquisition in children with Down syndrome. Poster presented at the Symposium on Research in Child Language Disorders, University of Wisconsin—Madison.

Miller J, Stoel-Gammon C, Leddy M, Lynch M, Miolo G (1992b): Factors limiting speech development in children with Down syndrome. Miniseminar presented at the annual meeting of the American Speech-Language-Hearing Association, San Antonio, TX.

Miolo G, Sedey A, Murray-Branch J, Miller J (1992): Prelinguistic vocalizations and lexical development in children with Down syndrome. Poster presented at the annual meeting of the American Speech-Language-Hearing Association, San Antonio, TX.

Sedey A, Rosin M, Miller J (1991): A survey of sign use among children with Down syndrome. Poster presented at the annual convention of the American Speech-Language-Hearing Association, Atlanta, GA.

Sedey A, Miolo G, Murray-Branch J, Miller J (1992): Hearing status and language development in children with Down syndrome. Poster presented at the annual meeting of the American Speech-Language-Hearing Association, San Antonio, TX.

Linguistic Variability in Persons with Down Syndrome:
Research and Implications

Anne E. Fowler

In studies of persons with Down syndrome, as in classrooms and homes, two areas of cognitive function stands out as being of particular concern: the ability to hold verbal information in mind (verbal memory), and the acquisition and use of syntactic and morphological aspects of language (linguistic structure). These often constitute relative weaknesses in contrast to relative strengths in social communication, receptive vocabulary, and visual–spatial function (e.g., Fowler, 1990; Miller, 1987, 1988). At the same time, however, there is tremendous variability within the syndrome with regard to language function. For example, although normally developing children produce their first words between 6 and 14 months, children with Down syndrome begin producing words anytime between 9 months and 7 years; normally developing children put words together into simple sentences somewhere between 14 and 32 months, whereas children with Down syndrome make their first two-word combinations somewhere between 18 months and 8 or even 11 years. These onset measures vary individually from within the normal range to delays that are nothing short of frustrating (Stray-Gunderson, 1986). This extreme variability is evident as well in ultimate language attainments: although language is often limited (e.g., Wisniewski et al., 1988), there are many highly fluent adults to provide exception to that generalization (e.g., Rondal, 1994).

Why do so many persons with Down syndrome experience disproportionate difficulty in language and memory, and why are ultimate levels of language attainment so much greater in some individuals than in others? Is it the case that having Down syndrome puts a child "at risk" for language difficulties or do linguistic successes in even some individuals argue against that?

Two caveats are in order. First, it must be acknowledged that we have only just begun to tap the potential of persons with Down syndrome. For too long, expectations imposed at birth have limited this group, depriving them of educational opportunity and often of homes. With some of these barriers removed, there are now scores of young adults with Down syndrome who have violated all prior expectations, and the children growing up today may exceed even these attainments. A second caveat concerns the scope of what is meant by "language." Here the focus is on the structural rule-governed aspects of language—the formal system by which sounds are combined into words (phonology), and words into grammatically well-formed sentences (morpho-syntax). Whether assessed in comprehension or production, it is these structural aspects of language that appear to be disproportionately affected in Down syndrome, relative to other aspects of cognitive function. With these caveats firmly in place, three questions may be asked: 1) what is the nature of the difficulty; 2) what are the underlying sources of linguistic variation; and 3) how can we respond to the information we have?

WHAT IS THE NATURE OF THE DIFFICULTY?

Evidence for a specific difficulty with language derives from three different kinds of comparisons: verbal versus nonverbal processing; linguistic versus nonlinguistic communication; and syntax and grammar versus lexical knowledge.

Comparisons of Verbal and Nonverbal Processing

It has consistently been noted that linguistic processing abilities in persons with Down syndrome lag behind nonlinguistic processing abilities (e.g., Bilovsky and Share, 1965; Marcell and Weeks, 1988; Varnhagen et al., 1987). In a recent study it was found that even in young adults recruited on the basis of "good" verbal skills, sequential (largely verbal) abilities lagged significantly ($p < .05$) behind nonsequential (largely visual–spatial) abilities in 18 of 33 cases (Doherty, 1993; Fowler et al., 1993); there was at least a trend in that direction in 79% of all subjects. In contrast, only two (6%) of these adults showed a significant verbal advantage ($p < .05$). In the same study, subject scores on a visual–spatial task qualified as significant *strengths* relative to the composite *weaknesses* in 18 of 33 cases; performance overall on visual spatial processing was significantly better than performance on each of three different measures of sequential processing. Lest these results be construed as indicating a general difficulty with sequential processing, it should be added that the subjects achieved significantly higher age-equivalent scores when asked to replicate a series of hand shapes (which can be encoded visually, motorically, or linguistically) than when asked to retain strings of digits or common names (Doherty, 1993; for similar findings, see also Pueschel, 1988). Verbal memory was assessed without necessarily requiring a verbal output; in some cases, subjects could indicate an appropriate response by sequential pointing.

That verbal processing is a specific area of weakness is also evident in a direct comparison of the same young adults with Down syndrome with normally intelligent adults and much younger children matched on verbal memory. In this case, verbal span was based on the number of digits that could be recalled in the correct sequence, and visual–spatial span on the number of tapped blocks that could be reproduced sequentially without error. (To discourage the use of verbal encoding strategies, the blocks were identical in color and size and randomly scattered on a board.) It is generally the case that subjects perform better on the verbal measure, and this was the overall result in this study as well [$F(1,47) = 15.58; p < .001$]. However, there was a significant interaction between task and group. For both groups with Down syndrome, the word span exceeded the block span (see Fig. 1); for the case of the young adults with Down syndrome, there was a slight trend in the opposite direction (Racette, 1993). Interestingly, this pattern of verbal weakness seems to be more a function of the fact that these young adults have Down syndrome than it is a reflection of their overall cognitive difficulties. Quite different profiles are evident in other well-studied forms of congenital retardation. For example, in persons with fragile X syndrome, processing deficits extend to all kinds of sequential pressing, linguistic or not, suggesting that the underlying problem may be more attentional than linguistic (Dykens et al., 1993). And in persons with Williams syndrome, it is the verbal processing abilities that significantly and consistently exceed performance on visual–spatial abilities (e.g., Bellugi et al., 1988).

Dissociations within the Language System

Within the broader language system, it often seems that a lot more is being communicated than objective measures of morpho-syntactic structure would suggest. Although it is not easy to assess communicative (pragmatic) function quantitatively, several studies suggest that clinical intuition may be accurate. For example, there is now evidence that children with Down syndrome at the one- and two-word stage of spoken language development display conversational skills not yet evident in normally developing children at that same language level; they engage in complex imaginative play sequences and have mastered such conversational rules as turn-taking, making appropriate responses to questions, and making repairs when they are not understood (e.g., Beeghly et al., 1990; Coggins and Stoel-Gammon, 1982; Greenwald and Leonard, 1979; Mahoney et al., 1981; Peskett and Wootton, 1985). Children with Down syndrome also appear to have better social understanding than would be expected on the basis of developmental level (e.g., Baren-Cohen et al., 1992). In adults too, studies of communicative function (including gestures and turntaking) suggest that there is much communication going on even in those persons who are essentially nonverbal (Price-Williams and Sabsay, 1979).

The acquisition of morpho-syntax also appears to be generally less well-developed than conceptional aspects of lexical knowledge, at least as assessed via receptive vocabulary measures (Fowler, 1990; Miller, 1987, 1988). For instance, in Fowler et al. (1993), adolescents had receptive vocabulary levels equivalent to a six-year-old, but functioned more like three-year-olds in terms of the complexity of the sentence structures they could produce and understand. Performance on standardized receptive vocabulary measures exceeded performance on standardized measures of syntactic comprehension in 31 of 31 cases. (See Chapman et al., 1993, for similar results using a large sample of children 5–20 years of age.) What is of particular interest in all these studies is the fact that although actual levels of language structure vary tremendously, the profile remains relatively constant even in those functioning at the highest levels.

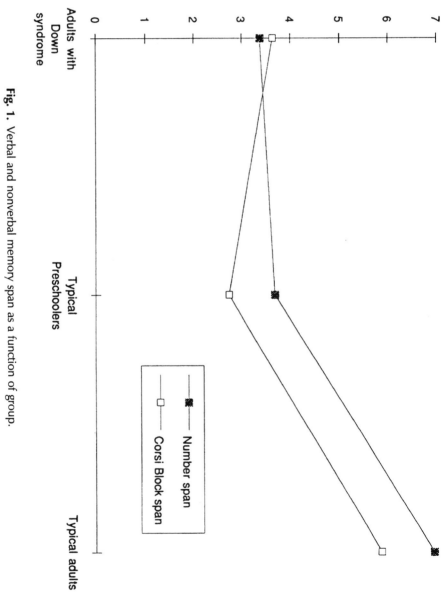

Number of items recalled

Fig. 1. Verbal and nonverbal memory span as a function of group.

WHAT UNDERLIES DIFFICULTIES IN VERBAL MEMORY AND MORPHO-SYNTAX?

Although there is strong evidence that verbal memory and morpho-syntactic structure are areas of relative weakness in Down syndrome, it is less clear why this should be so. Why too is there such wide linguistic variability? Several possibilities present themselves; it should be noted that multiple factors may be operating to the same effect.

Environmental Factors

It is demonstrably the case that environmental factors have an important effect on overall levels of cognitive function. Persons with Down syndrome benefit from loving homes, early intervention, appropriate educational services and medical care, and positive expectations communicated by family, school, and the broader community (e.g., Hodapp and Zigler, 1990). On the other hand, structural linguistic skills may be markedly delayed even when other environmentally more labile abilities (such as receptive vocabulary) indicate environmental advantages. If environment does play a role, it will more likely be in terms of a very specific linguistic environment. For example, it has often been hypothesized that parents of children with Down syndrome speak inappropriately to them, perhaps pitching their speech at too high a level in light of the age of their child, or perhaps, at too low a level, being cognizant of the mental retardation (e.g., Cardoso-Martins et al., 1985; Jones, 1980). However, other studies suggest that parents speak to their children with Down syndrome much like they address normally developing children functioning at the same language level (Rondal, 1977). Similarly, despite its plausibility and popular appeal, the idea that variation in language input will explain differences in the acquisition of language structure has not received much support even in the normal case (e.g., Newport et al., 1977; Gleitman et al., 1984). Neither have input differences succeeded in explaining the phenomenon of specific language impairment in normally intelligent children (e.g., Johnston, 1988).

Environmental factors may play a role in explaining some of the variability in ultimate language function. Impoverished language input may create the language deficit to some extent, but enhanced language input may serve to ameliorate the difficulties (e.g., Meyers, 1988; Buckley, 1985). It may well be that some of the linguistically more advanced children benefit from particularly successful and appropriate interventions, but if adults are considered it is impossible to carefully determine the content (or even the fact) of relevant interventions retrospectively. Further systematic research in this area is critical.

The Role of Hearing Impairment in Explaining Language Deficits

A common explanation for the increased incidence of language problems in Down syndrome relates to the increased incidence of middle ear infection—and resulting hearing loss. Studies indicate that 40% of the Down syndrome population have mild hearing loss; 10–15% have a more severe hearing loss. Although hearing problems will surely exacerbate a problem in learning language, and must be treated, they do not tell the whole story. In persons with Down syndrome, as in normally intelligent children with specific language impairment, language problems may also be evident even when no hearing problems are evident. Furthermore, even in samples of people with Down syndrome which do include those with hearing impairment, the pattern of language difficulty does not match the error patterns that typically stem from hearing impairment (Wisniewski et al., 1988). Finally, it should be noted that the many studies of otitis media and language impairment in children without Down syndrome have led to equivocal results at best (Kavanagh, 1986). In sum, although hearing impairment surely contributes to the language problem in the many persons with Down syndrome, it is unlikely to explain the whole problem.

Difficulties with Rule Learning

In an effort to understand why language structure was so difficult, Fowler (1988) and Fowler et al. (1993) looked closely at the language-learning process itself, including longitudinal studies in which children were visited on a monthly basis over many years. The hypothesis was that perhaps some specific inability to make linguistic generalizations such as "plurals are marked by a final morpheme s, the phonetic specification of which is to be determined by the final segment of the noun being marked" would be found. It was thought that children with Down syndrome might make shallow rather than deep generalizations, learning items piecemeal, rather than learning rules that applied across the lexicon. No evidence was found to support this hypothesis. Rather, two major conclusions were reached.

First, both the sequence of language development, and the structures acquired, are absolutely *normal*. Although, as mentioned above, syntax and vocabulary may get out of synchrony, no child has been known to simply skip over a step in the language-acquisition process. Similarly, despite numerous attempts to find evidence of deviant language structures, no unambiguous cases of deviance have been observed. Indeed, in several studies where the language output of persons with Down syndrome are matched with the output of normally developing youngsters half their age, the two are indistinguishable in all regards. This appears to be true at both low and high language levels.

Second, even the *rate* of development can be normal for periods (indicating acquisitions of a general rule) and yet lead ultimately to low language levels. Fowler et al. (1994) suggests that progress in language does not proceed at a slow continuous pace over childhood. Instead, it appears that progress is most rapid (and indeed can, for short periods, proceed at a near normal rate) from 4–7 years of age; these "spurts" are offset by long—sometimes interminable—periods where there is very little growth. What does characterize language learning in Down syndrome is inconsistent application of a rule after it has apparently been acquired. In the normal case, once the plural has been mastered, it is never deleted; in Down syndrome, the plural may be here today, gone tomorrow, and back again the following day.

In sum, persons with Down syndrome are not unable to acquire language rules, and when they do, the rules appear to take much the same form as in normally developing children. However, it does seem that many persons come to a point in linguistic development where they cannot make the next forward step. It is also the case that they are unable to consistently maintain and apply the rules they have acquired.

A Shutdown in Development?

The findings might suggest that the extreme disparities between language structure and other aspects of cognitive function stem from a shutdown in the language learning sometime in middle childhood (see also Chapman, 1993). Although plateaus are often lengthy, it is not the case that language learning ceases altogether beyond that 4–7-year-old spurt. There is evidence for growth in language structure in late adolescence, years after any progress had taken place (Fowler, 1988). In a recent study looking at the interpretation of novel verbs (Naigles, Fowler, and Helm, in press), adolescents with Down syndrome applied in same strategies to interpret novel verbs as were used by very young children, demonstrating more linguistic flexibility than normal adults. From the clinical sector, too, there are reports that even older adolescents with Down syndrome are responsive to language intervention; both Meyers (1988) and Buckley (1993) report significant growth in grammatical morphology upon introduction to written language.

The Potential Role of Phonology in Explaining Deficits in Memory and Morpho-Syntax

The hypothesis currently being explored is that the difficulty so many people with Down syndrome experience in fully mastering the morpho-syntax of English may relate to more basic difficulties at the phonological level, both in *perceiving* speech and in *encoding* incoming acoustic information into a representational format that can be accurately, and readily, retrieved to serve memory, production, and comprehension. Because speech perception and articulation have been found to be closely related to phonological encoding in memory in the normal population, no attempt will be made to distinguish between them here. The general point is that verbal memory ultimately depends on the quality of phonological representations; if these are weak, phonological memory is compromised (Baddeley, 1986; Brady, 1991; Hulme and MacKenzie, 1992). Because much of grammatical knowledge is clued by acoustically nonsalient elements (Gleitman et al., 1988), it may be that phonological limitations (especially in perception) may lead to grammatical problems as well.

The hypothesis under investigation is that as phonological perception and production skills vary, so will verbal memory and grammatical–syntactic function. Although the phonological hypothesis is still new and largely untried as an explanation for linguistic weaknesses in Down syndrome, it is currently being pursued as an important explanation for language/memory deficits in normally intelligent children with specific language impairment (Gathercole and Baddeley, 1989), and in children with specific reading disability (e.g., Brady, 1991; Fowler, 1991; Liberman et al., 1989; Stanovich, 1988). Although the overall levels of function are higher in these groups, the shape of cognitive profiles (with verbal scores lower than nonverbal scores) is similar to the profile observed in Down syndrome.

Preliminary evidence suggests that variation in phonological skill may provide an important piece of the puzzle in Down syndrome as well. Not only are both memory and grammatical morphology relative weaknesses in Down syndrome, but there is evidence that each may stem from phonological deficits. For example, there is evidence for an important relation between more basic measures of phonology (e.g., articulation accuracy) and verbal memory (Racette, 1993). Similarly, a simple test of articulation correlated significantly $[r(31) = .73, p < .00001]$ with the correct imitation of grammatical markers, a measure that, in turn, is an accurate index of language production. Although grammatical morphology was also related to general cognitive level $[r(31) = .40, p < .01]$, the articulation scores explained an additional 37% of the performance in grammatical morphology over and above what had been explained by general cognitive level alone. Although there is much research to be done to explore possible links between perception, memory, grammar, and morphology, at least one study has observed a direct correlation between phonological and syntactic development in persons with Down syndrome (Crosley and Doweling, 1989).

If phonological factors are causally related to syntactic weaknesses, then intervention studies focusing on phonology should yield positive effects. Again, more research is required, but there is reason to believe that those intervention programs that are successful may be succeeding because they do enhance phonological salience. In normal children, the one factor in parental speech that enhanced grammatical development was a preference for making requests with an interrogative (Will you pick up your peas?) rather than imperative constructions (clean your room), thereby placing otherwise nonsalient verbal auxiliaries (will, have, are, is) into the front, stressed position. Children receiving this input produced verbal auxiliaries earlier than those hearing a preponderance of imperatives. Similarly, we would argue that these same auxiliaries can be rendered salient by presenting them in written form, as was done by Meyers (1988) and by Buckley (1985).

IMPLICATIONS

If language problems are to be relegated to the most fundamental aspects of perception, it might seem futile to even think about what might be done to facilitate language acquisition. However, having a better understanding of the source of the difficulty should aid immeasurably in the treatment. Some of the ramifications of current research on language learning, providing goals that parents and teachers should work together to attain, based on what we know to date are:

1. *Developmental normalcy.* Both the process and products of language learning in persons with Down syndrome appear to be normal in all respects. Therefore, communicate in a normal fashion, just as with all other children at that same language level.
2. *Keep the developmental sequence in mind.* Language learners are not going to skip a step, whatever the chronological age, so focus your efforts on the next challenge.

3. *Make the next step salient.* Hyperarticulate overlooked syllables and words in your own speech, use question commands, keep a close check on hearing.
4. *Signed language and written language will not interfere* with progress in spoken language, and may even aid it.
5. *Different domains* within language *proceed independently.* Feel free to push on one (articulation, reading, vocabulary, comprehension) even if progress in another (syntax, production) is currently stalled.
6. *Invest in speech therapy,* keeping in mind that articulation is more susceptible to training than syntax. It has its own merits for teaching, and will provide your child with a greater sense of power to be understood.
7. *Nurture forward progress,* especially during age 4–7, but remember that the potential for language growth continues into adulthood.
8. *Be easy on yourself.* The difficulties are genuine and each success is to be treasured.

REFERENCES

Baddeley A (1986): Oxford: Oxford University Press.

Baren-Cohen S, Tager-Flusberg H, Cohen D (eds.) (1992): "Understanding other minds: Perspectives from autism." New York: Oxford University Press.

Beeghly M, Weiss-Perry B, Cicchetti D (1990): Beyond sensorimotor functioning: Early communicative and play development of children with Down syndrome. In Cicchetti D, Beeghly M (eds.): "Children with Down syndrome: A developmental perspective." Cambridge: Cambridge University Press, pp. 329–368.

Bellugi U, Marks S, Bihrle A, Sabo H (1988): Dissociation between language and cognitive functions in Williams syndrome. In Bishop D, Mogford K (eds): "Language development in exceptional circumstances." London: Churchill Livingstone, pp. 177–189.

Bilovsky D, Share J (1965): The ITPA and Down's Syndrome: An exploratory study. Am J Ment Defic 70:78–82.

Brady SA (1991): The role of working memory in reading disability. In Brady SA, Shankweiler DP (eds): "Phonological processes in literacy." Hillsdale, NJ: Lawrence Erlbaum, pp. 129–151.

Buckley S (1985): Attaining basic educational skills: Reading, writing and number. In Lane D, Stratford B (eds.): "Current Approaches to Down's Syndrome." New York: Praeger Press.

Buckley S (1993): Developing the speech and language skills of teenagers with Down's syndrome. In Buckley S (eds.): "Down's Syndrome Research and Practice." Portsmouth, England: University of Portsmouth, pp. 63–71.

Cardoso-Martins C, Mervis CB, Mervis CA (1985): Early vocabulary acquisition by children with Down syndrome. Am J Ment Defic 90:177–184.

Chapman R, Ross DR, Seung H-K (1993): Longitudinal change in language production of children and adolescents with Down syndrome. In "Sixth International Conference for the Study of Child Language." Trieste:

Coggins TE, Stoel-Gammon C (1982): Clarification strategies used by four Downs Syndrome children for maintaining normal conversational interaction. Ed and Train Ment Retarded 17:65–67.

Crosley P, Doweling S (1989): The relationship between cluster and liquid simplification and sentence length, age, and IQ in Down's syndrome children. J Commun Dis 22:151–168.

Doherty BJ (1993): Relationships between phonological processes and reading ability in young adults with Down syndrome. Masters thesis. Bryn Mawr College.

Dykens EM, Hodapp RM, Leckman JF (1993): "Behavior and development in fragile X syndrome." Newbury Park, CA: Sage.

Fowler A (1988): Determinants of rate of language growth in children with Down syndrome. In Nadel L (eds.): "The Psychobiology of Down Syndrome." Cambridge, MA: MIT Press.

Fowler A (1990): Language abilities in children with Down syndrome: Evidence for a specific syntactic delay. In Cicchetti D, Beeghly M (eds.): "Children with Down Syndrome: A Developmental Perspective." New York: Cambridge University Press, pp. 302–328.

Fowler AE (1991): How early phonological development might set the stage for phoneme awareness. In Brady SA, Shankweiler DP (eds.): "Phonological Processes in Literacy." Hillsdale, NJ: Erlbaum, pp. 97–117.

Fowler A, Doherty B, Boynton L (1993): Phonological prerequisites to reading in young adults with Down syndrome. Unpublished manuscript.

Fowler A, Gelman R, Gleitman R (1994): The course of language learning in children with Down syndrome: Longitudinal and language level comparisons with young normally developing children. In Tager-Flusberg H (ed.): "Constraints on Language Acquisition: Studies of Atypical Populations." Hillsdale, NJ: Erlbaum.

Gathercole S, Baddeley A (1989): The role of phonological memory in normal and disordered language development. In Euler CV, Lundberg I, Lennerstrand G (eds.): "Brain and Reading." New York, MacMillan.

Gleitman L, Gleitman H, Landau B, Wanner E (1988): Where learning begins: initial representations for language learning. In Newmeyer FJ (ed.): "Linguistics: The Cambridge Survey, Vol. III. Language: Psychological and Biological Aspects." New York: Cambridge University Press, pp. 150–193.

Gleitman L, Newport E, Gleitman H (1984): The current status of the Motherese hypothesis. J Child Lang, 11:43–79.

Greenwald CA, Leonard LB (1979): Communicative and sensorimotor development of Down's Syndrome children. Am J Ment Defic 84:296–303.

Hodapp RM, Zigler E (1990): Applying the developmental perspective to individuals with Down syndrome. In Cicchetti D, Beeghly M (eds.), "Children with Down Syndrome: A Developmental Perspective." New York: Cambridge University Press.

Hulme C, MacKenzie S (1992): "Working Memory in Mental Subnormality." Hillside, NJ: Erlbaum.

Johnston J (1988): Specific language disorders in the child. In Lass N, McReynolds L, Northern J, Yoder D (eds.): "Handbook of Speech–Language Pathology and Audiology." Philadelphia: B Decker, pp. 685–715.

Jones OHM (1980): Prelinguistic communication skills in Down's syndrome and normal infants. In Fields TM, Goldberg S, Stern D, Sostek AM (eds.): "High Risk Infants and Children: Adult and Peer Interactions." New York: Academic Press.

Kavanagh JE (ed.) (1986): "Otitis Media and Child Development." Parkton, MD: York Press.

Liberman IY, Shankweiler D, Liberman AM (1989): The alphabetic principle and learning to read. In Shankweiler D, Liberman IY (eds.): "Phonology and Reading Disability." Ann Arbor, MI: University of Michigan Press, pp. 1–34.

Mahoney G, Glover A, Finger I (1981): Relationship between language and sensorimotor development of Down syndrome and nonretarded children. Am J Ment Defic 86:21–27.

Marcell MM, Weeks SL (1988): Short-term memory difficulties and Down's syndrome. J Ment Defic Res 32:153–162.

Miller JF (1987): Language and communication characteristics of children with Down syndrome. In Pueschel S, Tinghey C, Rynders J, Crocker A Crutcher C (eds.): "New Perspectives on Down Syndrome." Baltimore: Brookes Publishing, pp. 233–262.

Miller J (1988): The developmental asynchrony of language development in children with Down Syndrome. In Nadel L (ed.): "The Psychobiology of Down Syndrome." Cambridge, MA: MIT Press.

Naigles L, Fowler A, Helm A (in press): Syntactic bootstrapping from start to finish with special reference to children with Down syndrome. In Tomasello M, Merriman W (eds): "The Acquisition of Verbs." Englewood Cliffs, NJ: Erlbaum.

Newport EL, Gleitman H, Gleitman L (1977): Mother I'd rather do it myself: Some effects and non-effects of maternal speech style. In Snow CE, Ferguson CA (eds.): "Talking to Children: Language Input and Acquisition." Cambridge: Cambridge University Press.

Peskett R, Wootton AJ (1985): Turn-taking and overlap in the speech of young Down's syndrome children. J Ment Defic Res 29:263–273.

Price-Williams D, Sabsay S (1979): Communicative competence among severely retarded persons. Semiotica 26(1/2):35–63.

Pueschel S (1988): Visual and auditory processing in children with Down syndrome. In Nadel L (ed.): "The Psychobiology of Down Syndrome." Cambridge, MA: MIT Press, pp. 199–216.

Racette K (1993): Phonological bases of memory in normal preschoolers and young adults with Down syndrome. Masters thesis, Bryn Mawr College.

Rondal J (1977): Maternal speech in normal and Down syndrome children. In Mitler P (ed.): "Research to Practice in Mental Retardation, vol. 2. Baltimore: University Park Press.

Rondal J (1994): Exceptional cases of language development in mental retardation: The relative autonomy of language as a cognitive system. In Tager-Flusberg H (ed.): "Constraints on Language Development: Studies of Atypical Children." Hillsdale, NJ: Erlbaum, pp. 155–174.

Stanovich KE (1988): The right and wrong places to look for the cognitive locus of reading disability. Ann Dyslexia 38:154–180.

Stray-Gunderson K (1986): "Babies with Down syndrome: A new parents guide." Rockville, MD: Woodbine House.

Varnhagen CK, Das JP, Varnhagen S (1987): Auditory and visual memory span: Cognitive processing by TMR individuals with Down syndrome and other etiologies. Am J Ment Defic 91(4):398–405.

Wisniewski KE, Miezejeski CM, Hill AL (1988): Neurological and psychological status of individuals with Down syndrome. In Nadel L (ed.): "The Psychobiology of Down Syndrome." Cambridge, MA: MIT Press.

Perspectives on Grammatical Development in Down Syndrome

Jean A. Rondal

Approximately fifty years of systematic research studies have yielded a picture of language functioning and language development in persons with Down syndrome that is beginning to have a reasonable degree of accuracy. Very briefly, we know that persons with Down syndrome have developmental difficulties and lasting problems, of unequal gravity, however, with each one of the major components of language:

1. phonetics and phonology (speech perception and sound articulation)
2. lexicon (receptive and expressive vocabulary, organization of the mental lexicon)
3. thematic semantics (particularly, the apprehension and the combination of elementary semantic relations into complex semantic structures associated with clause and sentence processing)
4. grammatical morphology (word inflections marking gender, number, case, tense, and aspect features)
5. syntax (phrase, clause, and sentence organization)
6. discourse (paragraphic and textual organization; cohesion)
7. pragmatic regulations (for example, anchoring new information to knowledge shared with the interlocutor; using one's previous knowledge to retrieve some information or associative link left unspecified by the interlocutor)

For detailed review of this literature, see Fowler, 1988, 1990; Miller, 1987; and Rondal, 1985, 1988a, 1988b, 1994a.

An interesting question, and one that has practical importance, is: Does the development of language in Down syndrome differ from that seen normally, beyond the delays and the final incompleteness of this development? Any sound answer to this question, sometimes referred to, in general terms, as the delay-difference problem, has to be given language component by language component, for the reason just stated. It would appear that, for each major language component, children with Down syndrome develop language by passing mostly through the same steps and sequences of steps as typical children. Most of the time, their language evolution, similar to that of corresponding mentally retarded children of other etiologies, is characterized by delays, synchronies, limitations of various sorts, and incompleteness (Rondal, 1988a; Miller, 1988; Fowler, 1990). But in spite of these serious limitations, the language of persons with Down syndrome is meaningful, relevant, and has communicative value. The above indications should not be taken to mean, however, that linguistically (or otherwise) people with Down syndrome are simply comparable to young typical children or that their language development is just a "slow-motion picture" of normal language development. The delays and asynchronies existing between language components make language development in children with Down syndrome and mental retardation particular, even if grounded in the same logic and exhibiting similar processes as language development in typical children. This last statement must be qualified in one important respect. Regarding phonetic and phonological development, on one hand, and morpho-syntactic development on the other, it is not fully clear, at the present time, whether specific limitations or even abnormal processes in language processing exist in children with Down syndrome and mental retardation of etiologies other than Down syndrome on top of the developmental delays observed in these subjects. Further research is needed on these points.

Judging from what precedes and pending additional investigation on the exact dynamics of the phonetic–phonological and morpho-syntactic evolutions in people with Down syndrome, it would seem that the immediate-past and present-day practices in language intervention with children with Down syndrome, consisting in having these children recapitulate normal development as much and as early as possible (cf. Rondal, 1987), are basically sound. It should be added, in keeping with the intervention topic, that such interventions should be conceived in a "modular way," as sequences of developmental steps, the logic of the remedial work, and its specific contents, vary substantially from language component to language component. Indeed, there is no reason to expect that educating or reeducating some particular aspects of language (e.g., lexicon) will automatically lead to noticeable improvements in other aspects (e.g., morpho-syntax). Also, the intervention programs should be allowed (and be designed in such a way as) to continue throughout adolescence and even early adulthood, as people with Down syndrome may very well progress in some aspects of language until relatively late in life (Rondal and Lambert, 1983; Fowler, 1990).

Most interestingly, cases of exceptional language development (particularly from the point of view of phonology and morpho-syntax) have been recently described in the specialized literature. These people (see Rondal, 1994b, 1994c for discussions of such cases) present a most astonishing contrast between their moderate and/or severe general cognitive limitations and the levels reached in language (particularly phonology and morpho-syntax, as indicated) that are much beyond what is usually observed in persons showing signs of retardation. Table 1 briefly summarizes some of these examples.

I was fortunate enough to be able to study in detail one such case, a woman with Down syndrome with regular trisomy 21, named Françoise. Table 2 gives some information on the case (described in detail, in Rondal 1994b).

Table 1. Exceptional Cases of Language Development in Subjects showing Signs of Mental Retardation

1. Exceptional written language development in a man with Down syndrome (Paul, studied between ages 13–41) (Seagoe, 1965).
2. Hyperlinguistic mentally retarded adolescents with Williams syndrome (Van, age 11; Cristal, age 15; Ben, age 16) (Bellugi et al., 1988).
3. Hyperlinguistic (from a phonological and grammatical point of view only) subjects showing signs of mental retardation of unknown etiologies (Antony, age 6; Rick, age 15; Laura, age 16) (Curtiss, 1988; Yamada, 1990).
4. Exceptional language development in a woman with Down syndrome (Françoise) (Rondal, 1994b).
5. Hydrocephalic mentally retarded subjects with exceptional language capabilities (several subjects, particularly D.H., an adolescent girl with spina bifida and arrested hydrocephalus, and Christopher, age 29, performance IQ 67, presenting a good level of ability in translating into English from three languages—French, German, and Spanish) (Anderson and Spain, 1977; Cromer, 1991; O'Connor and Hermelin, 1991).
6. Trilingual hyperlexia (Dutch, French, and English) together with severely reduced oral language in a microcephalic mentally retarded adolescent (Isabelle) (Lebrun et al., 1988).

A full discussion of such (and possibly similar instances to be discovered and documented) is beyond the scope of this presentation. But let me stress a few points. First, such observations indicate that advanced or even normal phonological and morpho-syntactic developments are possible (even if they have been exceptional until now) together with severe cognitive retardation (particularly, markedly reduced operational development, reduced short-term memory, etc.). This, incidentally, demonstrates that phonological and morpho-syntactic developments are somewhat autonomous processes with regard to general cognitive development, even if it is the

Table 2. A Brief Summary of Françoise's Case (Rondal, 1994b).

1. Chronological age: 32–36 at the time of the study
2. Mental age (EDEI)[a]: nonverbal: 5 years 9 months; verbal: 9 years 10 months
3. IQ (WAIS): performance: 60; verbal: 71
4. Cognitive development: intermediate between preoperational and operational level (according to Piaget's scheme)
5. Auditory–vocal word span: 4
6. Sentence (word) span: 14
7. MLU (mean length of utterance): 12.24 (sd 9.65; range 1–58; upper bound 58)
8. Conceptual aspects of language (lexicon, semantics, pragmatics): in line with (nonverbal) cognitive development level
9. Computational aspects of language (phonology, grammar): expressively as well as receptively normal (or close to normal)

[a]Epreuves Différencielles d'Efficience Intellectuelle (Perron-Borelli & Mises, 1974)

case that some level of cognitive functioning is necessary in order to "trigger" grammatical development. It can be stated, therefore, judging from the exceptional examples mentioned above, that serious problems with grammar (and articulation and sound discrimination) may not be a requisite of Down syndrome. We must find out why and how such cases exist, and, based on this knowledge, try to make "exceptional" language development possible in as many children with Down syndrome as possible. Research is currently in progress on some aspects of this important problem.

REFERENCES

Anderson E, Spain B (1977): "The Child with Spina Bifida." London: Methuen.

Bellugi U, Marks S, Bihrle A, Sabo H (1988): Dissociation between language and cognitive functions in Williams syndrome. In Bishop D, Mogford K (Eds.), "Language Development in Exceptional Circumstances," pp. 177–189. London: Churchill Livingstone.

Cromer R (1991): "Language and Thought in Normal and Handicapped Children." London: Blackwell.

Curtiss S (1988): The special talent of grammar acquisition. In Obler L, Fein D (Eds.), "The Exceptional Brain," pp. 364–386. New York: Guilford Press.

Fowler A (1988): Determinants of rate of language growth in children with Down Syndrome. In Nadel L (Ed.), "The Psychobiology of Down Syndrome," pp. 217–245. Cambridge, MA: MIT Press.

Fowler A (1990): Language abilities in children with Down syndrome: Evidence for a specific syntactic delay. In Cicchetti D, Beeghley (Eds.), "Children with Down syndrome. A developmental perspective," pp. 302–328. New York: Cambridge University Press.

Lebrun Y, Van Endert C, Szliwowski H (1988): Trilingual hyperlexia. In Ober L, Fein D (Eds.), "The Exceptional Brain," pp. 253–264. New York: Guilford Press.

Miller J (1987): Language and language communication characteristics of children with Down's syndrome. In Pueschel S, Tingey J, Rynders J, Crocker A, Crutcher D (Eds.), "New Perspectives on Down Syndrome," pp. 233–262. Baltimore: Brookes.

Miller J (1988): The developmental asynchrony of language development in children with Down syndrome. In Nadel L (Ed.), "The Psychobiology of Down Syndrome," pp. 167–198. Cambridge, MA: MIT Press.

O'Connor N, Hermelin B (1991): A specific linguistic ability. Am J Men Retard 95:673–680.

Perron-Borelli M, Misés R (1974). "Epreuves Différentielles d'Efficience Intellectuelle." Issy-les-Moulineaux: Editions Scientifiques et Psychologiques.

Rondal JA (1985): "Langage et Communication Chez les Handicapés Mentaux." Brussels: Mardaga.

Rondal JA (1987): "Le Developpment du Langage Chez l'Enfant Trisomique 21. Manuel Pratique d'Aide et d'Intervention." Brussels: Mardaga.

Rondal JA (1988a): Language development in Down's syndrome: A life-span perspective. Int J Behav Develop 11:21–36.

Rondal JA (1988b): Down's syndrome. In Mogford K, Bishop D (Eds.), "Language Development in Exceptional Circumstances," pp. 165–176. London: Churchill Livingstone.

Rondal JA (1994a): "Language in Mental Retardation. Theory, Evaluation, and Intervention." London: Whurr.

Rondal JA (1994b): "Exceptional Language Development in Down Syndrome. A Case Study and Its Implications for Cognition–Language and Other Language-Modularity Issues." New York: Cambridge University.

Rondal JA (1994c): Exceptional language development in mental retardation. Natural experiment in language modularity. Int J Psych, to appear.

Rondal JA, Lambert JL (1983): The speech of mentally retarded adults in a dyadic communication situation: Some formal and informative aspects. Psychologica Belgica 23:49–56.

Seagoe M (1965): Verbal development in a mongoloid. Excep Child 6:229–275.

Yamada J (1990): "Laura. A Case for the Modularity of Language." Cambridge, MA: MIT Press.

V. Education

Perspective

Andy Trias

From age 3 until I was 7, I went to a parish school near my home. One day I asked my mother why children in my class were age 4 and I was the only one age 5. And she told me that I had a problem that made learning more difficult. But she said that the children are all different and learn if they make the effort. Then I went to special schools where I learned to read and many other things. I learned to help children who have more problems than I. When I was 11, my teachers and my parents decided that I was ready to go to a regular school. It was a very large school and we were 30 in a class. Most of them were two years younger than I. I stayed until I was 17. In those 6 years I learned many things.

I have made my education work. The effort has been worthwhile for myself and for other people. Each one of us with our own differences can find a place in the world. What I disliked most was leaving the class for individual support, and what I liked best was history, which has always interested me very much. I was very lucky with my friends and I learned a lot from them. And they always treated me like one of them. And I cannot forget my teachers who helped me very much.

At home they treated me the same as my brothers and sisters. And I quarrelled quite often with the sister near me in age.

One day I was asked what I felt when I discovered that I had Down syndrome. At first, I did not like to know this. Or at least, I should have been told when I asked my mother why my classmates were two years younger than me. They took a long time to tell me. This is something that my friends complain about regarding their parents, also. I would have preferred to know sooner.

I would like to ask all the parents of persons with Down syndrome not to worry and to have confidence in us. We need the confidence in order to progress because we are like everyone else. Although we have Down syndrome, this does not mean that we don't feel the same as any other normal person. I have never given any importance to the Down syndrome of my friends. I have always wanted to help those that need help.

To finish I would like to ask teachers to give a lot of importance to our education, and our parents to have confidence in us.

Inclusion in Education and Community Life

Lou Brown

In 1929, the life expectancy of a person with Down syndrome in the United States was 9 years. It was very, very hard to keep children with Down syndrome alive then. In many parts of the world, we've gotten better and better since then at helping people who are in biological distress live longer. The big push came during and after World War II, when many countries put a lot of time, effort and money into trying to help people who were hurt in the war. Many of those people who were involved in that effort later pursued careers in the helping professions. We also had a big baby boom after the war. A lot of these babies would have died had they been born before the war, but with more people in the helping professions and better information and techniques of helping people in biological distress, they lived longer.

Many of those children who were born had Down syndrome or other severely disabling conditions. After 3 or 4 years of living with these children parents started to say, "You know, it's not good for me to be with this child 24 hours a day, 7 days a week. And it's probably not good for the child either." What help was available for them? Basically, nothing. People who had a lot of money found a private place to send their child—a nice, clean place, usually in a country environment. Not many people had that kind of money, nor did they necessarily want to send their child away. Other people put great pressure on the government to build more institutions, more special places. More and more young people were put in institutions in my country. That was a horrible disaster.

Most people who had children with Down syndrome kept their children at home. They met others in the same circumstances and said "Look, what if you take my child this weekend and I'll take your child next weekend?" Then they heard about other parents with children with disabilities, and they set up a little group. Often they found a place, usually a little place in a religious facility of some kind—a synagogue, a temple or a church—and they set up a day program. A special place for their children who were disabled, who could not go to regular schools, to go during the day. And this movement—the private day care center phase, or day center phase—spread all across the U.S.

Every once in a while, one of these parents would say, "I'd like to enroll my child in the public school." We'd say, "We don't serve kids like yours in the public schools, but there's a nice program over there." Those parents went, and found other parents in the same boat; they found understanding and acceptance.

But there were parents who said, "We go to a public beach and there's no problem; we go to a public park and we have no problem; we go to a public concert and we have no problem; we come to a public school and we have a problem. Why is it that the only public place we have a problem getting into is a public school?"

In 1975 the parents got this law passed that said that in the United States *all* children have a right to a tax-supported education. We had no experience with these kids with disabilities, so we looked around and said, "Well, the parents put up these special places for them; that's what we'll do." We set up special schools for people with severe intellectual disabilities. And I thought it was a great idea. In my community, Madison, Wisconsin, we put our services in a special school, and we built this school up to over 160 students, who were happy. Things were going really well.

In 1976, we closed our handicapped-only school—the last one in my community. What did we do, when we were under orders from the school administration to close the last of our special schools? We set up these little special areas in other schools around the city. Why did we do that? Well, one reason we offered in those days was that we couldn't afford to spend the money to make every public school building barrier-free. We spent our money to make some buildings barrier-free, and then we bused kids there. Whether they needed a barrier-free environment or not was irrelevant; we wanted them in there.

The second reason we set up these special areas in different schools was because we found out that there was tremendous professional pressure for special education teachers to be with each other.

The third reason we set up these special areas for kids with disabilities, including kids with Down syndrome, was because in 1976 we felt that regular education professionals were just not ready to serve these children.

And then one day this parent walked in and said, "I would like to enroll my son, Andre, in the regular public schools." We said, "Madam, we would have to assess him first." She said, "Fine." So she signed a paper and we assessed him on Monday, Tuesday, Wednesday, and Thursday—it was very complicated. On Friday, we sat the family down, and we said, "Madam, Sir, your son Andre is medically fragile and profoundly retarded." The mother looked at her husband, looked at us, and said, "You know, I could have told you that last Sunday." And I said, "We are going to enroll Andre at Shade School." And she said, "Now, Shade School, where is that?" Shade School is the next elementary school over from this school, which is where her other children go. She said, "You see, we take Andre to the park, and he can't play with normal kids, but he learns more, he looks, he watches, he is getting to know the kids in the neighborhood. And the babysitters, because, you know, it's very important for us to have some help with Andre, and we want the kids to know him, so they can come babysit with us. And he goes to religious services there. So I thought, maybe Andre can go to school with the kids in the neighborhood." And we said, "Madam, you have to try to understand this. You see, we don't have enough kids like Andre to make a class of kids like him in the school in your neighborhood. You got that?" She said, "Yeah. Now you are going to try and understand this. I don't want Andre in a class with kids like Andre. When you put Andre with kids like Andre, he bites the back of the seat. When you put him with normal kids, he looks, he watches, and he tries to do the same as them. I want Andre to go to school with normal kids."

We had a meeting to ask "What point is she trying to make, and how are we going to counter that and what points are we going to make?" We couldn't reach a conclusion. At the end of the meeting of the 20 people, 16 thought she was still crazy, two were undecided, and two thought she had some pretty good points. So we had to meet again. And then it was a 10–10 split. Then we had to meet again, and we said, "Oh, they did it to us again. Now we are going to have to change again."

So it is a very, very difficult process of converting from cluster schools to a natural distribution where the child goes to the same school she or he would go to if not disabled. That's what we call the home school.

Now many of us bus for racial balance, or to a magnet school, so we don't say neighborhood school, because lots of kids don't go to school in their neighborhood; but they go to school, and the key issue for us is to forget all the word games. The key critical issue is, your child goes to school with a preponderance of students in his or her own neighborhood. That's the issue.

Why are we doing this? Why are we going through all of this? This is a question that was really never asked for years because we didn't know how long disabled people were going to live. Now we are talking average lives of 45–50 years and who knows what it's going to be 10 years from now?

What's the purpose of an education program? We say, to prepare people to live, work and play in an integrated society. We tried preparing people to work in a segregated society, institution ward, shelter workshop, group home, activity center. It's terrible. It's just not good enough. It is better than nothing, perhaps, but it's just not good enough.

So whatever it is that helps prepare a person with disabilities to function in integrated society, to live, work and play in the real world, we do. And you know, if we do that, and the system interferes with it, we have to do something about the system.

The environment in which people with significant disabilities function matters. The more complicated, challenging, and stimulating their environment, the more they achieve and the higher quality of their life.

So the question for us is, if we know environments matter, what environments do we put people with disabilities in? What environments do we want to create for them? Our position is that every child with disabilities should have the right to attend the same schools and the same class as anyone else. And then we negotiate. Should the child spend 100% of the time in the same classes? I think not. If you are severely disabled intellectually, it means something. And that argues against 100% of the time. Maybe 90% of the time, or 80%? I don't know. When children are young, it should be 100%. But as chronological age increases we have to start thinking about preparing people to live, work, and play in an integrated society. The purpose of the school program is not to prepare people to live, work, and play in a school program.

We are in the midst of this fascinating, complicated, challenging, difficult process of arranging for children with a wide array of significant disabilities to attend regular education classes. We walked into one school and said to the principal, "There is a young child with Down syndrome who lives right around the corner from the school. We send a bus to her house, pick her up, and bus her to a school an hour away. She doesn't know anybody there. She comes home at 4 o'clock, and she is just alone. It's not good. So, what we'd like to talk to you about is, maybe next year this child should be going to the school right down the street." He said, "You know, come back in a couple of weeks, we'll check it out." So we came back in a couple of weeks and said, "Well, Sir, what do you think?" He said, "Well, we had a staff meeting, and we took a vote, and we voted no."

Can you imagine, in this day and age, these responsible educators, voting no on people with disabilities?

Here's a real example—the mother and father of Rachel Holland in Sacramento, California. To make a long story short, Rachel Holland was 7 years old, she had Down syndrome, and her family wanted her to go to school with normal children, in a normal class. And the school district said no. There ensued a court case with witnesses here and appeals. The Sacramento school district, as best as we can tell, spent $750,000 dollars to keep one child with Down syndrome out of a regular education class. One child. And they lost. Incidentally, there is an opening as a special education director in Sacramento.

And then there is Raphael Alberti, a 7-year-old with Down syndrome in Clementine, New Jersey. His parents went to hearings, and state appeals, and in federal court they won. They won in appeals court, too. That district probably spent about $200,000 trying to keep one child out. So you figure, "Wow, think about that!" And money is supposed to be scarce, particularly school money! And why is it that if you try to take a normal child out, people will spend a million dollars fighting you. But if you try to get a child with disabilities in, they spend a million dollars trying to keep your child out. Think about that.

When you segregate people with obvious disabilities, you rob them of the opportunity to be individuals. They become the disabled, the handicapped group. Generally, the people that we focus upon are the lowest intellectually functioning one or two percent of the population. But the fact that a person is significantly disabled intellectually is not a justification for excluding them from growing up with a regular education.

I say to you, parents of young children, if you don't watch it, if you don't do something about it, your children are going to lead horribly constricted lives. So one of the basic purposes of educational programs is to prepare your child to function in a normal array of rooms, places, streets, parks, shops, stores, and workplaces.

How many people do you come into contact with if you are disabled? First there is your family; then you get a babysitter, and a therapist, or a teacher. Who is with your child? Who's going to be with them the rest of their lives? Family and people you pay money to. Unless we do something about it.

We have this thing we call "The Madison Social Relationship Inventory." It's one of our versions of assessment. We sit down with parents and say, "Look, we'd like to talk to you about your child's social life." We want to know, to get some basic information. If we ask you questions that you think are none of our business, say it. We don't want to violate your privacy. But we want to ask you some questions. We want to know who your child eats with. That, at first, sounds really strange to a parent. Then we want to know who your child travels with. Then we want to know if your child has any relationships with normal children in a regular education classroom. You see, our thesis is that the regulation education, classroom of today is the integrated workplace of tomorrow. And we want to know if the child has any tutors, people who really know how to help him. More often than not, the child is involved in school-sponsored extracurricular activities. Who is your child with after school, or after work, and (the toughest one), does your child have a friend? Basically, we want to know that.

If your child goes to a segregated school, can you build eating relationships with normal people? No! That's a service that's not available, an extremely important service that your child needs. If your child goes to a clustered school, it's a regular school, but it's not the one where the kids in the neighborhood go. Can you build relationships with normal people in school? Of course you can. Can they then eat together after school, on weekends, summers, holidays? No! So then you've got to pay people to eat with them, or you've got to be there yourself. Now, if the child goes to a school with a preponderance of students in the neighborhood, can you build relationships at school and then make sure that they occur after school and during nonschool times? Yes! These are some of the reasons that neighborhood schools are better.

Our thesis is that when people with disabilities are distributed as they would be distributed if they weren't disabled, they do better than if you group or cluster them. It's relatively easy to build a relationship if there is one person with Down syndrome in the group, and 9 to 15 nondisabled people. The more people with disabilities you put in the group, the lower the probability of building relationships with normal people. So we spend a lot of time arranging it so that people with disabilities are distributed, not grouped. And when you start distributing, then you start getting some people who will come over, be next to, talk to, look at, and eventually touch, and it's touch that we want. Touch is critical.

We had a belief that people with significant disabilities should be integrated. We tried segregation, and it is just not good. It doesn't mean that integration is perfect right now, in all cases, but at least we have a chance to beat the other options. We have laws that say children should be educated in the least restrictive environment. Well, who knows what that is? Schools should be close to home—how close is close? We have all these things that people play tricks with, but parents are taking our school districts to court, and judges are saying, yes it makes sense. We are winning cases all over the country. They say, "Yes, children should go to school with normal children, brothers and sisters, friends and neighbors." So we are winning through the law. Now schools all over this country have to serve children—I hate to even say that, "have to"; they should want to—with significant disabilities in regular education settings. So now we have to figure out how to make it work.

We have a couple of rules. What we want to do is to give you ammunition for when you go back to your neighborhood school. What you want to do is to take the heat off the other person. So, upfront you say, "We are not the least bit interested in interfering with the educational achievement of normal children." You have to tell people that or they'll say, "What about. . . . " And then you say "The other thing we want very badly is for a person with disabilities to learn something meaningful. Not just put them in class, hire an aide, be with them, and do dumb stuff. No, that's a waste of time, that's not what we call education. We have to figure a way to have a person with a significant disability learn something meaningful, without it interfering with the achievement of nondisabled people."

One thing we can do is take a person with Down syndrome and put her or him in a regular education classroom and do nothing. We call that "dumping." In this day and age it's not a good strategy. The other thing we can do is go into a class and say, "Look, we've got this person coming in who is disabled. We want you to change everything you are doing, just because that person is there." Well, it often doesn't sell well. But in some cases it works.

Now, another thing you want to do is say, "Look, the normal kids will get everything they were going to get if this person wasn't there. But, because of this person, they are going to get something, well, a little bit different. They are going to be in the same group, doing the same activity, but we are going to modify it just for this person. These children are studying customs in foreign lands; well, this person who is disabled might be doing something else." We come up with an alternative, in the same classroom, for the child. That's meaningful. And then, if we can't figure out a way, to make it something meaningful, we get out of there.

Here is another story, about Jamin. The normal kids in Jamin's class were involved in planning their weekend; they were reading, they were experiencing, they were negotiating with other people, they were writing a journal, so they were learning some really good skills in this particular community. They decided where to go, who to go with, what the dress codes were, how much money you needed, how you were going to get there, what to do if you got lost. And they were writing down all these things. Parents liked it, teachers liked it. It was a good, practical use of a lot of skills. And there was Jamin, who was just not involved. He couldn't do all that. And you don't want to have them stop doing that just because of Jamin. After a while, the teacher started watching and studying it. And what they did was make pictures for Jamin. They made stamps with writings on them, and then they got kids to interact with him; then they came up with a way in which he could be involved in that activity. It was different, it was modified for him, but he was involved in that activity. And that's the key. So he would then have a stamp that said "Would you like to?" and a picture of a swimmer, and a picture of him. He could then ask "Would you like to go swimming with me?" and the other kids could say yes or no. And they worked it out from there.

The next thing is for the teacher to get out of there. You don't want to have a hired one-to-one all the time. Where does that lead? In adult services, a lot of the people are 21 or 22 years old. They have finished school. Are you going to have to hire someone to be with them for the rest of their life? No! So it's OK to go in with sophisticated, relevant, meaningful specialized help, but then get out; get out and let these relationships take over.

There is another option. Here is a problem—math. There is tremendous variation, tremendous range in the functioning of people with Down syndrome. They are not all alike. Take Dan for example. He is 15 years old with six more years of school to go and he can't make change for a dollar yet. For a portion of the day, he gets math instruction, trying to make change for a dollar. But we also hedge our bets. We get some direct math instruction in the instructional material center, and then we have real math. Not school math, real math. Here is how it works. Dan works as part of his school program. He leaves school and goes downtown; he is working. He makes money. Fit and good, right? And we want him to buy a snack. Now, he has Down syndrome, so he can't eat what I eat. He has to have something nutritious, not fattening. So we guide him away from fattening stuff, and he goes and gets grapes. He has 79 cents in his pocket. Grapes are $1.19 a pound. He starts putting grapes in his bag. He's got a real math problem, not a school math problem. Basically, you work it out like this. Grapes are $1.19 a pound and he has got 79 cents in his pocket, which I doubt that he can even count. All he knows is he's got money in his pocket. How many grapes can he put in his bag? Let me ask this question. How many people in the supermarket can figure that out? So what do you do? Do you wait until he does real shopping, until he gets mathematically up to the point where he can do all the math that's necessary to shop? He is going to be 647 years old before he can buy a grape. How do you solve this problem? It's very simple. You say, "Dan, look. You put as many grapes in that bag as you want. You take that bag of grapes to the counter, you put the grapes on the counter, and you put your money on the counter, and you let her figure it out."

There used to be a line separating special education from regular education. In the old days, we were on this side of the line, the other people, there. We didn't bother with them. We weren't concerned with what they were doing, because we wanted our kids to be separate, sheltered, and protected. It can't be that way anymore. We tried that. It didn't work, so we have to cross that line.

In the process of crossing that line we are learning, or we are looking at what goes on in regular education classes a little bit differently than even people in regular education look at it. One of the things to look at is the way regular education teachers group their students. This is extremely important for the success of people with disabilities. Individuals with significant disabilities learn nothing by themselves. They may practice what they know, but they learn no new things. People with severe disabilities learn nothing in a large group. They have a learn how to act in a large group, but they don't learn anything in a large group. They learn most interacting with another person, in a small group.

Our thesis is: The regular education class of today is the integrated workplace of tomorrow. Who is in the regular education class today? The physicians, the engineers, the workers of tomorrow.

There is a two-person group. We think that people with significant disabilities learn much from two-person interaction. Very much. But the problem is, we dominate them with people who are paid to be with them, with professionals, and we minimize relationships with peers. So we spend a lot of time developing two-person interactions with people.

We used to have a special school, and it was absurd. So then we started taking the people off the school grounds to real environments—nonschool environments. And then we went to special classes, and we could still leave the special class and go downtown. And now we come into regular classes and we don't want to give up instruction in the real world, because it's been so valuable for us. So we ask, "Gee, does full inclusion mean never ever, ever, not one single minute, leaving your regular class?" No, not at all. We don't want to give up our community instruction, our off-school or nonschool instruction.

Well, how can you have it? Can you have your cake and eat it? The answer is, I really think so. What we have to do is build relationships at school, and then make sure those relationships are expressed in nonschool environments. Some of that requires taking normal kids off school grounds with us to learn things in the real world.

Why do we want two-person interactions? We want an outcome, after 21 years of learning, that another person's not disabled; we want a partnership and a sharing in a contributory way. A lot of work environments are two-person in nature—you have a work buddy, work partner. It is critically important that you function as an individual in the presence of others so that you can work in the real world. It is very important that you can work as a partner, with another person.

We want to orchestrate these things, these regular education activities, so everybody learns a little bit. Certainly we have to practice some things we already know to get to the things that we really need to learn. And, of course, the next phase, as always, is to fade out. To get out of there. We don't want to hire somebody to be with somebody 100% of the time. We want to get out.

A large group is tough. A large group is a problem. There's no doubt that people with significant disabilities have to learn to function in large groups. That's why experiences like coming to this conference are wonderful. You see these kids avoiding moving objects, waiting in line and anticipating the door closing on their faces because nobody can see them. You know, you watch them and it's great. So you have to learn to function, but I am not sure you learn much more than how to function in a large group.

When you put kids with significant disabilities in regular education settings, normal children do better academically. We've been tracking the standardized academic achievement scores of nondisabled children in the Madison Public Schools since 1971. And every year since 1971 they've gone up. Last year, they were rated the seventh highest academic achievement scores of any public school in the U.S. Every year in the national standardized tests, the kids from Wisconsin, Minnesota, and Iowa score the highest in the U.S. *Why?* The answer is, every year we put more and more kids with severe disabilities in regular education settings with them. The more kids we put in those classes, the higher the achievement scores of non disabled kids go.

We have this problem. We want our kids to go to school with normal children, brothers and sisters, friends and neighbors, and other people don't. It's new, it's different. It presents stress, conflict. And so what we'd like to do is find out what they are worried about, get it out in public, and talk about it. Maybe if we see legitimate things we'll deal with them. We'd like to go through some of the reasons people have given us why they don't want your children to go to school with normal kids. One is, of course, academic achievement. There is absolutely no credible information to suggest that disabled kids would interfere with the academic achievement of normal people.

There's a fellow, Jack Giordi, who is doing a dissertation on all the kids in Madison who did and did not go to school with kids with severe disabilities to see if there is any difference in achievement. He can't find any yet.

Another reason they give can be summed up by a question such as "Will my daughter be a doctor if she goes to school with these kids." Well, we are following up long term normal kids who went to school with disabled kids to see if they are making different choices than kids who didn't go to school with kids with severe disabilities. One mother asked me, "You know, if my daughter's friends see her tutoring a disabled classmate would they still be her friends?" We don't know the effect on friendship of interacting with a person with a disability. We're following that up. What about hiring decisions? Maybe people are going to say, "You know, I went to school with them. I don't want to work next to them." Or maybe they'll say, "You know, I went to school with kids with Down syndrome. We had fun, we travelled together, we ate together. It'd be fine. I have no problem. It'd be great."

In the past, we overloaded environments with people with disabilities. And it denied them many things. It segregated them from society and developed bad attitudes. We did it with good intentions. Now we want a natural distribution. In the past, we allowed people with disabilities to have a collective identity: the crippled, the retarded, the emotionally disturbed. Now we want an individual identity. In the past, we believed in homogeneous grouping. Now we want heterogeneous grouping. In the past, we taught in simulated environments and assumed that children would learn it there and then do it in the real world. The problem is, they don't generalize well. We have to teach as much as we can in the real world.

So I have a rule for you. It's better to teach a few skills in many environments than it is to teach many skills in a few environments. The purpose of school is to prepare people to live, work and play in an integrated society.

Peer-Related Social Competence and Inclusion of Young Children

Michael J. Guralnick

The study of young children's social competence has become a major area of investigation in recent years. It is an interesting construct, both from conceptual and developmental perspectives, and is even becoming a more prominent feature in our assessments of the effectiveness of early intervention programs (Guralnick, 1990a).

A component of that broader construct, social competence with peers, has received almost unprecedented attention in recent years. Along with growing evidence that failure to establish productive relationships with peers in the early years signals potentially significant difficulties in future life adjustment, we have every reason to believe that relationships with peers is a vital developmental process. For example, many researchers and theorists have suggested that peer relationships foster the socialization of aggressive tendencies, contribute to moral development, promote language and communication, and facilitate the development of prosocial behaviors and social–cognitive processes (Bates, 1975; Garvey, 1986; Hartup, 1983).

Although none of the research that has led to these conclusions has been carried out with children with disabilities, there is every reason to believe that the significance of these developmental processes is similar for both children who are typically developing and children with disabilities. In fact, we do know that it is the relationship of adults with disabilities with their peers and coworkers that pose the most serious threats to productive employment and to their quality of life in general.

SOCIAL COMPETENCE OF CHILDREN WITH DISABILITIES

For the last few years, I have been directing a line of research attempting to understand the peer-related social competence of preschool-age children with general developmental delays, including a substantial number of children with Down syndrome (for characteristics of the children see Guralnick and Bricker, 1987). This research has taken two major directions: (1) understanding the peer competence of developmentally delayed children, primarily through descriptive cross-sectional and short-term longitudinal studies, and (2) efforts to understand the nature and extent of peer interactions as they occur when one's companion is a nonhandicapped child.

This line of research has, I believe, a number of important implications for a variety of overlapping issues. First, these are important issues in the field of child development—basic processes of social exchange and development. This is especially the case for understanding relationships between children with and without disabilities, but it also relates to the basic design of preschool environments to establish conditions for the growth of peer competence. The third issue of interest relates to public policy concerns. Peer relations and our understanding of interactions among diverse groups of children have much to contribute to an empirical base for the concept of inclusive environments and how children with disabilities are involved in the community, especially considering that early childhood programs may be their first formal experience in community-based activities.

Descriptive Studies of Peer Relations

Over the past few years, I have collected information with regard to the social/communicative interactions of primarily mildly and moderately delayed preschool-age children (e.g., Guralnick and Groom, 1985, 1988; Guralnick and Weinhouse, 1984). For the most part, the settings have been community programs, usually specialized. Overall, I am comfortable with the representativeness of the samples, drawing upon approximately 250 children served by the primary service provider in the community and carefully defining those samples. In another instance, I have looked at children in mainstreamed settings, typically in contrived playgroups (see subsequent discussion). Observation time varied, ranging from 30–100 minutes per child, depending on the situations.

Measures

Two peer interaction scales have been used. The first is a variation of the Parten scale (1932), characterizing the overall quality of play. It is not a perfect scale (there are some concerns about its sequential and hierarchical nature), but it has been used extensively and is sensitive to developmental changes, environmental variables, familiarity, same and mixed-age groups, and in identifying nonhandicapped children at risk. Usually it employs a 10- or 20-second observational interval followed by a recording interval for classroom observations or just 10-second segments for videotapes. Nested within the solitary, parallel, or group-play categories are four measures of cognitive play: 1) functional; 2) constructive (uses materials, creates something); 3) dramatic (pretend), and 4) games with rules.

A second set of measures is nonsequential as well, but it was selected because it provides more specific information to enable us to determine some component behaviors of peer interactions and also gain some sense of the qualitative nature of social exchanges. This set is based on the White/Watts scale but has been substantially modified by us and others over the years (see Doyle et al., 1980). Fourteen major categories are coded whenever they occur. Eleven component categories record the social interactions of a focal child as directed to peers (who were recorded). Two categories are responses of the focal child to peers, and the final category is the extent to which the focal child served as a model to a peer. The scale contains a small sequential feature, tracking the success of children for certain categories.

In addition, in a number of studies, the communicative interactions of the participants were painstakingly transcribed and then analyzed in a number of different ways (Guralnick and Paul-Brown, 1989). In general, for both utterance-by-utterance analyses and instances in which a series of utterances or turns were tracked, analyses could be categorized as follows: 1) structural–syntactic measures such as utterance complexity (MLU and other measures); 2) functional—how utterances were used; and 3) discourse and speech-style measures, based to some extent on the sociolinguistic literature.

Summary of Peer Interactions

Although this series of studies revealed a substantial number of findings, the most significant patterns are as follows:

1. Developmentally delayed children engage in limited amounts of group play, far less than expected for developmentally matched younger, nonhandicapped children. This conclusion is based on comparisons of delayed children in specialized programs to nonhandicapped children at similar developmental levels and to groups matched carefully in terms of mental age (Guralnick and Groom, 1987a).

2. Social interaction figures with peers are actually worse than it appears on the surface. Specifically, fully 33% of children engage in social interaction less than 5% of the time in free-play; alternatively, 20–25% of children accounted for 50–60% of the peer interaction. Many children had great difficulty going beyond simple initiation–response sequences.

3. Cross-sectional studies revealed minor changes over the preschool period (3–6 years). Peer interaction did improve over the course of a year, but apparently new playmates or summer disruptions caused returns to baseline.

4. Absence of directive/organizing interactions, such as positive-leads or use of others as resources, were notable. Limited evidence was observed for children's abilities to positively influence their peers in a goal-directed manner.

5. Delayed children did discriminate among peers, and when they did interact they tended to prefer one or another playmate. These unilateral friendships were rarely reciprocated, however, as few playmates whom they chose, chose them in return. In addition, in contrast to appropriately matched groups of nonhandicapped children, the delayed children failed to take advantage of even their unilateral friendships, as play was not more complex or sophisticated with "friends" versus "nonfriends."

6. Data on directive episodes of delayed and nondelayed children are currently being analyzed, examining the processes children use in this important social task. Preliminary findings suggest major social process differences that may be associated with delayed children's poor peer relations. For example, in comparison to appropriate nonhandicapped groups, requests tend not to be mitigated, often setting up a

confrontational atmosphere. There is little variation in follow-up requests, compromise and negotiation occur rarely, and delayed children do not tend to accept alternative proposals. These processes contrast sharply with those of nonhandicapped children.

Effect of Inclusion

Given this set of circumstances, how is it possible to alter the quantity and quality of peer interactions of delayed children as well as those with other disabilities? One approach is to consider the social environment of the children with disabilities in classrooms. Most of the data on peer interaction difficulties were obtained when disabled children were in specialized settings; i.e., all children in the setting manifested similar difficulties.

What might we expect if the social environment were changed to include nonhandicapped peers? One possibility is that the nonhandicapped children would take over some of the directive functions not exhibited by delayed children. That is, like parents or teachers, they might take some control over the situation just in those deficit areas of delayed children and perhaps allow for some building of extended exchanges. Nonhandicapped children may have an intermediate status between adults and true peers that produces asymmetries but still contains some peer-like characteristics.

Some evidence can be cited suggesting that this is a reasonable hypothesis. In dyadic situations in which children are systematically paired with one another to allow comparisons with partners who are either delayed or nondelayed, substantial increases in the peer interactions of the delayed children occur. These increases appear to be stimulated by the directive abilities of the nondelayed peers (Guralnick and Groom, 1987b). The fact that delayed children prefer to interact with nonhandicapped peers, and the demanding nature of these mainstreamed environments also suggest that the availability of nonhandicapped children may have some positive impact.

Results of Recent Research

What happens when comparisons are made in group-play situations between specialized and integrated settings? Actually, very limited differences are obtained. Some studies have revealed slight increases in peer interactions or some reduction in inappropriate play but, by and large, very few differences have been observed.

Given reasonable expectations for more substantial positive effects, why aren't the findings more significant? It is possible that the quality of the integrated environment is poor, i.e., very isolated delayed children with little contact with nonhandicapped classmates. Alternatively, we need to look at characteristics of the nonhandicapped peers and the social environment itself as a possible source. It is important to note that virtually all of these minimal-effect observational studies had two characteristics in common: 1) nonhandicapped children were about a year younger; and 2) the primary program was designed for delayed children who were integrated into various play settings that included nonhandicapped children or settings in which a few non-handicapped children were invited. Since delayed children prefer nonhandicapped peers, are more socially interactive when participating with similar-age rather than younger nonhandicapped children, and even in group settings, are found in most advanced play with similar-age nonhandicapped children, it is possible that minimal effects could be due to the availability of only younger same-age nonhandicapped children. Also, it is possible that since most studies occurred in an integrated setting, with the dominant peer group still being the delayed children, the demands and social climate were still those of children with disabilities.

Support for these explanations comes from a study in which delayed children's peer interactions were compared when interacting in mainstreamed settings (i.e., the primary program was designed for nonhandicapped children but included full-time a few similar-age delayed children) in comparison to a specialized setting (all delayed children). Although not entirely an unflawed study, strong evidence was found that, during free play, peer interactions as well as the quality of cognitive play, particularly more constructive play, improve substantially in the mainstreamed setting (see Guralnick and Groom, 1988). In our current work, we have replicated these findings in experimental playgroups. In fact, the increased level of peer interactions occurring in inclusive as compared to specialized settings appears to hold for samples of children with cognitive delays and communication disorders.

Despite positive findings, it is important to note that the quality of play, as measured by the group-play category on the Parten scale, did not vary with the setting. It suggests that mainstreamed settings may be a necessary but not sufficient condition for building peer interactions.

In fact, it is becoming increasingly clear that a peer–social competence curriculum that is highly individualized is essential (Guralnick 1990b). As a consequence, I have recently developed an assessment instrument designed to serve both educational and clinical purposes (see Guralnick, 1992). It is educational in the sense that it is intended to communicate the idea that forming successful peer relations is an integrative process, one that depends extensively on fundamental developmental abilities and skills associated with cognitive, language, motor, and affective domains. An evaluation of the social–communicative skills that emerge from this integrative process, such as the ability to direct others, to request permission, to express disagreement, or acknowledge requests, constitutes Level I of the assessment. However, this integration of abilities and skills goes further, requiring children to apply those social–communicative skills in various contexts to achieve specific interpersonal goals. Social tasks such as entering a group or resolving a conflict constitute important contexts or events for children. While engaging in these tasks, children must transform their social–communicative skills to social strategies while considering various factors including the specific context of the situation as well as the skills, abilities, and status of their companions. Strategies children use may include negotiating, insisting, mitigating a directive, or threatening a companion. The effectiveness and appropriateness of the strategies selected by children during this integrative process constitute the core of socially competent interactions with peers. Level II, the level of Social Strategies and Social Tasks, is intended to assess children's peer-related social competence within this higher-order framework.

This assessment instrument is also a clinical tool in that it is designed to help organize how educators and clinicians think about the complex factors that influence young children's peer relationships. In essence, the assessment process is intended to guide clinical judgment to assist in formulating the most likely hypotheses with regard to why children may be experiencing difficulties in peer relationships. Having accomplished that, this clinical information can be used as a basis for designing intervention programs. The link between assessment and intervention and the processes associated with that task are part of a new intervention program based on this approach.

Taken together, inclusive early education in conjunction with specific assessment–intervention programs in the domain of peer relations may well be necessary to maximize the peer-related social competence and inclusion in community life of children with Down syndrome and others with general developmental delays.

REFERENCES

Bates E (1975): Peer relations and the acquisition of language. In Lewis M, Rosenblum LA (Eds.): "The Origins of Behavior: Friendship and Peer Relations" (Vol. 4), pp. 259–292. New York: Wiley.

Doyle A, Connolly J, Rivest L (1980): The effect of playmate familiarity on the social interactions of young children. Child Dev 51:217–223.

Garvey C (1986): Peer relations and the growth of communication. In Mueller EC, Cooper CR (Eds.): "Process and Outcome in Peer Relationships," pp. 329–345. Orlando, Florida: Academic Press.

Guralnick MJ (1990a): Social competence and early intervention. J Early Intervent 14:3–14.

Guralnick MJ (1990b): Peer interactions and the development of handicapped children's social and communicative competence. In Foot H, Morgan M, Shute R (Eds.): "Children Helping Children," pp. 275–305. Sussex, England: Wiley.

Guralnick MJ (1992): A hierarchical model for understanding children's peer-related social competence. In Odom SL, McConnell SR, McEvoy MA (Eds.): "Social Competence of Young Children with Disabilities: Nature, Development, and Intervention," pp. 37–64. Baltimore: Brookes.

Guralnick MJ (in press): Developmentally appropriate practice in the assessment and intervention of children's peer relations. Top Early Child Spec Educ.

Guralnick MJ, Bricker D (1987): The effectiveness of early intervention for children with cognitive and general developmental delays. In Guralnick MJ, Bennett FC (Eds.): "The Effectiveness of Early Intervention for At-Risk and Handicapped Children," pp. 115–173. New York: Academic Press.

Guralnick MJ, Groom JM (1975): Correlates of peer-related social competence of developmentally delayed preschool children. Am J Ment Defic 90:140–150.

Guralnick MJ, Groom JM (1987a): The peer relations of mildly delayed and nonhandicapped preschool children in mainstreamed playgroups. Child Dev 58:1556–1572.

Guralnick MJ, Groom JM (1987b): Dyadic peer interactions of mildly delayed and non-handicapped preschool children. Am J Ment Defic 92:178–193.

Guralnick MJ, Groom JM (1988): Peer interactions in mainstreamed and specialized classrooms: A comparative analysis. Except Child 54:415–425.

Guralnick MJ, Paul-Brown D (1989): Peer-related communicative competence of preschool children: Developmental and adaptive characteristics. J Speech Hear Res 32:930–943.

Guralnick MJ, Weinhouse EM (1984): Peer-related social interactions of developmentally delayed young children: Development and characteristics. Dev Psychol 20:815–827.

Hartup WW (1983): Peer relations. In Hetherington EM (Ed.): "Handbook of Child Psychology: Socialization, Personality, and Social Development" (Vol. 4), pp. 103–196. New York: Wiley.

Parten MB (1932): Social participation among preschool children. J Abnorm Soc Psychol 27:243–269.

Inclusion of Students with Disabilities in Public Schools and Classrooms with Their Nondisabled Peers

Mary Falvey

Educational programs for students with disabilities have dramatically changed in the United States over the years. At one time, children with disabilities were not allowed access to public schools. Finally, laws were passed and children and adolescents with disabilities were allowed to go to public schools; however, these schools were typically segregated; that is, only students with disabilities attended. Gradually, these segregated schools made way for special segregated classes on "regular" education campuses with varying amounts and types of interactions with their nondisabled peers. All forms of school segregation, partial or complete, are being questioned and criticized today in many educational and legal arenas. Full inclusion of students with disabilities, that is, students attending the same public school they would attend if they did not have a disability while receiving the necessary supports to be successful, is the current best practice for several reasons. First, the research has demonstrated that students with disabilities are more successful when educated with their nondisabled peers. In addition, students without disabilities are more likely to develop positive attitudes towards their peers with disabilities when they go to classes and school together. Second, Public Law 94-142 requires that school districts create inclusive educational models. Specifically the law states:

> ... That to the maximum extent appropriate, handicapped children, including those children in public and private institutions or other care facilities, are educated with children who are not handicapped, and that special classes, separate schooling, or removal of handicapped from the regular educational environments occurs only when the nature or severity of the handicap is such that education in regular classes with the use of supplementary aids and services cannot be achieved satisfactorily.

Third, several court cases have supported inclusive educational services and have made forced segregation illegal. The first case that defined and clarified the principle that separate is not equal was Brown vs. Board of Education:

... [S]eparate educational facilities are inherently unequal. This inherent inequality stems from the stigma created by purposeful segregation which generates a feeling of inferiority that may affect their hearts and minds in a way unlikely ever to be undone. [Segregation] generates a feeling of inferiority as the [child's] status in the community that ... affects the motivation of a child to learn ... [and] has a tendency to retard ... educational and moral development." (Chief Justice Earl Warren, United States Supreme Court, May 17, 1954)

Two recent court cases in the United States that have applied principles of the Brown decision to children with disabilities are Holland vs. Sacramento Unified School District (Court of Appeals, decision pending) and the Oberti vs. Clementon School District (Court of Appeals, decision rendered May, 1993). Both of these cases have asked the courts to clarify school districts' responsibility with regard to inclusive education and, in both cases, the courts have required school districts to create inclusive educational opportunities for Rachel Holland (Holland case) and Raphael Oberti (Oberti case).

In addition to legal interpretations supporting inclusive education, friendship development is more likely to occur in inclusive settings than segregated settings. Segregated settings are often outside of the students' neighborhoods and are located in schools that are not typically attended by their brothers, sisters, and neighbors. According to research, a prerequisite to friendship development is close proximity and frequent opportunities. Stated another way, in order for children and adolescents to develop friendships they must have frequent opportunities to interact with their peers, which is facilitated by close proximity. Students attending schools outside their neighborhood will have more difficulty forming friendships with their neighbors since they will not have school, school activities, and school related activities in common.

Another reason for creating inclusive educational opportunities is that schools are a microcosm of society and must reflect values we want for the greater society. If we want, as a society, to value all of its members, then we must teach through our words and efforts that no individual or group should be segregated or rejected. Segregated schools and classes teach nondisabled children that some forms of segregation and rejection are appropriate. These children will grow up with these values, and it is likely to effect them as adults, their relationships with others, and their outlook on life.

Although the reasons for creating inclusive educational opportunities may be extremely compelling, the strategies to create such inclusive schools requires hard work. The following strategies can be used to facilitate the development of heterogeneous classrooms. First, schools must use relevant and meaningful assessment procedures, which include:

Family interviews/MAPs
Performance assessment
Portfolio or "authentic" assessment systems

Curriculum-based assessment
Ecological and student repertoire inventory
Frequency counts
Functional analysis

Second, personalized and individualized instructional strategies for each student must be determined and used. Multilevel instruction, where students learn at their own level together, is an important element of individualized instruction. Teachers should anticipate students' difficult behaviors ahead of time and try to prevent them from occurring. Teachers should find ways for students to become increasingly self-directed and self-reflective to avoid an overreliance on instructional interventions. Teachers must always demand quality work from students and not assume that if they have a disability they cannot "measure up" and do the work of their non-disabled peers. When choosing a general education classroom for a student with a disability, teachers who use activity-based instruction that engages students as active learners (e.g., simulation, applied-learning stations, role play and demonstration, community-referenced and community-based projects, cooperative groups, games) should be given serious consideration.

Third, instructional arrangements can also be used as effective strategies for facilitating inclusive educational opportunities. Using cooperative groups, writing workshops, individualized math and writing folders, individualized task completion, whole language, and team teaching are but a few examples. Rotating student groups, modifying instructional presentations, skills, skill sequence, rules, and motivation/reinforcement, and collaborating within an integrated related-services model (e.g., occupational therapy, physical therapy, and speech therapy) can be successful instructional arrangements. Providing accessibility and reasonable accommodations in the delivery of instructional arrangements is essential.

The fourth strategy is to create curriculum adaptation strategies. Although there are several strategies for adapting the curriculum, teachers should allow students to access the curriculum without adaptations if at all possible. Adapting the curriculum when the student does not need adaptations could make it more difficult for the student to participate in all aspects of life both within and outside of school. However, when a student is unable to access the curriculum as is, strategies for adapting the curriculum include:

Providing physical assistance
Adapting materials
Multilevel curriculum
Curriculum overlapping
Substitute curriculum

It is critical that students are provided with a relevant curriculum, teaching strategies that reflect students' individualized learning styles, and inclusive settings. The next decade will involve the creation of hundreds of thousands of inclusive schools that will be better prepared to effectively educate all students.

SUGGESTED READINGS

Ainscow M (Ed.) (1991): "Effective schools for all." Baltimore: Brookes.

Armstrong T (1987): "In their own way." Los Angeles: Jeremy P. Tarcher, Inc.

Biklen D (1992): "Schooling without labels." Philadelphia: Temple University Press.

Derman-Sparks L, The A.B.C. Task Force (1989): "Anti-bias curriculum: tools for empowering young children." Washington, D.C.: National Association for the Education of Young Children.

Falvey MA (1989): "Community-based curriculum: instructional strategies for students with severe handicaps," 2nd ed. Baltimore: Brookes.

Falvey M (Ed.) (in press): "Heterogeneous and inclusive education: assessment, curriculum, and instruction." Baltimore: Brookes.

Giangreco M (1993): "Choosing options and accommodations for children: a guide to planning inclusive education." Baltimore: Brookes.

Glasser W (1992): "The quality school: managing students without coercion." New York: Harper Collins.

Male M (1994): "Technology for inclusion: meeting the special needs of all students." Boston: Allyn & Bacon.

Oakes J, Liptom M (1990): "Making the best schools: A handbook for parents, teachers, and policymakers." New Haven, CT: Yale University Press.

Sailor W, Anderson JL, Haverson AT, Doering KF, Filler J, Goetz L (1989): "The comprehensive local school: Regular education for all students with disabilities." Baltimore: Brookes.

Teaching Children with Down Syndrome to Read and Write

Sue Buckley

INTRODUCTION

I began investigating the reading skills of children with Down syndrome in Portsmouth, U.K., in 1980 after receiving a letter from a father describing how he had discovered that Sarah, his daughter with Down syndrome, began to learn to read at the age of three. She was just beginning to imitate and to use single words in her speech. He taught her to read on flashcards the words that he wanted her to use in her speech and he observed that she began to use the words she had learned from the printed form at a faster rate than those in the spoken form. By 1989 Sarah was 12 years old and being educated in a local comprehensive school. She had received all but one year of her education in mainstream schools and was considered to be exceptionally able for a child with Down syndrome. The father believed that her exceptional progress had been the result of teaching her to read early and that other children might be helped in the same way.

His experience suggested that preschool children with Down syndrome could learn to read and that reading might be a "way-in" to language for these children. In 1979 children with Down syndrome were not thought capable of learning to read at all by most professionals and there was very little research into the reasons for their spoken language difficulties. With a grant from the Down's Syndrome Association in the United Kingdom, I was able to appoint a teacher and set up a research study to begin to investigate these hypotheses. We followed the progress of 15 preschool children for three years while they received a regular home-teaching program from us based on the Portage Programme (Shearer and Shearer, 1972).

Joanna, the first child that we tried teaching to read in 1980, learned 30 words in a month at 2 years of age. It was immediately clear that Sarah's experience might well apply to other children with Down syndrome, and the Joseph Rowntree Foundation agreed to fund our work for a further year. The results of that first project have been published in full elsewhere (Buckley, 1985a), as has an evaluation of the "parents as teachers" aspect (Buckley 1985b). We also published a videotape illustrating this work in 1983, which is still available.*

EARLY READERS

We now know that many children with Down syndrome show an ability to begin to learn to read at an unusually early age. Our own early findings have been confirmed in published studies by Greene (1987) in Ireland and by Norris (1989) in the U.K. We also receive many letters and reports from parents and practitioners who have successfully taught preschool children to read by following our advice. Our experience suggests that the majority of children with Down syndrome can learn to read single words by three to four years of age, some even earlier.

Some of the other children whose early progress we have recorded read their first words at the following ages: Digby at 25 months, Emma and Daniel at 28 months, Zoe at 3 years 5 months and Jamie at 3 years. These children were all at the single-word stage of speech (beginning to use a small number of single words appropriately) except for Digby. Digby began to learn to read before he could produce any spoken words. He demonstrated his comprehension by reading the flashcard and pointing to the correct object or picture. All the children named above have continued to make steady progress with both reading and spoken language skills. They all have greater skills in these areas than is usually expected for children with Down syndrome, and all started school at 5 years of age in ordinary primary schools.

IMPORTANT OBSERVATIONS

Reading Errors

In the 1980 research project we recorded the children's progress with their reading and, while, initially, we were most surprised by the speed and accuracy of their performance, we were even more surprised by some of the errors we began to see. We expected the children to make visual errors, i.e., to confuse words that look similar such as *hair* and *rain* or *this* and *shoe*. These are the sorts of errors seen in the early performance of all beginning readers taught in this "look and say" way (Seymour and Elder, 1986) and we found them in our children's performance. We did not anticipate the other consistent type of error that we observed when the children were reading single words, the semantic error. Here the word the child says has the same meaning as the one they are looking at but has no visual similarity. For example, the child looks at the printed word *shut* and says *closed* or looks at *sleep* and says *go to bed*. These semantic errors excited us at the time for two reasons.

First, they suggested that the children were decoding the print for meaning and not just "barking at print" in a meaningless way as some critics were suggesting. They were reading single words on flashcards, so they had no available clues to meaning, such as might be provided by pictures or the rest of a sentence. They must have decoded the printed word for meaning and then thought of a word that was linked by meaning to the target word on the card. Second, the errors demonstrated that the brain could go straight from print to meaning, without changing the visual image of the word to its spoken form first and then accessing the meaning. In 1982, reading

---

*The Sarah Duffen Centre, University of Portsmouth, Portsmouth PO5 INA, U.K.

theorists were still arguing about whether the brain could actually do this. Our children were demonstrating that it could.

Signing

In 1982, signing was just beginning to be introduced to the younger children in special schools in the United Kingdom, and some of the children we were working with learned signing at school, after we had taught them to read. We noticed two interesting effects of learning sign. First, some of our children were able to sign the correct responses to flashcards without any extra teaching. We felt this was another clear illustration that they were not simply "barking at print" but were reading the print for meaning and able to replace the spoken response we had taught them with a sign entirely on their own initiative. Second, for some of the children signs were an easier and faster response mode than speech. They would look at a flashcard and appear to be concentrating on producing the correct spoken response, meanwhile their hands were already making a correct sign. This additional time needed to produce speech suggested to us that the children might have some sort of specific production difficulty with speech. Even when they knew what they wanted to say, they had difficulty in saying it.

This was one of the first clues we had to indicate that not all the language delay typical of children with Down syndrome could be blamed on general cognitive delay. In fact, the way in which the children substituted similar-meaning words and signed when reading encouraged us to feel that they were more intelligent and had more understanding of language than they were being given credit for. What was beginning to emerge was the possibility that the children's language development was being delayed by a series of specific language-learning difficulties in addition to the effects of any general cognitive delay.

Pantomime

When we watched the videotapes on which we recorded the children's reading progress, we noticed that we had captured a number of sequences in which a child was trying to describe an experience or explain something to his mother for which his spoken language skills were inadequate. The child would resort to the combined use of single keywords and mime to try to convey his message. We were convinced again that the children knew what they wanted to say but could not express themselves in speech.

There are a number of possible hypotheses which could be generated to explain these observations. For example, the child may not have mastered enough grammar to be able to construct the sentences that were being implied by the combination of words and gesture. Alternatively, we could postulate that the child was thinking in sentences but could not execute them in speech.

Either way, we were fairly confident that the childrens' cognitive development was more advanced than their expressive language development. This has since been confirmed by several studies. For example, Cunningham and his colleagues demonstrated a lag between mental age and language age, with expressive language falling even further behind than receptive language as children get older (Cunningham et al., 1985). Other studies have confirmed these findings (Miller, 1988).

READING ENHANCES SPEECH

Our own observations and those of many other parents and teachers suggest that the original hypothesis was right and that reading is a "way-in" to their first language for these children. Daniel's progress recorded by his home-teacher illustrates the typical effect of early reading on speech development.

Daniel's first spoken words were "Daddy," and "teddy" at 14 months and he was using some 50 single words at 27 months. He was introduced to flashcards by his home-teacher at 28 months and reading 10 flashcards at 2 years. He was reading two-word phrases at 2 months later and these rapidly transferred to his speech. Two months after this he was reading 22 words and a month later he was reading six three-word phrases, which rapidly transferred to his speech. At 3 years 4 months he was reading 66 words and many two- and three-word combinations of these. At 3 years 5 months he was reading simple books and the words "and" and "a" appeared in his speech. At 3 Daniel was reading four-word sentences and at two months later he had a sight vocabulary of 116 words and was speaking in six-word sentences. [Data taken from the records of Daniel's home teacher (Norris, 1989).]

In summary, the main benefits reported for speech are:

1. New words learned from flashcards soon begin to emerge in the child's speech and may do so more quickly than words the child is only hearing.
2. Practicing two- and three-word utterances in reading accelerates their emergence in the child's speech.
3. Practicing proper sentences in reading leads to the use of function words and increasingly correct grammar and syntax in speech. Mastering the rules of grammar and syntax is difficult for youngsters with Down syndrome and many authors have drawn attention to this (see Fowler, 1990 for a review).
4. The children who read early in this way achieve higher levels of literacy and linguistic competence than has hitherto been expected in children with Down syndrome. Their "reading ages" are frequently close to their chronological ages up to 8 or 9 years of age.
5. Reading practice improves phonology and articulation, possibly because the letters in words provide the cues the child needs to sound all the phonemes. Many children with Down syndrome have clearer articulation when reading than when speaking.

WHY READING MAY HELP SPEAKING

Research has moved on since our original study and it is now possible to begin to build up a picture of some of the specific learning difficulties that delay the language development of children with Down syndrome. As you read the following sections, I think you will begin to see why learning to read may help these children overcome some of their difficulties.

Hearing Loss

In the last ten years, a number of studies report a high incidence of significant hearing loss in young children with Down syndrome that may be affecting the language development of as many as 80% of infants and toddlers (Cunningham and McArthur, 1981). Such losses, even if transitory due to otitis media, will obviously make learning language from listening difficult for the child.

Specific Modality Effect

A number of studies have demonstrated that children with Down syndrome perform better when tasks are presented visually rather than auditorily and when the response can be made manually by pointing or selecting rather than orally (see Pueschel, 1988 for a review). This general finding indicates that impairments in auditory processing due to hearing loss, poor auditory discrimination, and limited auditory memory and impairments in the complex mechanisms of speech production are limiting the children's performance.

Auditory Short-Term Memory

Recent studies have demonstrated poor development of auditory short-term memory span relative to cognitive development throughout childhood for children with Down syndrome (Mackenzie and Hulme, 1987, 1992). This makes sentence processing and, hence, the learning of grammar and syntax from listening particularly difficult and may explain why most children with Down syndrome still speak in immature keyword utterances even in their teens. Recent research has highlighted the importance of this memory function for most aspects of language acquisition in children (Gathercole and Baddeley, 1993).

Visual Memory

Children's visual memory may be more effective than their auditory memory for short sequences of information. For most children auditory memory is better than visual memory, but the reverse is usually the case for children with Down syndrome (Marcell and Armstrong, 1982; Marcell and Weeks, 1988). This may be one reason why children with Down syndrome enjoy learning to read and learning with a computer—both activities present information visually.

We think that another benefit of computer-aided learning is that it is under the child's control, so it provides as much time as needed to think and organize responses, before assuming failure or asking another question as an adult might. The computer also always rewards success and never gets irritated! Computer programs designed to teach speech have received a lot of attention in the United States (see Meyers, 1988, 1990). There are also many useful programs to teach reading and writing skills.

Speech Production

Various authors are drawing attention to speech–motor delay and difficulty, which affects the child's ability to speak clearly. The progress of early signers, who often sign extensively for some months before they begin to speak, suggests a specific word production problem (LePrevost, 1986). The growing gap between the level of language comprehension and expressive ability in most children with Down syndrome has also been reported by Miller (1988) and by Jenkins (1993); Jenkins suggests that there are continuing production difficulties as they get older.

BEGINNING LATER

The range in normal reading development is wide, with some children starting in their preschool years and others not until they are eight or nine. We would expect the same range in children with Down syndrome. Children who start later may make rapid progress and become good readers.

Symbol systems such as Rebus or Makaton symbols can be used for the children who are not able to master print and should bring the same benefits for speech development. However, we always try print with a child first and only use symbols if he or she cannot master print. Symbols are not a stepping stone to print, they are an alternative and different system and most children do not need to learn them. The earlier the child can make a start with reading, the greater the benefit for their speech and language skills, but there will be language benefits whenever they start.

HELPING TEENAGERS

The advantage of reading for language learning has been demonstrated in our own work with older children. In a study designed to investigate the possibility of improving the spoken language skills of a group of teenagers, two teaching methods were compared. The methods and materials used were identical except for the addition of printed sentences on the picture cards used in the "reading" condition (Buckley, 1993). The teenagers learned faster and more accurately in the "reading" condition for every structure taught. Contrary to our expectations, the advantageous effect of the "reading" condition was most dramatic for some of the least able teenagers. They learned twice as fast in this condition even though they were nonreaders at the outset of the study. There seem to be two reasons for this. These teenagers had very poor short-term auditory memories and some were, therefore, simply not able to remember and repeat the sentences they were learning if they only heard them. A further experiment indicated that the effect of the print was due to storing the visual image of the word, not just to the enhanced practice possible in the visual condition.

TEACHING READING TO TEACH LANGUAGE

While the idea of teaching reading to teach spoken language still meets with resistance from some teachers, it has been used successfully for more than 25 years in some areas of special education in the United Kingdom, and I would urge all teachers to read Ella Hutts' detailed and insightful account of this approach (Hutt, 1986). We have made extensive use of her methods and "Language through Reading" materials since 1982.

Teaching Principles

We use exactly the same principles to develop teaching programs whatever the age of the child. The methods are based on experience and findings of research into the development of reading skills in ordinary children and adults (see Gathercole and Baddeley, 1993 for a review).

Reading Readiness

We have found no way of predicting a child's potential for reading or readiness to read. In our view both concepts are meaningless. Many of the children we know who have made great progress with reading would have failed all the usual readiness tests at the outset. The only way we know of determining whether a child with a learning disability is able to learn to read is to try teaching them in the ways we suggest. The only way to find out how far they may progress is to continue to teach them.

If you use the errorless learning approach that we advocate below and make the tasks fun you can do no harm by trying some reading activities with any child. If they make no progress after a few games, leave it and try again in a month or two. Meanwhile, keep reading interesting stories to the child and keep labels on everyday items and names on hooks, etc., so that print is a natural part of their world.

Establish a Sight Vocabulary

The first words chosen for flash cards are usually family names and then words that we know the child comprehends and uses. The words are printed neatly on flashcards by hand in lower case and without any pictures. Our own experience and that of researchers working with ordinary children shows that the children learn to read words faster without pictures to distract them (Wu and Solman, 1993). They are all taught to read their first words by a carefully structured behavioral approach that emphasizes the importance of task analysis, teaching in small steps, using an errorless learning method, and social reinforcement.

Matching, Selecting, and Naming

The children learn first to match the words by playing matching games with the flashcards, then to select them when asked for spoken name, and, finally, to "name" or read them. As the children's sight vocabularies grow, so does their understanding of the complete task and they become increasingly able to learn to read new words without the need to break the task into the three steps. We break the early reading task into its component parts deliberately, in order to help the child understand each step in the task. In so doing, we will be able to see the reason for the child's failure from the step in the task that he or she cannot master.

Errorless Learning

We also advocate errorless learning as the best way of building success and self-confidence. Errorless learning simply means teaching children to complete the new task by guiding them through each step correctly with prompts and not allowing them to fail. As the child becomes more confident, the teacher fades the prompts until the child can do the whole task without help. In our early work, we found that it seemed to be difficult for children to correct wrong responses—more difficult than for ordinary children—so it was important to prevent wrong guesses in the initial stages of learning. Jennifer Wishart's research on aspects of early cognitive development in children with Down syndrome has drawn attention to this sensitivity to failure and lack of consolidation strategies when learning. She also advocates errorless learning as the preferred teaching method (Wishart, 1988).

New Words for Phrases and Sentences

Once we know that the children are able to establish a sight vocabulary in this way, we introduce words into their flashcard vocabulary that they do not yet comprehend or use in their speech. For these words, games are played and activities devised to teach the meanings. These words are chosen to enable us to build phrases and sentences for the children to practice. The choice of phrases and sentences is determined by the child's level of spoken language use. In this way, we use reading to enable the child to practice the words, phrases, and sentences needed to develop spontaneous speech skills and master the rules for grammar and syntax.

The Meanings of Words

The reading work does not go on in isolation from a whole range of other games and activities designed to help the child learn the meanings of words and how to use them in communicative interactions. For all children, an understanding of the meanings of words and the ways in which they are used grows slowly. At first, "cat" will be used as a label for the child's own cat. It will take time and experience of many different cats before the child realizes it's a label for a class of objects. Indeed, even as adults we add to our knowledge of the cat family and thus extending the concept behind the label. Childrens' understanding of words grows with using them and then having their utterances expanded or corrected.

Understanding Sentences

It is easy to teach a sight vocabulary so that children can read a sentence aloud correctly, but they may not comprehend it, as the grammar and syntax may be too advanced for them. Once the teacher is aware of the level of the child's language comprehension skills, stories can be chosen that use grammar and syntax that is within their current comprehension level. We encourage parents and teachers to make simple books based on the child's own experiences and to write sentences with the child's spoken language needs in mind so that they are reading words, phrases, and sentences that will help them to talk more clearly.

Phonics

We encourage early success and confidence in this "look and say" whole-word way and then move on to give children a more sophisticated understanding of the reading process by pointing out the letter–sound correspondences in the words that they can already read correctly. Knowledge of letter sounds enables children to work out an unfamiliar printed word by themselves. We draw their attention to the initial or onset sounds by finding two words in their sight vocabulary with the same initial or onset sounds. Recent work has suggested that children break the words into onset and rhyme, such as "str" and "ing" for "string," "str" being the onset and "ing" the rhyme (Goswami and Bryant, 1990). Early readers break the words up in this way for themselves as their experience with reading words grows.

Research suggests that once a printed word is familiar, the brain recognizes it as a whole word and goes straight from print to meaning (Ellis and Young, 1988), so a child can learn to read successfully without having any understanding of letter–sound correspondences at all, providing someone is on hand to teach every new word. There is no limit to the size of the vocabulary that can be established in this "look and say" way. However, most children with Down syndrome are able to learn some letter–sound rules and therefore help themselves to tackle new words in their reading and also to spell when writing. Some researchers believe that phonic knowledge is more important for spelling than reading (Frith, 1980, 1985). Frith suggests that most children learn to understand and use phonics from their own experience as they progress with their reading and writing, in particular as a result of engaging in the activity of writing and spelling words. Teaching letter sounds as an activity isolated from the actual reading, writing, and spelling tasks is less likely to help the child realize the relevance of the knowledge.

Any reader interested in recent research into reading and spelling development in children would find Margaret Snowling's book "Dyslexia" (Snowling, 1987) a readable introduction containing information relevant to teaching any child to read.

WRITING

We teach writing as soon as we begin teaching reading, in order to develop the children's motor control and also to draw their attention to the letters in words from the outset. At first, we encourage tracing over words the child can read by placing the flashcard words in a book with plastic film on the pages, such as a photograph album. If the child uses a water-based pen to trace, the film can be wiped clean for more practice. As the child's control improves, we fade the prompts, reducing the word outlines gradually to dotted letters and then encouraging copying of words on a line below. Other activities, including finger painting, tracing over letters with fingers, and drawing in sand are all encouraged to improve fine motor coordination in preparation for writing, but the best way to develop writing skills is to keep practicing writing.

By encouraging writing from the start, we can also help the child to see how reading is relevant to their everyday lives as we write messages for them to take home to read and make diaries recording their daily activities. We make use of simple word-processor programs on the computer to enable the children to compose their own sentences before their writing is legible. Such programs are usually highly motivating.

READING AND TALKING

Young children with Down syndrome can learn to read and talk at the same time, the two skills interacting and informing each other, as indeed they do for all children. As Garton and Pratt point out, "the development of written language skills influences spoken ability, as new language structures and functions are learned for writing which in turn are adopted for speaking" (Garton and Pratt, 1989, p. 2).

Down children exposed to reading at a much earlier stage in their language development than normal are more dependent on direct and accurate visual decoding skills and use the direct visual route to the meaning of words more than the ordinary five year old, as they do not have enough knowledge of spoken language to guess an unfamiliar printed word from the context provided by a sentence or a picture. They may also not have enough knowledge of phonics to "sound out" words initially. The way in which any child tackles a new task will vary according to the knowledge and skills that they have available to them.

TEACHING IN THE UNITED KINGDOM

In the United Kingdom, most children with Down syndrome are still being educated in special schools for children with learning difficulties, though the situation is changing fast. In many areas the younger children are joining mainstream schools. The teaching of reading is not a priority in the early curriculum of most special schools, though this situation is beginning to change.

The children in mainstream schools are more likely to be learning to read, though the teachers may not have access to advice regarding the need to take account of the child's language comprehension level or the way in which reading can be used to improve speech. At present, parents are often the driving force and teach their child to read at home. All the children mentioned earlier in this chapter were taught by their parents, following our advice. The following extracts from a letter from a parent describes the benefits she observed for her daughter.

> I started to teach Emma to read after hearing you talk in Bristol seven years ago. She was then two years and four months of age. Emma is now nine years old and an able and avid reader. She attends our large local mainstream primary school and holds her own well in the second year junior class. She seems to develop in leaps and bounds. Being able to read has done so much for her.
>
> It helped her speech. For example, when she began to read at age two, she spoke understandably but imperfectly as she left out the definite and indefinite articles, prepositions, etc. The change came when she was able to sentence-build in flashcards. Today her speech is mature and her teacher commented at the last parents evening that the extent of her vocabulary and her turn of phrase would leave many in the class standing.
>
> It helped in the way other children regarded Emma and not least her own self-esteem. They knew and she knew that in reading she was

amongst the best in the class. This apparently less able child wasn't so less able after all.

Emma is now an independent reader and books give her so much. She wakes early and reads for at least one hour every morning. She makes her own choice of book but everything she reads fulfills her—she chuckles when reading "The Twits" and cries over "Heidi." These are her two favorite books at the moment and she reads them over and over again. Equally, however, she will read poems or her atlas, history book, nature book, etc., from which she teaches herself. She loves her Bible. She is very proud when her five year old sister carries the newspaper to her and asks "What time is————on the television?" She is always able to tell her and I feel Sarah, who I feel senses rather than knows of Emma's differences, is thrilled with the sense of her big sister having the "big sister" image for once.

REFERENCES

Buckley SJ (1985a): Attaining basic educational skills. In Lane D, Stratford B (eds.) "Current Approaches to Down's Syndrome." Eastbourne, UK: Holt Saunders.

Buckley SJ (1985b): Teaching parents to teach reading to teach language. In Wolfendale S, Topping K "Parental Involvement in Childrens Reading." London: Croom Helm.

Buckley SJ (1993): Language development in children with Down's syndrome: Reasons for optimism. Down's Syndr Res & Prac 1(1):3–9.

Buckley SJ, Emslie M, Haslegrave G, LePrevost P (1993): The Development of Language and Reading Skills in Children with Down's Syndrome, 2nd ed. Portsmouth, UK: University of Portsmouth.

Cunningham CC, Glenn SM, Wilkinson P, Sloper P (1985): Mental ability, symbolic play and receptive expressive language of young children with Down's syndrome. J Child Psychol & Psychiatry 26(2):255–265.

Cunningham C, McArthur K (1981): Hearing loss and treatment in young Down's syndrome children. Child Health Care & Devel 7:357.

Ellis AE, Young AW (1988): "Human Cognitive Neuropsychology." Hove, UK: Erlbaum.

Fowler A (1990): Language abilities in children with Down's syndrome: evidence for a syntactic delay. In Cicchetti D, Beeghly M (eds.) "Children with Down Syndrome." Cambridge: Cambridge University Press.

Frith U (1980): "Cognitive Processes in Spelling." New York: Academic Press.

Frith U (1985): Beneath the surface of developmental dyslexia. In Patterson KE, Marshall JC, Coltheart M (eds.) "Surface Dyslexia." Hove, UK: Erlbaum.

Garton A, Pratt C (1989): "Learning to be Literate: The Development of Written and Spoken Language. Oxford: Blackwell.

Gathercole S, Baddeley A (1993): "Working Memory and Language." Hove, UK: Erlbaum.

Goswami U, Bryant P (1990): Phonological Skills and Learning to Read. Oxford: Blackwell.

Goswami U (1992): Phonological factors in spelling development. J Child Psychol & Psychiatry 33(6):967–976.

Greene K (1987): Involving parents in teaching reading: A project with nine children with Down's syndrome. Mental Handicap 15:112–115.

Hutt E (1986): Teaching Language-Disordered Children: A Structured Curriculum. London: Edward Arnold.

Jenkins C (1993): Expressive language delay in children with Down's syndrome—a specific cause for concern. Down's Synd Res & Prac 1(1):10–14.

LePrevost P (1986): The use of signing to encourage first words. In Buckley S, Emslie M, Haslegrave G, LePrevost P. The Development of Language and Reading Skills in Children with Down's syndrome. Portsmouth, UK: Portsmouth Polytechnic.

MacKenzie S, Hulme C (1987): Memory span development in Down's syndrome, severely subnormal and normal subjects. Cog Neuropsy 4:303–319.

MacKenzie S, Hulme C (1992): Working Memory and Severe Learning Difficulties. Hove, UK: Earlbaum.

Marcell MM, Armstrong V (1982): Auditory and visual sequential memory of Down syndrome and non-retarded children. Am J Ment Defic 87(1):86–95.

Marcell MM, Weeks SL (1988): Short-term memory difficulties and Down's syndrome. J Ment Defic Res 32:153–162.

Meyers L (1988): Using computers to teach children with Down's syndrome spoken and written language skills. In Nadel L (ed.): "The Psychobiology of Down's Syndrome." New York: NDSS.

Meyers L (1990): Language development and intervention. In Van Dyke DC et al. (eds.): "Clinical Perspectives in the Management of Down's Syndrome." New York: Springer-Verlag.

Miller J (1987): Language and communication characteristics of children with Down syndrome. In Pueschel SM et al. (eds.): "New Perspectives on Down Syndrome." Baltimore: Paul Brookes.

Miller J (1988): The developmental asynchrony of language development in children with Down syndrome. In Nadel L (ed.): "The Psychobiology of Downs Syndrome." Bradford, UK: NDSS.

Norris H (1989): Teaching reading to help develop language in very young children with Down's syndrome. Paper presented at the National Portage Conference.

Pueschel S (1988): Visual and auditory processing in children with Down syndrome. In Nadel L (ed.): "The Psychobiology of Down Syndrome." New York: NDSS.

Seymour P, Elder L (1986): Beginning reading without phonology. Cog Neuropsy 3:1–36.

Shearer MS, Shearer DE (1972): The Portage project: A model for early childhood education. Exceptional Children 36:210–217.

Snowling M (1987): "Dyslexia." Oxford: Blackwell.

Wishart J (1988): Early learning in infants and young children with Down's syndrome. In Nadel L (ed.): The Psychobiology of Down Syndrome. New York: NDSS.

Wu H-M, Solman R (1993): Effective use of pictures as extra stimulus prompts. Br J Ed Psyc 63(1):144–160.

Curricular Adaptations:
Reconfiguring Teaching Practice to Support Students with Disabilities in General Education Classrooms

Alice Udvari-Solner

Increasing numbers of students with mild, moderate, and severe disabilities* are receiving daily instruction in general education classrooms in their neighborhood schools. The term inclusive education has emerged to describe this practice. The philosophy underlying inclusion is that all children can learn together, and the multiplicity of learning styles found in diverse groups of children is valued (Biklen, 1985; Forest, 1987; Stainback and Stainback, 1992). Instructional practices in inclusive classrooms reflect the beliefs that individual differences can be accommodated and learning outcomes will vary based upon each child's educational priorities. These issues of equity, diversity, and individualization are integral elements of the current elementary and secondary educational reform and restructuring movements.

As the population of students in general education becomes more and more diverse, there is a growing realization that general education practices, particularly those that rely heavily upon teacher-directed whole-class learning, must be adapted, modified and shaped in order to accommodate all learners. The purpose of this chapter is to outline definitions, techniques, and strategies that professionals and parents may use to generate curricular adaptations that are responsive to the learning needs of students with a range of intellectual abilities.

CURRICULAR ADAPTATIONS: A DEFINITION

Adaptations can be defined as any adjustments or modifications in the environment, instruction, or materials used for learning that enhance the person's perfor-

*Throughout this chapter the phrase "student with disabilities" will be used to refer to school age children with moderate to severe handicaps. This population includes students with intellectual disabilities, dual sensory impairments, and multiple physical disabilities. It should be noted that the general process described in this paper for adapting curriculum can be applied to students with a range of learning needs; however, the student examples presented here represent individuals with disabilities that require significant curricular modifications.

mance or allow at least partial participation in an activity. The purpose of an adaptation is to assist the individual to compensate for intellectual, physical, or behavioral challenges (Nisbet et al., 1983). An adaptation allows the individual to use his or her current skill repertoire while promoting the acquisition of new skills. More specifically, curricular adaptations serve the important function of preventing a mismatch between the student's skills and the lesson content (Giangreco and Putnam, 1991).

Embedded in this definition is the concept of partial participation—at least some degree of active involvement in a task or activity (Baumgart et al., 1982; Ferguson and Baumgart, 1991). The principle of partial participation acknowledges that many students, particularly those with severe disabilities, might never learn the skills to perform an activity with complete independence. Partial participation is central to the involvement of students with disabilities in general education classrooms because it reinforces the idea that a student should not be excluded from an activity due to the fact only a portion of the required skills can be performed.

STRATEGIES TO RECONFIGURE GENERAL EDUCATION PRACTICES

Curricular adaptations make the difference between a student merely being present in the classroom and being actively involved in daily school life. When collaboratively engineered, curricular adaptations minimize the differences between students with a range of abilities. Curricular adaptations serve three important functions: (1) to increase the student's opportunity to be an initiator, (2) to reduce the level of abstraction of curricular content, and (3) to make classroom content relevant to the student's current and future life.

Successful modifications individualize the lesson content and help create a match between the student's learning style and the instructor's teaching style. Therefore, most adaptations employed in the general education classroom address either the way instruction is arranged and delivered or the way the student takes part in an activity. In many ways these two factors are interrelated, because the way instruction is delivered directly affects how the student is expected to respond and participate.

If a student with disabilities is unable to participate in a general education activity as it has been originally constructed, changes may need to be made in one or more of the following instructional conditions:

• instructional groupings or arrangements
• lesson format
• teaching style or delivery of instruction
• curricular goals and learning outcomes
• environmental conditions
• instructional materials
• level or type of personal assistance

A change in one or more of these instructional components is considered a curricular adaptation. If adjustments in these seven areas still do not allow the student to participate in an educationally relevant way, then an eighth option may be employed:

design an alternative activity for the student with disabilities and a small group of peers. Each curricular adaptation is described in more detail below.

Change the Instructional Grouping or Arrangement

When a lesson is planned the teacher must select the instructional arrangement that is most appropriate for the lesson content. For any given activity there are a number of instructional arrangements from which to choose. Alternatives for student groupings include:

1. large-group or whole-class instruction
2. teacher-directed, small-group instruction
3. cooperative learning groups
4. student-directed small group or peer partners
5. peer tutor or cross-age tutor
6. one-to-one teacher/student instruction
7. independent seat work

One instructional arrangement is not necessarily superior to another. In fact most instructors use a combination of these groupings throughout a day. However, by nature, whole-class and independent seat work arrangements often pose the most problems for students with disabilities. When whole-class instruction is used students receive information in much the same manner and are expected to keep pace with the instructor. A high degree of attention and effective listening are usually expected. For many students with disabilities who have difficulty processing, understanding, and integrating information, it is difficult, if not impossible, to assimilate and make sense of all the information. By nature of their size, large-group arrangements offer fewer opportunities for students to respond and stay actively involved. Furthermore, students who are unable to sit attentively for an extended period may also have difficulty remaining focused in larger groups.

Long periods of independent seat work can pose similar difficulties. Students are expected to perform in a quiet, self-reliant manner while working independently at their desks. In many cases, students with disabilities often require prompts, cues, and assistance to interpret classroom material used during independent seat work. While many students have acquired skills to work independently, others need supervision and instruction to perform independently or semi-independently. Generally speaking, instructional arrangements that incorporate peer interaction, division of responsibilities, and interdependence among children allow many more options for participation by a student with disabilities (Johnson and Johnson, 1986). These arrangements also have "built in" support systems—the presence of other classmates.

It is virtually impossible for the instructor to eliminate all whole-group or independent seat work. However, the instructor should be aware that the participation of a student with disabilities will be affected in these arrangements. When it is possible to transform large-group or independent work into cooperative, small-group, or partnership structures, the teacher should do so. When large-group or independent work is necessary, steps should be taken to individualize material and match the presentation of information with the student's learning style.

Change the Lesson Format

Tied closely to instructional arrangements is the lesson format. Teachers may use one or a combination of the following techniques to organize a lesson and impart information to students and engage them in learning:

1. *Lecture/demonstration/practice.* This traditional teaching format is one of the most frequently used models (Callahan and Clark, 1988). Also referred to as the expository mode of teaching, the instructor provides an explanation of a concept or topic, then supports verbal information with an illustration or model. A lecture/demonstration format is often followed by students participating in a class discussion, or engaging in independent practice of the concepts covered by the teacher.

2. *Whole-class inquiry or discussion.* After exposure to verbal or written information, students are engaged in a question and answer exchange. Students are called upon or volunteer answers. Class members are encouraged to ask additional questions or elaborate on the topic. The teacher usually directs and manages the discussion.

3. *Games, simulations, role playing, presentations, and activity-based lessons.* Activities are arranged that reinforce or extend the lesson content and encourage students to apply the information that has been previously taught or discussed. This type of lesson format is characterized by students (a) being actively engaged, (b) participating in the planning process, (c) learning by discovery, and (d) constructing their own knowledge. These activities are relatively short in duration, usually one class period or a portion of a class period. For example, after a brief introduction to a science chapter on genetics, the class is divided into small groups. Each group conducts a mini-survey to record the prevalence of certain genetic traits in the sixth grade student population. After surveys are completed each team presents its findings to the class.

4. *Experiential lessons.* This type of lesson format uses real-life activities to apply or enhance skills. Activities can take place in the classroom or nonschool environments. For example, the students in a beginning architectural drawing class must design and build a small storage shed at a local park. In the context of this activity, which lasts for 10 weeks, the students draw a feasible plan, order appropriate materials, and utilize construction skills. Experiential lessons are also appropriate in lower grade levels. For instance, in a first grade classroom, students are asked to bring simple recipes for healthy snacks and beverages from home. On a weekly basis during language arts, a small group of students plan and cook a healthy snack that is shared with the class. The students write their own recipe, make a grocery list, calculate the correct amount of money needed, purchase the groceries, and prepare the snack. As a result of this year-long activity a student-generated recipe book is developed. Experiential lessons can be as short as one class period, employed over a number of weeks, or occur on a regularly scheduled basis throughout the year.

5. *Community-referenced instruction.* Community-referenced instruction is char-

acterized by students applying skills in nonschool settings that have some relationship, relevance, and purpose to their lives, now or in the future. Instruction may relate to vocational, domestic, community, or recreation curricular domains. This lesson format differs from experiential lessons because it takes place exclusively in the community and occurs on a regularly scheduled basis across the year.

The value of activity-based, experiential, and community-referenced lessons is becoming more evident as the school population becomes more and more diverse. These lesson formats offer options to assign different roles to students, delegate tasks that are matched to the student's ability level and knowledge base, individualize the presentation of information, and differentiate the materials more effectively than in lecture/demonstration or whole-class inquiry format. Furthermore, learning is arranged in concrete and applied ways, resulting in education that is a dynamic interaction between the student and the environment (Sharon and Sharon, 1976).

Change the Teaching Style or Delivery of Instruction

Another influential factor affecting the inclusion of students with disabilities is the teaching style employed. By making subtle changes in the teacher's delivery of instruction, a complementary match may be achieved with the student's learning style. A few simple guidelines that educators can follow to modify their teaching style or delivery of instruction include:

- Tell the student exactly what you want him/her to learn or accomplish.
- Simplify instructions and demonstrate what you want completed.
- Use concrete materials/examples that relate to the student's life.
- Try to reduce irrelevant details and stick to the essential attributes of concepts.
- Divide material to be learned into smaller tasks and sequence learning tasks from simple to complex.
- Provide repeated opportunities to practice the skill(s) of concern.
- Provide regular and frequent feedback throughout a lesson when initially teaching new information; monitor and provide feedback and intervention before errors are made to establish a pattern of success.
- Incorporate learning games and the use of mnemonic devices to recall information.
- Desensitize the student to stressful situations by moving through a series of progressively more demanding steps.
- Model and encourage self advocacy skills (e.g., requesting an alternative presentation style, stating when material is too difficult/confusing, etc.).
- Back up oral information with alternative methods of input such as headset/tape player, highlighted information, written directions.
- Elaborate or shape a student's response to correspond with the context of the lesson.
- Include a higher frequency of verbal prompts and direct physical assistance when necessary for a student with more significant disabilities.

Change the Curricular Goals or Learning Outcomes

To match the unique needs and skills of students with disabilities within the context of a general education activity, it may be appropriate to individualize the learning objectives. Also referred to as multilevel or flexible learning objectives, the instructor may vary the goals and outcomes of the lesson for one or more students (Giangreco and Putnam, 1991; Stainback et al., 1992).

In a heterogeneous classroom, learners will acquire and apply knowledge at different levels and rates. Bloom's taxonomy of instructional objectives outlines six levels of learning (Bloom, 1956). These levels include knowledge, comprehension, application, analysis, synthesis, and evaluation. Educational goals can be individualized based upon the student's learning priorities at each of these levels. For example, a group of three students must create a story about Alaskan wildlife that will be presented orally to the class. One of the group members has severe intellectual and dual sensory impairments. The students have the option to develop audiovisual materials to communicate their story, select music to complement the presentation, or act out the story line dramatically. This particular group decided to make a diorama to represent Alaskan terrain and clay figures to depict the animals in the story.

The learning objectives for the two students without disabilities relate to applying and synthesizing past information, composing a sensible story, utilizing correct grammar, and employing accurate handwriting skills. The curricular objectives for the student with disabilities focus on using fine motor skills to participate in the creation of the diorama figures, following tactile signs from his classmates, and making choices within the context of the activity. These objectives represent learning at the knowledge and comprehension level.

An objective to practice group cooperation skills is expected for all of the students in the group regardless of ability level. For the two students without disabilities this means using encouraging statements and gentle physical touch. For the student with dual sensory impairments group cooperation skills translate to accepting guidance from a friend without resisting physical touch. Individualizing the curricular goals, attending to each student's level of learning, and acknowledging the value of each child's educational priorities, allows the three students to work successfully in a heterogeneous group.

Changes in curricular goals may be significant, as illustrated in the above example, or they can be as minor as allowing the impaired student more time to complete an assignment, perform fewer test items per page, or master only the highest priority material from a unit. When taking a flexible or multilevel orientation to curricular goals, it is also important to remember that "academics" per se or mastery of skills related to traditional content areas may not be the primary concern or fundamental reason for the student's inclusion in a specific subject area. The social aspects of the activity and the skills that facilitate interpersonal relationships may be considered of equal or greater importance and therefore should be regarded as viable learning outcomes (Stainback and Stainback, 1992; York et al., 1988).

Change the Environmental Conditions

Circumstances in the learning environment can affect any student's ability to acquire information. When lessons are designed with students in mind who have sensory impairments, physical handicaps, information-processing difficulties, or alternative-communication methods, modifications in environmental conditions may be particularly warranted. Environmental conditions refer to such things as lighting, noise level, visual and auditory input, physical arrangement of the room or equipment, and accessibility of materials.

A student who requires adaptive materials or devices may need additional space for an expanded work area. Placing the student's desk next to a large work table, or providing a bookshelf that is easily accessible provides a simple accommodation. A student who has difficulty sitting for any period of time may be equipped with more than one desk in the room, allowing the child to move to different locations in the room when needed without disrupting the class. Other environmental adaptations may include space for maneuvering a wheelchair or a private area for a student to stretch out on the floor when a break from sitting in a wheelchair is required. Alternative locations for group work may also be appropriate. Using space in the hallway, library, or outdoors may enhance the functioning of the student with disabilities by reducing distractions. These alternative spaces may be considered as long as their use does not unduly segregate the student with disabilities. Occasionally, changes in the social climate or social rules of the classroom are needed to accommodate a student with disabilities. This might involve allowing a higher noise level in the room for a student who occasionally makes loud vocalizations or allowing partners to read to one another when other students are expected to read silently.

Change the Instructional Materials

Teachers use an assortment of materials for instruction, including standard-curriculum texts, magazines, newspapers, trade books, filmstrips, movies, manipulatives, games, art supplies, computers, and objects used in daily life (Callahan and Clark, 1988; Ferguson and Jeanchild, 1992). Students with disabilities may benefit from using the same materials as other students in class, require slight variations, or need alternative materials. Materials may be changed or created to be more manipulable, concrete, tangible, simplified, and matched to the student's learning style or comprehension level.

In a high school contemporary affairs class, a syndicated news magazine is used as the primary text. To accommodate a student with disabilities who is unable to read, the class materials were modified in two ways. Classmates without disabilities were enlisted to read selected articles, then record themselves on audio tape while paraphrasing the content. In addition, the student with disabilities was asked to videotape three airings of news each week. These film clips were shown and discussed in class. Both of these adaptations matched the student's individual learning style without being stigmatizing and illustrated the reciprocal contributions of students with and without disabilities.

Change the Level or Type of Personal Assistance

In the classroom, the teacher provides direct instruction, facilitates learning among students, or monitors behavior and performance. Spontaneous assistance is provided when requested by the student, needed by the student to perform correctly, or required to maintain classroom control. Many students with disabilities need higher levels of assistance or intervention than are provided to typical students. The need for assistance may range from periodic spot checks to close, continuous supervision. Assistance may vary from day to day or be required at predictable times. Providing prompts, verbal cues, gestures, or physical assistance can support the student's participation on a temporary or ongoing basis.

Personal assistance can be provided by a variety of individuals in the school environment, including peers, cross-age tutors (i.e., coaching from an older student), the general educator, special educator, related service personnel, classroom volunteers, or instructional assistants (i.e., paraprofessionals, teacher aides). To facilitate inclusion and independence, an underlying goal should be to reduce the need for paid or specialized assistance over time. Consequently, it is preferable that natural supports (supports that are provided by the teacher and peers) be employed to the greatest extent possible.

Regular prompts, cues, and even physical assistance that do not interfere with the instruction or the learning of others in the classroom can often be incorporated as inconspicuous elements of the teaching sequence. The intervention or assistance from someone "outside" of the classroom structure can sometimes cause the student to be stigmatized and reduce spontaneous interactions from peers in the environment. Therefore, assignment of a full-time assistant should be assessed cautiously and arranged only when absolutely necessary.

Create an Alternative Activity

Establishing an alternative activity is a curricular adaptation that can be employed when changes in the previous seven instructional conditions cannot be made. An alternative activity is most often activity-based or experiential in nature and in some instances may be community-based. By design, the activity should include the student with disabilities and a partner or small group of nondisabled peers.

Learning centers that offer alternatives to the typical curriculum can be established in elementary and middle school grades within the classroom so that more than one activity can occur in the same environment. For example, when a fifth grade class is taking a reading test during language arts, Jessie, a student with disabilities, and a small group of classmates who have mastered the test material, work on a classroom newsletter. Jessie uses a tape player to record his classmates' ideas for a news article and plays back the tape a paragraph at a time, while a classmate uses a computer to transcribe the information.

At the high school level, alternative work areas might be established in the classroom, commons, or library. In secondary subject areas, research teams can be formed to investigate student's interests. As students generate questions related to the course topics they are encouraged to write their ideas in a shared notebook. When the opportunity arises, a small research team of two or three students, including the student with disabilities, can investigate the topic using the school or public library. The written and multimedia information gathered is then utilized or presented in class the following day. Student-directed learning is fostered for the typical class members as they are allowed to explore their own interests. When this type of alternative activity was implemented in a local high school, a student with severe disabilities was an integral part of the team, obtaining slides and magazine articles that reinforced the content area. She participated in the presentation by using an adaptive switch to activate the slide projector.

Optimally, alternative activities should be: (a) similar or related to the curricular content of other students in the class (e.g., language arts, science, health, etc.); (b) meaningful for all of the students involved; and (c) arranged so that additional supervision from an adult is not necessarily required. Merely arranging one-to-one instruction with an instructional assistant in the same room does not constitute an alternative activity. By definition, the arrangement must include peers without disabilities.

There are many ways to categorize and conceptualize curricular adaptations. The eight curricular adaptations that have been discussed provide a framework from which to make decisions. For any given activity a student with disabilities may require no modifications at all or a combination of several adaptations. The process to select and utilize appropriate adaptations can be operationalized as an eight-component decision-making model. This eight-component model summarized in Table 1 is framed by a series of questions to facilitate communication between general and special educators *before* instructional decisions have been made for the entire class. The adaptation strategies move from the least intrusive means of modification to more intrusive systems. Educators are guided to consider changes in the structure of instruction, demands and evaluation criteria of the task, learning environment, the way the task is done, changes in the student's support structure, and, finally, the use of alternative activities. To facilitate and streamline communication between team members a Curricular Adaptation Planning form is offered in Table 2.

A commitment to the principles of inclusion brings with it new roles for educators and new expectations for teaching practices. Well-conceived curricular adaptations can maximize abilities and minimize discrepancies in performance between students. Adaptations should promote opportunities for face to face interactions with peers, increase the student's opportunities to be an initiator and active participant, and reduce the level of abstraction of information while making activities more concrete and meaningful to the student's current and future life.

Selecting the right adaptations is still an imprecise "science." There are no definitive sources to say "If you experience this type of disability, then you need this precise adaptation." Good adaptations come from the thoughtful, collective observations and foresight of parents, peers, and professionals. Albert Einstein was quoted as saying, "Imagination is more important than knowledge." This statement rings true when developing adaptations. Team members must allow themselves to think and

Table 1. Eight-Component Decision-Making Model for Designing Curricular Adaptations

Examine the Structure of the Instruction

1. Can the student actively participate with the lesson as is? Will the same essential outcome be achieved?
2. Can the student's participation be increased by arranging the lesson in:
   - Cooperative groups?
   - Small groups?
   - Partner learning?
   - Peer tutors or cross-age tutors?
3. Can the student's participation be increased by changing the lesson format?
   - Activity-based lessons, games, simulations, role-plays
   - Experiential lessons
4. Can the student's participation and understanding be increased by changing the delivery of instruction or teaching style?

Change the Demands of the Task

5. Will the student need adapted curricular goals?
   - Adjust performance standards
   - Adjust pacing
   - Same content but less complex
   - Similar content with functional/direct applications
   - Adjust the evaluation system (grading)
   - Adjust management techniques

Examine the Learning Environment

6. Can changes be made in the classroom environment or lesson location that will facilitate participation?
   - Environmental/physical
   - Social
   - Lesson location

Change the Way the Task is Done

7. Will different materials be needed to ensure participation?
   - Same content but variation in size, number, format
   - Additional or different materials/devices

Change the Support Structure

8. Will personal assistance be needed to ensure participation?
   - From peers or general education instructor?

Arrange Alternative Activities that Foster Participation and Interaction

9. Will a different activity need to be designed and offered for the student *and* a small group of peers?
   - In the classroom
   - In other general education environments
   - In community-based environments

Table 2. Curricular Adaptation Planning Form

GENERAL INSTRUCTIONAL PLAN Date: _____	DO CHANGES NEED TO BE MADE IN:		
Content Area/Subject: Instructor: Estimated Time: Activity:	Instructional Arrangement?	Lesson Format?	Delivery of Instruction Teaching Style?
Materials:	Curricular Goals (Academic & Social)?	Social/Physical Environmental Conditions or Lesson Location?	Instructional Materials?
	Level of Personal Assistance?	An Alternative Activity or Any Other Adaptations?	

create beyond the confines of traditional teaching conventions . . . when this happens the result is beneficial for all learners.

REFERENCES

Baumgart D, Brown L, Pumpian I, Nisbet J, Ford A, Sweet M, Messina R, Schroeder J (1982): Principle of partial participation and individualized adaptations in educational programs for severely handicapped students. J Persons Severe Handicaps 7:17–43.

Biklen D (1985): "Achieving the Complete School: Effective Strategies for Mainstreaming." New York: Teachers College Press.

Bloom BS (1956): "Taxonomy of Educational Objectives: Handbook I. Cognitive Domain." New York: McCay.

Callahan J, Clark L (1988): "Teaching in the Middle and Secondary Schools: Planning for Competence" (3rd ed.). New York: MacMillan.

Ferguson D, Baumgart D (1991): "Partial Participation Revisited." (Available from Schools Projects Specialized Training Program, University of Oregon, Eugene, Oregon 97403.)

Ferguson D, Jeanchild L (1992): It's not a matter of method: Thinking about how to implement curricular decisions. In Stainback S, Stainback B (eds.): "Curriculum Considerations in Inclusive Classrooms: Facilitating Learning for All Students," pp. 159–174. Baltimore: Brookes.

Forest M (1987): "More education/integration: A further collection of readings on the integration of children with mental handicaps into regular school systems." Downsview, Ontario: G. Allan Roeher Institute.

Giangreco M, Putnam J (1991): Supporting the education of students with severe disabilities in regular education environments. In Meyer L, Peck C, Brown L (eds.): "Critical Issues in the Lives of People with Severe Disabilities," pp. 245–270. Baltimore: Brookes.

Johnson D, Johnson R (19860: Mainstreaming and cooperative learning strategies. Excep Child 52:553–561.

Nisbet J, Sweet M, Ford A, Shiraga B, Udvari A, York J, Messina R, Schroeder J (1983): Utilizing adaptive devices with severely handicapped students. In Brown L, Ford A, Nisbet J, Sweet M, Shiraga B, York J, Loomis R, VanDeventer P (eds.): "Educational Programs for Severely Handicapped Students," Vol. XIII, pp. 101–145. Madison, WI: Madison Metropolitan School District.

Sharon & Sharon (1976): "Small Group Teaching." Englewood Cliffs, NJ: Educational Technology Publications.

Stainback S, Stainback W (1992): "Curriculum Considerations in Inclusive Classrooms: Facilitating Learning for All Students." Baltimore: Brookes.

Stainback W, Stainback S, Moravec J (1992): Using curriculum to build inclusive classrooms. In Stainback S, Stainback B (eds.): "Curriculum considerations in Inclusive Classrooms: Facilitating Learning for All Students," pp. 64–84. Baltimore: Brookes.

Vandercook T, York J (1990): A team approach to program development and support. In Stainback W, Stainback S (eds.): "Support Networks for Inclusive Schooling: Interdependent Integrated Education." Baltimore: Brookes.

York J, Vandercook T, Caughey E, Heise-Neff C (1988): Regular class integration: Beyond socialization. In York J, Vandercook T, Macdonald C, Wolff S (eds.): "Strategies for Full Inclusion," pp. 117–120. Minneapolis: Institute on Community Integration, University of Minnesota.

The Basis of Reading Skill in Young Adults with Down Syndrome

Anne E. Fowler, Brian J. Doherty, and Laura Boynton

Not long ago, reading skill was a rare and celebrated achievement among persons with Down syndrome. The diary written by Nigel Hunt (Hunt, 1966) was an exception to the more general rule that children with Down syndrome do not learn to read and write, and therefore should not be taught. For the past 20 years, however, there have been dramatic changes in the lives of people with Down syndrome that could make an important difference in reading outcome. There is better medical treatment, earlier and more professional language intervention, and greater access to systematic reading instruction in and out of school. Perhaps most importantly, the expectations of parents, teachers, society, and the young people themselves have changed dramatically. Consistent with these changes, it is now estimated that a substantial proportion (40%) of adolescents with Down syndrome acquire at least some reading skill; and there is a small but growing pool of documented success stories (see Buckley, 1985, for an extensive review). In the study presented here, we seek first to document the incidence of reading under these more nearly optimal conditions. We then go on to explore just what factors contribute to reading success. In particular, we investigate the claim that successful readers with Down syndrome somehow bypass the usual, phonological, route to reading.

We begin with the hypothesis that successful readers with Down syndrome should meet the same prerequisites for reading that have been established in extensive research involving children without Down syndrome. According to that research, children who more readily learn to read are not necessarily more intelligent than less-skilled readers of the same age (or even older); they do, however, show specific strengths in phonological awareness, in verbal short-term memory, and in the accuracy and speed of word retrieval. By phonological awareness, I refer to the oral language ability to consciously attend to the sound structure of the language without regard to meaning. Phonological awareness is required to detect rhyme (e.g., that *coat* goes with *goat,* but not with *bat*), to segment words into their phonemic segments (e.g., *fun* into ffff-uuuu-nnnn), or to categorize words on the basis of shared segments (e.g., *c*at and *c*ough, ri*b* and cu*b*). In alphabetic languages, measures of phonological awareness correlate with reading success from kindergarten to adulthood, and serve as better kindergarten predictors of later reading success than almost any other measure (for a review, see Liberman et al., 1989). For children who lack phonological awareness, training programs that draw explicit attention to the internal structure of the word have significantly improved the prognosis for reading success. Although it is clear that reading instruction itself enhances phonological awareness (e.g., Morais et al., 1979), most research suggests that phoneme awareness is necessarily involved in achieving fully productive reading skill (Fowler, 1991). Phoneme awareness is most directly linked to decoding, the ability to apply letter–sound correspondences to sound out novel or unfamiliar words. Decoding skill is, in turn, an important component of word recognition, which refers to the ability to identify previously encountered, highly familiar real words (e.g., Gough and Walsh, 1991). Finally, although word recognition does not guarantee reading comprehension, it is, of course, an important component. Reading comprehension is a product of both decoding and listening comprehension; both must be in place for text to be understood (Gough and Tunmer, 1986).

Verbal short-term memory and facility with word retrieval are additional factors that co-vary with reading skill, although generally with less predictive power than phonological awareness. Verbal short-term memory refers to the ability to encode orally (or visually) presented material in a phonological store such that the material can be reproduced in exactly the same order that it was presented. A classic measure of phonological (or verbal short-term) memory is the digit span included on many intelligence tests. Word retrieval refers to the ability to rapidly and accurately retrieve the correct label when confronted with pictures of objects. Poor readers tend to respond more slowly and to make more errors (e.g., tornad*o* for volcan*o*). When assessed prior to reading instruction, both verbal short-term memory and word retrieval measures predict later reading skill (see Brady, 1991; Wolf, 1991, for an overview of these areas).

If phonological awareness is necessarily acquired prior to (or concomitant with) successful reading, successful readers with Down syndrome should be phonologically aware. Similarly, one should also expect that verbal short-term memory and word retrieval abilities would be important factors in reading success. Some investigators, however, argue that people with Down syndrome learn to read in a different way than most normal children. For example, Buckley (1985) suggests that phonological processes may not be relevant for the development of reading ability in those with Down syndrome because they learn to read words "as if they were an idiographic or picture language and had no print-to-sound relationships" (p. 327). As evidence, she points out that readers of her acquaintance never made phonological errors (e.g., *cat* instead of *car*), but did make semantic confusions (*go to bed* for *sleep*). She interprets these errors to suggest that children with Down syndrome, unlike typically developing children, go directly from the visual form to meaning. These findings, she suggests, cast doubt on the claim that "phonics" (i.e., explicit instruction in decoding) is essential to learning reading.

Contrary to common beliefs that learning phonics is essential for successful reading, it seems that it is a useful trick, i.e., given that you know the rules for converting print to sounds, you can work out how to pronounce new unfamiliar words and, conversely, you can work out how to spell words, but that this coding system is not used for normal reading. The reading performance of these young children shows that mastering phonics is not necessary for reading" (p. 327).

Because reading skill commonly exceeded oral language skill in the children she studied, Buckley suggests that learning to read is a completely different process for the child with Down syndrome compared to normal children, who have developed language abilities to aid in their acquisition of reading skills.

Whereas Buckley's subjects could recognize hundreds of words without evidence of productive decoding skills, this was not the case for a sample of 10 Italian-speaking schoolchildren with Down syndrome studied by Cossu et al. (1993). In their group, well-developed word recognition abilities were accompanied by correspondingly well-developed decoding skill, although in the context of poor reading and listening comprehension. However, they argue that proficient decoding skills had been acquired in the complete absence of phoneme awareness. To support this argument, they matched the readers with Down syndrome to a control group of normal children reading at the same level (mean age = 7.3 years) and compared the two groups on several different measures of phoneme awareness (segmentation, deletion, oral spelling, and synthesis). The children with Down syndrome performed consistently worse on all measures. On the basis of these results, it was argued that phoneme awareness is not a necessary precondition for, or even a consequence of, acquiring productive decoding skills.

Although there is disagreement about whether successful readers with Down syndrome will possess the prerequisites to reading that have been identified in normal children, there is more consensus regarding the need for instruction. It is the case that some very young precocious readers (without Down syndrome) come to read after only minimal exposure to the written language. Such children are characterized by highly developed memory skills. For example, this is the case for hyperlexic children studied by Healy (1982). However, because children with Down syndrome are typically characterized as having especially poor memory abilities (see Fowler, this volume), one would not expect to find naturally occurring precocity in this sample. And, in fact, none is found. In discussing case studies of superior reading skill among young people with Down syndrome, Buckley (1985) points out that the only "common factor . . . is that all the children received intensive structured teaching" (p. 317). Cossu et al. did not focus on instruction, but they note that all of their subjects had received standard formal reading instruction. Even those children reviewed by Buckley who had acquired only word recognition skills had participated in intervention programs focussed on reading. We expect, therefore, that instruction is a significant factor in reading success among persons with Down syndrome. We remain intrigued, however, by the large variability among people with Down syndrome in how much intensive teaching is required to achieve that success and in how much skill is ultimately achieved, even under optimal conditions. This variability has been noted by both Buckley (1985) and by Cossu et al. (1993).

In a study summarized here (Fowler et al., in progress), we first sought to document levels of reading skill in a cohort of young adults who have grown up in more improved conditions for reading success. In this study we explored the relationship between reading and phonological skill within our sample, rather than making comparisons across groups. As noted earlier, we were unable to directly assess the significance of instructional strategies for reading success due to the wide variety of programs experienced over a 20-year lifetime and the inevitable failure to recall the details of even a small portion of these in hindsight. We have, however, sought to further refine, on the basis of our data, what it is instructional programs should incorporate.

METHOD

Subjects

The study included 33 young adults with Down syndrome, full trisomy-21, between 17 and 25 years old, recruited from private and public schools, and through parent groups, in the Northeastern United States. None presented untreated hearing problems and most reported no history of hearing difficulty; all were monolingual speakers of English. Because we made a special appeal for adults who could read, the results of this study should be interpreted as reflecting the upper end of a distribution of persons affected with Down syndrome.

Each young adult completed 4 hours of individual testing, conducted either at our clinic at Bryn Mawr College, in their home, or at their school. Individuals were assessed on reading, on general ability, and on phonological skill, including measures of phonological awareness, verbal short-term memory, and word retrieval. Although multiple measures were taken in order to improve reliability and to avoid concluding too much from a single, potentially inappropriate task, only one measure for each area of function is presented here for the sake of brevity. (Full details are provided in Doherty, 1993, where it is shown that the measures presented here correlate well with other similar measures.)

Reading Measures

Woodcock Reading Mastery Tests—Revised (WRMT-R). All participants were given the Word Identification, Word Attack, and Passage Comprehension subtests of the WRMT-R (Woodcock, 1987). The WRMT-R is a widely used and highly reliable reading measure with age and grade norms from 5 years of age to adulthood. The Word Identification subtest consists of a series of real words (e.g., *is, sleep, gasoline,* and *spectacular*) to be read aloud; the Word Attack measure includes nonsense words that must be decoded using knowledge of letter–sound correspondences (e.g., *dee, plip, adjex,* and *monglustamer*). The Passage Comprehension measure includes sentences or a short paragraph missing a word or phrase; the participant must select from several (written) choices how best to complete the sentence.

General Cognitive Measures

Peabody Picture Vocabulary Test—Revised (PPVT-R). The PPVT-R is a widely used measure of receptive vocabulary with norms for persons from 2–18 years of age; it provides an age equivalent and a standard score, which correlates roughly with verbal IQ measures (Dunn & Dunn, 1981). In this test, the person points to which of four pictures best depicts a spoken word.

Kaufman Assessment Battery for Children—Mental Processing Composite (K-ABC). The K-ABC (Kaufman and Kaufman, 1983) is an individually administered instrument designed to assess mental processing (as opposed to acquired knowledge) in children between 2.5 and 12.5 years of age. We relied on age equivalent scores, to allow for meaningful comparisons across subtests. (Full details on modifications to the K-ABC testing and scoring procedure are presented in Doherty, 1993.)

Phonological Measures

Phoneme Awareness. To assess phoneme awareness, we relied on the Auditory Analysis Test (Rosner and Simon, 1971), for which participants are asked to repeat a whole word (e.g., "belt") and then to say only a portion of it—"Now can you say belt without the t?" Answer: bel(l). The test consists of 40 items, preceded by two practice items. The test is highly reliable (Yopp, 1988) and correlates with reading from kindergarten to adulthood. It yields a raw score and an approximate grade equivalent up to grade 6.

Verbal Memory Spans. To obtain verbal memory spans, we expanded the Number Recall subtest of the K-ABC, in which participants listen to a string of two or more digits and repeat them back in the same order. In our augmented version, participants had five opportunities to repeat strings at each length, after some practice with feedback. Subjects were given credit for a span of x when they could accurately reproduce x digits in the correct order in three out of five trials.

Word Retrieval. In the Boston Naming Test (Kaplan et al., 1983), originally developed for use with aphasic individuals, participants are presented with a line drawing and asked to provide, as quickly as possible, the name for the item depicted (e.g., *bed, toothbrush, harmonica,* and *abacus*). The number correct was compared to approximately age equivalents available in Guilford and Nawojczyk (1988).

Other Measures

Additional measures presented to young adults with Down syndrome were expected to be associated with reading, but not after controlling for general ability.

Visual Memory Span. The first of these was the Corsi Block Test, a nonverbal measure of sequential memory designed by Milner (1971) and often used as a measure of right-brain function in neuropsychological research. Variation in nonverbal visual memory has not proven to be a significant correlate of reading ability in normal IQ schoolchildren (e.g., Gould and Glencross, 1990; Rapala and Brady,

1990). In the Corsi Block test, the individual watches the examiner touch a sequence of randomly scattered identical blocks and then attempts to reproduce the same sequence. Calculation of a span paralleled procedures for verbal short-term memory.

Test of Auditory Comprehension of Language—Revised (TACL-R). The TACL-R (Carrow-Woolfolk, 1985) is a picture-pointing test standardized on children from 2–12 years. The test includes three sections, emphasizing individual lexical knowledge, grammatical morphology, and syntactic structures; we present the total age-equivalent score across all sections. This measure was included as a measure of oral language comprehension, predicted to be an important factor in reading comprehension, but not in decoding.

K-ABC Arithmetic. This subtest of the K-ABC Achievement Scales samples a student's knowledge of counting, ordering, terminology, and basic computation (addition, subtraction, multiplication, division). All questions are presented orally, and include a number of word problems. The task is designed to be appropriate for children 2.5–12 years. Although not as in-depth a measure as our extensive reading battery, it was a developmentally appropriate measure for this sample. We presented it to explore how school-based achievement measures would differ.

RESULTS

Reading Measures

Young adults with Down syndrome ranged widely in their reading skill, from kindergarten to 12th grade levels. They were classified into "reader groups" on the basis of their decoding scores on the Word Attack measure. Although every individual could recognize at least a few familiar words, those who could decode no more than two pseudowords were classified as "novice readers." Those who could decode 3–10 pseudowords had skills that were clearly "emerging" (first grade level), and those who could decode 11–29 pseudowords (second to fourth grade level) were considered to be "developing." Finally, those who could read at or above the 5th grade level (>29 pseudowords) qualified as "skilled" or productive decoders.

As can be seen in Table 1, these classifications based on decoding predicted performance on both Word Identification ($F(3,29) = 67.13$, $p < .0001$) and Passage Comprehension ($F(3,29) = 36.41$). Although the overall mean scores for Word Attack and Word Identification were close, the advantage for Word Identification was significant ($F(1,29) = 5.02$, $p < .05$). Of particular interest was a significant group-by-test interaction ($F(3,29) = 16.25$, $p < .0001$): whereas the less-skilled decoders showed a clear advantage for Word Identification, this pattern was reversed for the most skilled group.

As is often the case for persons with general cognitive impairment, reading comprehension lagged significantly behind single-word identification ($F(1,29) = 67.56$, $p < .0001$). This disparity became even more pronounced as decoding skill improved, as indicated by the significant task × reader group interaction ($F(3,29) = 10.76$, $p < .001$). Although decoding is clearly necessary for Passage Comprehension, it is not sufficient.

Table 1. Mean Age Equivalent Scores on Reading and Cognitive Measures for Four Groups of Adult Readers with Down Syndrome

Reader Group	n	Reading Measures			Cognitive Measures			
		Word Attack	Word Identification	Comprehension	PPVT-R	TACL-R	K-ABC	Arithmetic
Novice	12	5.7	6.7	5.6	6.1	5.1	5.0	5.7
Emerging	10	6.6	8.1	7.1	8.1	6.1	6.3	6.5
Developing	6	8.0	9.3	7.7	9.3	6.4	6.2	7.0
Skilled	5	16.0	12.7	8.4	11.1	7.8	7.1	9.0
Overall mean	33	7.9	8.5	6.9	8.1	6.1	5.9	6.7
(Standard deviation)		(3.8)	(2.3)	(1.3)	(2.3)	(1.4)	(1.2)	(1.4)

Association between Reading and Cognitive Measures

It can be observed by looking at Table 1 that reader group significantly predicts variation in vocabulary [PPVT-R, $F(3,29) = 12.74$, $p < .0001$], receptive language ability [TACL-R, $F(3,20) = 6.03$, $p < .01$], general cognitive ability [K-ABC, $F(3,29) = 7.16$, $p < .001$], and arithmetic achievement ($F(3,29) = 14.88$, $p < .0001$). It is especially interesting to observe the close correspondence in age equivalent scores for the Word Identification and the PPVT-R (both single-word measures) and for Passage Comprehension and the TACL-R (both sentence-level measures). Whereas decoding skill may, and in some individuals does, exceed either language comprehension measure, reading comprehension does not (cf. Gough and Tunmer, 1986, for the normal case). On the other hand, despite this apparent link between reading and acquired verbal intelligence, it is clear that our general ability measure (K-ABC) underestimates ultimate reading levels; this is consistent with findings from other studies of successful readers with Down syndrome and demands some explanation.

Although arithmetic function was not a major focus in our study, the link between arithmetic and reading is obvious. Indeed, looking at the adults on an individual basis, we observed some cases where reading exceeded arithmetic, but no cases of the opposite. The association may, of course, be exaggerated by the heavy reliance on language in the arithmetic measure.

Association between Reading and Phonological Skill

Whereas the overall mean age equivalent for Word Attack and Word Identification was 7.9 and 8.5 years respectively, participants were functioning at or below the 6-year-old level on the various phonological measures presented (see Table 2). At first blush, these results seem to support the claim that phonological factors are not relevant to reading acquisition in Down syndrome. These low scores, however, mask considerable variability in performance. In fact, when variation on the phonological measures was compared to variation in the reading measures, the correlations were highly significant, as evident in the third column. Most importantly, when we statistically controlled for the already high association between general ability and reading, the association between phonology and reading remained strong. For example, performance on number recall accounted for approximately 39% of the variance in decoding, and 38% of the variance in word recognition, over that accounted for by a general cognitive ability composite made up of the K-ABC and the PPVT-R. Similarly, performance on phoneme awareness accounted for 36% of the variance in word recognition, and 49% of the variation in decoding skill, after accounting for the variance accounted for by general cognitive factors. This means that phonological factors play an important role in predicting and explaining variation in reading skill beyond what can be attributed to general ability. Even the word retrieval measure explains variation in reading not explained by general cognitive factors; the fact that the association is somewhat smaller is consistent with findings from the general population.

The one unexpected result was the strong association between visual memory and

Table 2. Performance on Selected Phonological and Memory Measures

Phonological Measure	Raw Score Mean (Standard deviation)	Mean Age Equivalent (years)	Correlation with Decoding/Recognition	Partial Correlation with Decoding/Recognition
Phoneme awareness (AAT)	10.4 (10.4)	6.0	0.78*/0.72*	0.72[†]/0.60[†]
Verbal Span (K-ABC)	3.2 (0.76)	5.0	0.73*/0.72*	0.63[†]/0.62[†]
Visual Span (Corsi)	3.5 (0.90)	est. 6.4	0.65*/0.59*	0.50[†]/0.40[†]
Lexical Access (BNT)	28.5 (9.4)	est. 5.5–6	0.75*/0.77*	0.46[†]/0.49[†]

*$p < .001$.
[†]$p < .01$

reading evident from Table 2, suggesting that visual memory also explains reading variation not explained by general cognition. Indeed, even when verbal span was entered first together with general cognition, visual span explained an additional 8% of the variance in reading. At the same time, when visual span was entered together with general cognition; verbal span explained a unique 17% of the variance. This suggests that visual and verbal memory are both important, but distinct, contributors to reading skill in this group of young adults with Down syndrome. It does remain to be determined, however, just how visual memory plays a role.

A high correlation alone does not rule out the possibility, put forth by Cossu et al. (1993) that some persons acquire productive decoding skills without meeting the hypothesized phonological prerequisites. To explore this question more directly, we examined the actual scatterplot of how decoding skill maps onto phoneme awareness. The results, depicted in Fig. 1, indicate that no person in our study achieved decoding skills beyond the first grade level without answering at least 10 items correctly on our phoneme awareness measure, a feat that cannot be achieved by chance alone. More-

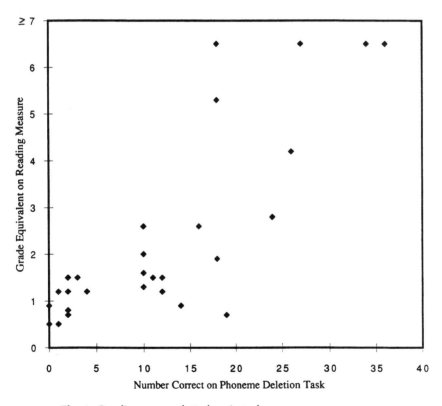

Fig. 1. Reading scores plotted against phoneme awareness scores.

over, no one achieved beyond the third grade decoding level without responding correctly to at least half of the phoneme awareness items. Although there are certainly cases of phoneme awareness that are not accompanied by reading skill, the opposite does not hold, as evidenced by the blank space in the upper left portion of the scatterplot. This result is consistent with the view that phoneme awareness is necessary but not sufficient for decoding success. In this group of English-speaking young adults, as in many groups of schoolchildren without Down syndrome, decoding skill does not develop in the complete absence of phoneme awareness.

As can be seen in Fig. 2, a surprisingly similar story can be told about verbal short-term memory. The plot indicates that all young adults with decoding skills at or above a grade level of 1.3 achieved a digit span of at least 3.0; and all six individuals decoding above the fourth grade level achieved a digit span of at least 4.0. As with phoneme awareness, it would appear that a minimum digit span is not sufficient for decoding skill (see data points in lower right), but is necessary (as evident in the lack of data points in the upper left).

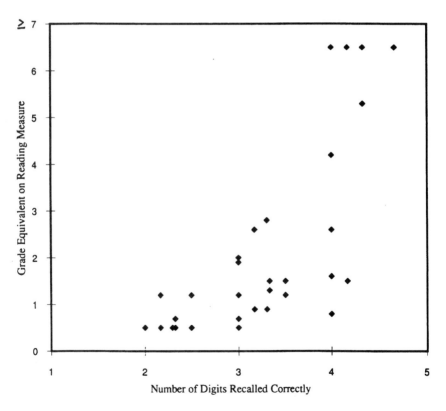

Fig. 2. Reading scores plotted against digit span measure.

DISCUSSION

In the study presented, young adults with Down syndrome varied greatly in reading skill, with scores ranging from kindergarten to adult levels. Although reading scores were linked with general levels of intellectual function, our results suggest that phonological skill explains additional variance that cannot be wholly explained by general ability. Below, we try to relate our findings to the questions raised earlier.

First, like Buckley, we find that even in today's more supportive educational climate, most persons with Down syndrome have not progressed beyond the early stages of reading. These early stages may, in any group, be achieved almost wholly via sight-word recognition, and it is clear that our less skilled readers relied almost exclusively on this strategy. However, in this group, as in any group, the lack of decoding skill severely restricts the reader's sight-word vocabulary.

The fact that many adults do not advance beyond the early stages of reading does not mean that different skills are required for reading success in persons with Down syndrome, only that they have not yet acquired the skills (or received the appropriate instruction) necessary to move forward. In fact, the third of our subjects who had made substantial progress in mastering orthographic decoding strategies were characterized by better-developed phonological skill. Although, as Cossu et al. (1993) found, productive decoders possessed less phoneme awareness than would be expected on the basis of grade-level norms, it was not the case that they possessed no phoneme awareness at all. Looking within the sample with Down syndrome, there was a direct correlation between phoneme awareness and decoding skill. These results suggest that young adults with Down syndrome can and do acquire productive decoding skills, and that their success depends on the same prerequisites implicated in any other group attempting to read. It is, in fact, promising that a little phoneme awareness goes such a long way. It should be acknowledged, too, that the fact that older people with Down syndrome possess so much less phoneme awareness than younger normal readers may have predictive implications: the younger normal readers stand a far better chance of rapidly becoming fully productive and automatic decoders.

In the present study, verbal short-term memory also proved to be a crucial component of reading success, even more so than in normally intelligent populations who vary in reading success. It may be that in most school-aged children, the minimal level of verbal short-term memory has already been met, and further variation does not have nearly as great an effect. Consistent with this interpretation, it can be seen in Fig. 2 that once the necessary prerequisite for decoding is met (here estimated at a digit span of 4.0), there is no longer any correlation with reading: those individuals with a digit span of 4.0 display the full range of reading skill evident in the sample. A higher span does not guarantee success, but a lower span apparently precludes it.

Although our evidence regarding instruction is necessarily limited, there are many reasons to believe that instruction was also a crucial component of the success achieved by our most skilled readers. Instruction could, for example, account for the variability among those young adults obtaining the highest digit span. Just as there is substantial evidence for the role of instruction in normally intelligent children with weak phonological skills, it would follow that the same kind of instruction would be equally, if not more, important for persons with Down syndrome. The most effective instruction focusses attention on the internal structure of the syllable (phonemes) before or simultaneous with the introduction of letters, which merely represent these phonemes (e.g., Bradley and Bryant, 1983; Lundberg et al., 1988; Ball and Blachman, 1990; see Adams, 1990; or Clark, 1988, for a review). Given the important association between phoneme awareness and reading in our group, the same instruction should prove helpful here as well. It is important, from a developmental perspective, to note that phoneme awareness training programs have been successful at the kindergarten level, yet retain their utility into adulthood; the programs can vary significantly without losing their effectiveness. Consistent with this, we were interested to learn that several of our most successful readers had spent several years beyond the preschool level in Montessori schools; the Montessori program does focus on the structural analysis of the syllable (Wilkinson, 1990).

The call for explicit and systematic instruction in phoneme awareness and decoding does not rule out the utility of other, additional, forms of instruction. Clearly, many factors contribute to reading success in this population. For example, Buckley (1985) focusses her attention on sight-word vocabulary in very young children (3–5 years of age). This could readily be combined with phonics instruction once a small repertoire of sight words is established. Sight-word training may, for example, be especially useful for helping children learn letter sound correspondences.

Finally, we wish to point out that our results provide no evidence that reading could not be introduced in adolescence and beyond; it may in fact be the optimal time. We observed considerable growth in reading skill in one young man first observed at 19 and later seen at 21 years of age; his family had recently hired a tutor. Although there is evidence from typical and atypical populations that oral language is most readily acquired in the first decade of life, reading differs importantly from speech and can be acquired at any time. If we are correct that minimal prerequisites in phonological memory must be achieved in order to experience real success in reading, it may be that many schools are giving up on reading instruction at just the time when it might actually prove effective.

ACKNOWLEDGMENTS

This research presented here was done in collaboration with Brian J. Doherty and Laura S. Boynton. This research was supported by a Science Scholar Award provided by the National Down Syndrome Society, by a Faculty Grant Award from Bryn Mawr College, and by an NICHD Program Project Grant to Haskins Laboratories (HD-01994). We are grateful for the unstinting involvement of families, schools, and parent organizations, and most especially for the dedication of the young adults who participated in our study. A very special thank you goes to Ceil Conner for all her efforts in recruiting participants and coordinating testing. The helpful comments of Donald Shankweiler on an earlier draft of this paper are much appreciated.

REFERENCES

Adams MJ (1990): "Beginning to Read: Thinking and Learning about Print." Cambridge, MA: MIT Press.

Ball E, Blachman B (1991): Does phoneme awareness training in kindergarten make a difference in early word recognition and developmental spelling? Read Res Quart 26:49–66.

Bradley L, Bryant P (1983): Categorizing sounds and learning to read—a causal connection. Nature 301:419–421.

Brady SA (1991): The role of working memory in reading disability. Brady SA, Shankweiler DP (eds.): "Phonological Processes in Literacy," pp. 129–151. Hillsdale, NJ: Erlbaum.

Buckley S (1985): Attaining basic educational skills: Reading, writing and number. In Lane D, Stratford B (eds.): "Current Approaches to Down's Syndrome." NY: Praeger.

Carrow-Woolfolk E (1985): "Test for auditory comprehension of language—Revised." Allen, TX: DLM.

Clark DB (1988): Dyslexia: Theory and Practice of Remedial Instruction. Parkton, MD: York Press.

Cossu G, Rossini F, Marshall JC (1993): When reading is acquired but phonemic awareness is not: A study of literacy in Down's syndrome. Cognition 46:129–138.

Doherty BJ (1993): "Relationships between Phonological Processes and Reading Ability in Young Adults with Down Syndrome." Unpublished masters thesis, Bryn Mawr College.

Dunn L, Dunn L (1981): "Peabody Picture Vocabulary Text—Revised." Circle Pines, MN: American Guidance Service.

Fowler AE (1991): How early phonological development might set the stage for phoneme awareness. In Brady SA, Shankweiler DP (eds.): Phonological Processes in Literacy, pp. 97–117. Hillsdale, NJ: Erlbaum.

Gould JH, Glencross DJ (1990): Do children with a specific reading disability have a general serial-ordering deficit? Neuropsychologia 28:271–278.

Gough PB, Tunmer WE (1986): Decoding, reading, and reading disability. Remed Spec Ed 7:6–10.

Gough PB, Walsh MA (1991): Chinese, Phoenicians, and the orthographic cipher of English. In Brady SA, Shankweiler D (eds.): Phonological Processes in Literacy, pp. 199–210. Hillsdale, NJ: Erlbaum.

Guilford AM, Nawojczyk DC (1988): Standardization of the Boston Naming Test at the kindergarten and elementary school levels. Language, Speech & Hearing Services in the Schools 19:395–400.

Healy JM (1982): The enigma of hyperlexia. Read Res Quart 17:319–338.

Hunt N (1966): "The world of Nigel Hunt." London: Darwen Finlayson.

Kaplan E, Goodglass H, Weintraub S (1983): "Boston Naming Test." Philadelphia: Lea and Febiger.

Kaufman AS, Kaufman N (1983): "Administration & Scoring Manual for the Kaufman Assessment Battery for Children." Circle Pines, MN: AGS.

Liberman IY, Shankweiler D, & Liberman AM (1989): The alphabetic principle and learning to read. In Shankweiler D, Liberman IY (eds.): "Phonology and Reading Disability," pp. 1–34. Ann Arbor, MI: University of Michigan Press.

Lundberg I, Frost J, Petersen O (1988): Effects of an extensive program for stimulating phonological awareness in preschool children. Read Res Quart 23:264–284.

Milner B (1971): Interhemispheric differences in the localization of psychological processes in man. Brit Med Bull 27:272–277.

Morais J, Cary L, Alegria J, Bertelson P (1979): Does awareness of speech as a sequence of phones arise spontaneously? Cognition 7:323–331.

Rapala MM, Brady S (1990): Reading ability and short-term memory: The role of phonological processing. Reading & Writing 2:1–25.

Rosner J, Simon DP (1971): The Auditory Analysis Test: An initial report. J Learn Dis 4:40–48.

Wilkinson K (1990): "A Study of the Emergence of Phonological Awareness As Influenced by Type of Nursery School Program, Parent Teaching, and Age." Unpublished doctoral dissertation, Bryn Mawr College.

Wolf M (1991): Naming speed and reading: The contribution of the cognitive neurosciences. Read Res Quart 26:123–141.

Woodcock R (1987): "Woodcock Reading Mastery Tests—Revised." Circle Pines, MN: American Guidance Service.

Yopp HK (1988): The validity and reliability of phonemic awareness tests. Read Res Quart 23:159–177.

Computer Learning in Early Elementary and Postsecondary Education

Joan Tanenhaus

EARLY ELEMENTARY EDUCATION

Computers can be a powerful tool in the education of young children with Down syndrome. They are highly motivational, allow children to be in control, build self-confidence and self-esteem, provide the much-needed opportunity for repeated success, and allow children to learn at their own rate, competing only with themselves.

The power of the computer lies in the selection of proper hardware and software, its effective use as a learning tool by creative parents, therapists, and teachers, and its integration with other learning.

For the very young, the computer is an interactive tool, with the child and teacher or parent working together. The child interacts directly with the computer and the adult is always there to guide, to direct, to explain, to model, to question, and, most of all, to enhance the experience. Computer learning must be integrated with other learning to be effective. Software should be selected so that language and vocabulary reflect learning in other educational settings. Always consider the motor and perceptual skills required to use the particular software. Print out pictures from the software programs and create off-computer activities such as lotto games and picture books. Select books from the library that deal with the same vocabulary and concepts that are in the software programs. Remember that the computer does not replace any other material or techniques; it just adds another tool for learning.

Children do not have to know how to use the keyboard in order to use the computer. Switches, Touch Windows, and expanded keyboards are some of the adaptive equipment that make it possible to introduce the computer before children are able to press keys or to recognize the letters of the alphabet. We are not teaching computer; we are using the computer to set a context for language and learning. With it, we can provide opportunities to improve visual perceptual skills, fine motor skills, and eye–hand coordination, provide readiness opportunities, improve reading, math, and academic skills while also giving the children control, practice, repeated success, self-paced learning and multisensory experiences. Voice output is a very significant

197

and helpful aspect of computer use for young children with Down syndrome. In the newest software, and especially the new CD-ROM technology, words are highlighted on screen as they are read aloud.

When trying to decide what kind of computer to purchase, always consider the software you will need and the adaptive equipment that might be necessary. For the very youngest children who will require switch use and basic cause-and-effect programs, the Apple II computer is the computer of choice. It can often be purchased second hand and therefore is very reasonably priced. It is easy to use and there is a wide selection of very simple software and extensive high-quality early education software available. It is a good choice for a beginning computer. The Macintosh also offers a wide selection of excellent software and can also run the Apple II software. It is able to be adapted, and has a built-in microphone that makes it easy to add voice to software programs. It is a newer computer and therefore will be able to take advantage of emergent technologies. However, it is the most expensive choice. The IBM compatibles have limited software for the very young child. Although they can be adapted for switch use, there are only a few very simple switch programs available. So although they are reasonably priced, they are limited in their application for very young children. Once the child is able to use the expanded or standard keyboard, they can be considered. IBM compatibles are more complex to use than either the Macintosh or the Apple II family.

In general, a color monitor is a must for young children. A printer is optional, but is valuable for creating off-computer activities that relate to software programs you are using. It also allows young children to print out pictures or text that they can then share with classroom teachers, classmates, peers, siblings, etc. If you can, consider one of the new color printers.

Once you have chosen a computer, it is important that you are careful about seating and positioning. Make sure that all wires are placed in the back of the computer and that no wires or cables are within reach of the child or on the floor in the walking or seating areas. Computer plugs should be placed into a surge protector. Don't place the computer near a direct source of heating or air conditioning.

Select a chair that is comfortable for your child. Make sure that the child's feet are on the floor and that the knee angle is approximately 90 degrees. If the table height is such that a higher chair is necessary, use a foot support of some kind so that the feet rest on it and the knee angle is maintained.

When your child is seated at the computer, make sure that the monitor is at eye level. Make sure that the screen is not too close and not too far away. Be especially careful if your child wears glasses or has a visual impairment. A CRT Terminal Valet allows you to clamp the computer monitor onto a platform that lets you raise and lower the monitor and also bring it closer or further away. Keyboard height should support a comfortable arm position.

Look at your child's posture as he or she is using the computer. If there is any unusual positioning (i.e., head tilted all the way up or down, arms elevated, etc.), you may need to reevaluate computer placement and seating or consult an occupational therapist.

Have adequate lighting. Make sure it is bright enough so that the screen can be seen easily. Be careful to place the light correctly so as to prevent glare on the computer screen. Look at the light during different hours of the day. Make sure there is good light on the keyboard or adaptive equipment. If you are using an external speaker, make sure that it is placed centrally, so that the source of sound is midline to the child.

Software has to be selected so that it is appropriate in concepts and vocabulary to the user's age and skill level. Look for clear graphics and, for older users, easy to read text. When educational programs are selected, make sure that rewards for correct responses are interesting and motivating. It is helpful if you can control as many options as possible, such as speed, sound, varied contents, amount of repetition, length of activity, etc. Look for an instructional manual that also includes suggestions for related activities. Always try to review the programs before purchase or try to locate a dealer that will allow returns if the software is not appropriate.

Some questions you can ask as you review software are:

1. Is the program easy to use and understand?
2. Does the user have the skills needed to use it?
3. Is it fun, interesting, and motivating?
4. Does the program provide a range of activities so that it can be used over a period of time and still be fun and interesting?
5. Does it have authoring capabilities (can we add our own words)?
6. If there is voice output, is the quality good?
7. Is the program free of stereotypes? Does it express positive values?
8. Does the program take advantage of the computer's unique abilities?

It is easy to see the educational value of programs that provide drill and practice for specific math, reading, and spelling skills. Become aware also of the educational and social benefits of some games and art and music programs. Think about how these software programs might help receptive and expressive language skills, eye–hand coordination, spatial concepts, turn talking, problem solving, sequencing, etc. Other areas to consider are development of independence and attention span and motivation.

Because of the relatively high cost of software, it is helpful to look for computer programs that offer special features. These include volumes that have options for controlling level of difficulty, speed of presentation, reinforcements, etc. Some programs come with data disks available so that additional activities can be added to the original program. Other programs have authoring capabilities in which the user's own vocabulary, spelling words, math problems, etc. can be entered for individualized work.

There are now specialized collections of public-domain software for education and language learning. These are free programs with only a minimal per-disk charge for duplicating, and they offer an excellent and inexpensive way to expand your computer software collection.

Very young children with Down syndrome can take advantage of the computer's capabilities before they are motorically, perceptually or cognitively able to use the standard keyboard. There are many alternate ways to provide computer access for them.

The easiest to use is a single switch that gets interfaced with the computer. Pressing and releasing the switch signals a response to the computer. There is no need to use the keyboard. With special software (much of which is public domain), cause-and-effect skills can be learned and/or reinforced. There are no right or wrong answers. Switches come in different sizes, shapes and colors—a simple plate switch can be 4 x 5" in bright red lucite.

The Touch Window is a touch sensitive screen that plugs into the Joystick port on the Apple II and IBM and into the ADB port of the Macintosh. It gets attached by Velcro to the computer monitor. The Touch Window allows young children to control the computer by touching the screen rather than using a keyboard. With the Apple II, you need special programs to use the Touch Window, but with the Macintosh, any program that works with a mouse works with the Touch Window.

Intellikeys is an expanded keyboard that lets you create keyboard overlays. These overlays are designed by the user to show only the specific keys needed by a particular program. For example, to run Stickybear Opposites, you could have two large arrow keys and a large space bar. When this overlay is placed on the Intellikeys, children press the symbol you have drawn to signal the computer. Intellikeys comes with 5 ready-made overlays and creating your own is very simple.

The Turbo Mouse is a commercially available version of the standard mouse. Instead of having to move the mouse all around, and hold it still while clicking, the Turbo Mouse stays in one spot. The children move the elevated Turbo ball with the palm or the fingers and then when the cursor is placed correctly, they can lift their hand from it and the cursor remains in the correct place. The click button can then be pressed.

These and other types of adaptive equipment allow children with special needs to join in and benefit from the new and unique applications of computers in the area of education and rehabilitation.

POSTSECONDARY EDUCATION

Computers can be an important learning tool throughout the lives of individuals with Down syndrome. Along with other work and life experiences, the computer has the potential to contribute to life-long learning in many ways including: specific subject areas such as social studies and science, general knowledge and vocabulary development, reading and math, motor skills, eye–hand coordination, memory strategies, and critical thinking skills. With the computer, learning can be in a recreational format that is fun while also helping to develop independence and self-esteem.

When you buy software, some will be able to be used independently immediately, and within the program there will be learning. You should also consider purchasing software that needs guided learning at first and then can be used independently after a while.

Guided Learning

We all have mentors who help us, especially computer users. These can be parents, siblings, teachers, or friends. Guided learning stretches the learning, because you can buy programs that need to be mastered before independent use. When doing guided learning, it is important to ask the right questions and give the right answers. For example, when the learner asks "What will happen if I press this," answer "Try it." When the learner asks "How do I get back to the other screen?" the person guiding the learning can respond with suggestions such as "What keys usually return us?" or "The escape key, the option key, and the command key sometimes work. Which should we try?" Then the next time, "Remember there were three keys . . . " This way the young adult learns to explore and to call upon previous experiences to solve problems.

Another technique I like to use is a guided learning sheet, used together with a talking word processor. Prepare an instruction sheet, along with the young adult, that gives step-by-step instruction to master the task. Make sure that she or he can follow the instructions and read the sheet. You can prepare the sheet as a word processing document of a talking word processor. Then the learner can pull up the document and hear the instructions as she or he is reading it.

If I could only say four words about choosing software, they would be "try before you buy." Ask for a 30-day review from software companies, and request the right to return if not appropriate. Ask your computer dealer if you can try the program in the store. Visit a computer resource center or join a user's group. Not all of these programs may be appropriate to the individual you are thinking of because their interests and skill levels vary. Look at some of the qualities of the programs: their open-endedness, which provides an opportunity to explore and think things out, their graphics, animation, and sound which provide excitement, motivation and encourage increased attention-span and focus. Look at the humor, the values portrayed, and the control they give the user.

APPENDIX

Software for Early Elementary Education (sources in parentheses—see below)

SINGLE SWITCH SOFTWARE
  For cause-and-effect, errorless early
    learning
      The New Cause & Effect (TLL)
      Switches, Pictures & Music (TLL)
      Switch Access Music (TLL)
      Switch Intro (DJDE)

  For timed activation—press switch
    when computer signals
      Scanning Game (TLL)
      Games 2 Play (DJDE)
      Children's Switch Progressions
        (RJ Cooper)
  For turn-taking, attention span
      Interaction Games (DJDE)
      Games 2 Play (DJDE)
TOUCH WINDOW
    Millie's Math House (Edmark)

Bailey's Book House (Edmark)
My House, My School, My Town
   (Laureate)
McGee (Lawrence)
INTELLIKEYS
Stickybear Opposites (Optimum)
OTHER EARLY EDUCATION
PROGRAMS
   Stickybear ABC (Optimum)
   Reader Rabbit Ready for Letters
      (Learning Company)
   Stickybear Reading Room (Optimum)
   Reading Maze (Great Wave)
   1,2,3, Sequence Me (Sunburst)
   Once Upon A Time (CompuTeach)
CD-ROM
   Just Grandma and Me (Broderbund)
   Arthur's Teacher Troubles
      (Broderbund)
   Silly Noisy House (Voyager)
   Word Tales (Warner)

Software for Postsecondary Education

SOFTWARE TO ENHANCE
EDUCATIONAL GOALS
   Where In the USA is Carmen San
      Diego? (Broderbund)
   Nigel (Davidson)
   Talking Academic Quiz Kid (Orange
      Cherry)
   SuperMunchers (MECC)
   Groliers Encyclopedia (Groliers)
   Math Blaster Mystery (Davidson)
   Story Starters: Science and Social
      Studies (Toucan/Queue)
   Geographic JigSaw (Eclat)
   Super Solvers Series (Learning Com-
      pany)
   The Oregon Trail (MECC)
SOFTWARE TO ENHANCE
LANGUAGE
   Banner Books (Toucan/Queue)

Crossword Magic (MindScape)
Big Book Makers (Toucan/Queue)
The Writing Center (Learning Com-
   pany)
Children's Writing/Publishing Center
   (Learning Company)
Intellitalk (Intellikeys)
Magic Typist (Olduvai)
Storybook Weaver (MECC)
SOFTWARE TO ENHANCE
TIME MANAGEMENT AND
ORGANIZATIONAL SKILLS
   In Control (Attain)
   What Are You Doing Today, Charlie
      Brown (Individual)
   DateBook Pro (After Hours)
SOFTWARE TO ENHANCE
RECREATION
   Print Shop (Broderbund)
   KidPix (Broderbund)
   Spelunx (Broderbund)
   Reunion (Leister)

Software Sources

Broderbund, 500 Redwood Blvd., Nova-
   to, CA 94948-6121, 800-521-6263
Compu-Teach, 16541 Redmond Way,
   Suite 137-C, Redmond, WA 98052,
   800-448-3224
Davidson & Assoc., P.O. Box 2961,
   19840 Pioneer Ave., Torrance, CA
   90509, 800-545-7677
Disney, 500 S. Buena Vista St., Bur-
   bank, CA 91521-6808, 818-567-5360
Don Johnston Inc., P.O. Box 639,
   Wauconda, IL 60084-0639, 800-
   999-4660
Edmark, 6727 185th Ave. NE, Red-
   mond, WA 98052, 800-426-0856
Educational Resources, 1550 Executive
   Dr., Elgin, IL 60123, 800-624-2926
Hartley, 3451 Dunckel Rd., Suite 200,
   Lansing, MI 48911, 800-246-1380

IntelliKeys (see IntelliTools)

IntelliTools, 5221 Central Ave., Suite 205, Richmond, CA 94804, 800-899-6687

Laureate Learning, 110 E. Spring St., Winooski, VT 05404-9818, 800-562-6801

Lawrence Productions, 1800 South 35th St., Galesburg, MI 49053-9687, 800-421-4157

Learning Co., 6493 Kaiser Dr., Fremont, CA 94555, 800-852-2255

MECC, 6160 Summit Dr., Minneapolis, MN 55430-4003, 800-685-6322

Mindplay, P.O. Box 36491, Tucson, AZ 85740-6491, 800-221-7911

Optimum Resource, 5 Hiltech Lane, Hilton Head, SC 29926, 800-327-1473

Public Domain Software (see TLL)

R.J. Cooper & Assoc., 24843 Del Prado, Ste. 283, Dana Point, CA 92629, 714-240-1912

Sunburst Communications, 39 Washington Ave., Pleasantville, NY 10570-2898, 800-628-8897

Switches, Interface (see TLL)

Technology for Language and Learning (TLL), P.O. Box 327, E. Rockaway, NY 11518-0327, 516-625-4550

Toucan/Queue, 338 Commerce Dr., Fairfield, CT 06432, 800-232-2224

Touch Window (see Edmark)

REFERENCE

Stainback S, Stainback W (1992): "Curriculum Considerations in Inclusive Classrooms: Facilitating Learning For All Students." Baltimore, Brookes.

VI. Clinical Care

Perspective

Marianna Paez

When Mom and Dad made me, some 25 years ago, there were no methods in our country by which to determine if a baby would have Down syndrome.

When Mom started labor pains on August 2, 1968, she went to the hospital. Some hours later the doctor said, "Come on, push. There's the head. Push a little more," and so I was born. The doctor told another doctor that I had Down syndrome. When Mom saw me, she cried a lot. My dad told her, "Calm down." Anyway, they registered me with my own name, Marianna.

Since I was very little, I had early intervention. Dr. Lydia Coreat, who was my doctor, would talk with my mother and would say, "Your daughter won't be very intelligent. But she'll have lots of things to do when she grows up, and she'll be able to choose what she wants. This much I can guarantee." I grew up and different professionals helped me to speak better, to think, to read, to write, to learn many things that would prepare me for life. My development was slow but sure.

I was integrated in a regular kindergarten and then attended ordinary primary school up to fourth grade. My fellow classmates were my friends and they lent me a hand. But they learned much quicker than I did. Each one chose his own life and I got on with mine. I continued my education up to adolescence in special education schools. I made new friends there.

My family, my friends shared these years with me. Little by little I discovered my true vocation, to be a professional cook. Right now I am attending the Rosario Vero Peñuloso School and this year I'll complete the work apprenticeship in the pasta factory. Once I leave school I'll start to work in another factory. I also go to the Institute Argentina de Gastronomia, where I am taking the first year course to become a professional cook. If everything goes well, next year I'll graduate at the same time as my classmates who do not have a handicap.

I would like to tell you that the people at the Institute, the principal and the secretaries, encourage me in my studies. In the different events in which I have taken part, and in which I have had to work until dawn, my classmates and the public that attended make me feel like them. They don't care that I have Down syndrome. My future project is to have my own food enterprise, even though I know that I need help. I'll work hard to make it work. I would like all young people like me to be able to feel the same, be able to find a decent job and earn money.

I would like to tell the parents who have a handicapped baby to let it enjoy their love and affection, to show it that it doesn't matter to have an extra chromosome. What matters is that we develop as individuals with the same right to live as anybody else, as a human being and to have a future of work with friends of the same age, whether they are normal or handicapped. What matters is that they may become a grown-up woman or man, and that when they finish work, they are able to go to parties to which they are invited, or to spend a night at a show, not to discriminate against them for being as they are.

Everyone should listen to our voice, understand it, and recognize our rights as citizens. Above all, I want to say that what matters most for me is that people value what I think. I want to be happy with my parents and siblings, but I also want to have my own home and family with Christian, my boyfriend, built on our love. I have come to terms with my handicap but I don't want to have to depend on my siblings when my parents are no longer with me. I work, I study, and with my friends we'll achieve a full life, even though with some support.

Handicapped people need help in order to carry on. Not everyone understands this. I've always said, those who laugh at someone who is handicapped are more handicapped than us.

I would like to finish by saying that it doesn't matter to have Down syndrome. It matters to be alive and to feel and hope like everyone else. It's true that we need help to carry on and fight in order to enjoy life, but the challenge is well worth it.

Early Interdisciplinary Specialized Care of Children with Down Syndrome

Benoit Lauras, Vincent Gautheron, Pierre Minaire,
and Benedicte DeFreminville

In France one of the first associations of parents and health care professionals aimed at a specific management of children with Down syndrome was created in St. Etienne 20 years ago. At present, more than 50 associations of this type exist in our country and form a national federation, FAIT 21 (Federation of the Associations for the Insertion of People with Down Syndrome).

From the beginning, it was important for us that the management of children should be started as early as possible and arise from a close cooperation between parents and professionals. We rapidly organized a flexible health care structure in which the physician is only one of the participants. A few comments about our experience follow.

INFORMING THE PARENTS OF THE CHROMOSOMAL ABNORMALITY

This is, in our experience, a fundamental moment in the management of Down syndrome. A few years ago, along with psychologists, we interviewed parents one to three years after the birth of their child. We were struck by the fact that the parents we met all talked about two distinct periods: before and after the disclosure of the diagnosis. We think it is a real medical act that requires a great deal of attention, care, precision, and timing. We think it is the first and probably the most important act of early management. After discussions among ourselves and with the families, we have decided on the following guidelines.

The parents should be informed of the diagnosis only when it is confirmed. In our country, the physical symptoms of Down syndrome elicit deep emotional reactions, and a diagnosis based only on these signs can be very disturbing for parents. We think it is necessary to have the diagnosis confirmed by chromosomal analysis. Therefore we have established an emergency protocol. Chromosomal analysis is made within four to five days, thus avoiding any delay in informing the parents. However, if during this period which allows the family to get acquainted with the baby, the parents are worried, we talk about the diagnosis, mentioning that we are awaiting cytogenetic confirmation.

The diagnosis should be announced when both parents are together. Otherwise, there is a risk that the first-informed parent becomes the bearer of the bad news for the other parent, and this is a situation that may create subsequent difficulties.

The announcement should be made in the presence of the child with Down syndrome. He or she is the one we are most concerned about, the one we are talking about; he or she must be present, in his or her cradle, or in his or her father's or mother's arms.

The physician must adopt a positive attitude. He or she must not conceal the truth nor deny forthcoming difficulties. However, it does no good to consider only the negative point of view. Therapeutic management must be rapidly considered. The potential that will have to be discovered and brought out in this different child, as in any child arriving in a family, will be discussed.

The individual and unique character of the newborn baby has to be preserved. Children with Down syndrome are too often considered as being all alike: loving children, musical. Every child is unique. This one has 47 chromosomes instead of 46, but he or she inherited these chromosomes from his or her parents, whom he or she will resemble. Of course, it is impossible to foretell the child's good and weak points, tastes, or skills, as it is impossible for any other ordinary child.

Finally, we think that the diagnosis must be announced by a physician who is familiar with this situation and who will take part in the subsequent follow-up of the child. Of course, it is not an easy task, but again, it is a real medical act whose consequences for the development of the child can be important.

Further information and support must be provided. During the first interview, most parents are overwhelmed at the news and do not remember the information provided. Another interview must therefore be planned in order to clarify some issues, and adapted documentation must be provided.

We think that *other parents of children with Down syndrome can most effectively support* the newly informed parents and help them mourn the loss of the nondisabled baby they were expecting. For this purpose, some parents have set up a service where they can rapidly welcome new parents. The latter are informed of this possibility as soon as diagnosis is confirmed.

SPECIFIC MEDICAL PROBLEMS

Some particular concerns need to be carefully addressed in the follow-up of children with Down syndrome. They can be split into 1)the initial assessment, 2) the follow-up.

Initial Assessment

Within days or weeks following birth, the following need to be checked:

1. Screening for malformations associated with chromosomal abnormality. Besides intestinal abnormalities, which are screened for very early (duodenal atresia), it is critical to screen for congenital heart disease, even in the absence of any clinical

symptoms, because of its frequency. An echocardiogram is thus performed in a systematic and careful manner. The development of early and irreversible pulmonary hypertension is a dramatic risk for children with Down syndrome. It is thus necessary to screen for possible congenital heart disease, and assess its consequences in order to plan future management, which, in our practice, often includes early surgical repair after studying blood pressure with a catheter.

2. In the first few days, hematological tests, renal echography and thyroid function evaluation are also performed.

3. Early detection, within the first months of life, of hearing impairment, which may affect the acquisition of language. Auditory evoked responses should be obtained in a systematic manner at the age of 6–9 months.

Follow-up

In our experience, children should be examined regularly (every year), and we have set up specialized clinics where physicians and ancillary medical professionals (physiotherapists, speech therapists, psychologists) are present and participate. The consultations take place at the hospital, where it is possible to perform the necessary examinations, including X rays and hormone dosing. Some conditions are carefully monitored:

1. *Growth.* The growth curve of children with Down syndrome is usually inferior to the curve of children with 46 chromosomes, but two issues need to be stressed. a) As with individuals with 46 chromosomes, there are variations in the Gaussian curve: both curves overlap and, therefore, children with Down syndrome can have normal or nearly normal height. b) What matters is that the child grows steadily and, as for any other child, a break in the growth curve must lead the physician to screen for an associated pathology (particularly thyroid deficiency).

2. *Weight.* Aided by dietary specialists, we try to prevent excess weight gain from the first years of life. We think that excess weight is a handicap for the child in his activities, and for the image he presents to others and to himself.

3. *Visual impairment.* Screening for refraction disorders (short-sightedness, long-sightedness), cataract, or squint is important in the first years of life. Though difficult, treatment of such impairments is important in order to prevent a secondary disability.

4. *Dentition.* Abnormal placing of teeth with inordinate tooth eruption is frequent. Such abnormalities, often aggravated by tongue hypertrophy, must be treated in time by orthodontic treatment.

5. *Immune status.* Deficiency of the defense factors often occurs (bactericidal disorders, thymus-dependent lymphocyte disorders). Therefore, the physician must be particularly careful with immunization schedules, and should not hesitate to recommend immunization against hepatitis B and, in fragile children, immunization against flu (influenzae vaccine) before the winter season.

6. *Thyroid function evaluation* as well as T3, T4 and TSH levels should be obtained and thyroid antibodies should be screened for every 2 years until the age of 8 or in case of delayed growth or major hypotonia. If necessary, a treatment is

introduced with thyroid hormone (rare in our experience). We particularly monitor the increase of TSH.

7. *Orthopedic concerns.* A visit with a specialist is proposed to parents in a systematic manner every 2 or 3 years. a) Cervical spine is particularly monitored because there are risks of atlantoaxial luxation. Generally, lateral X-rays centered on CI–CII in hyperflexion and hyperextension is obtained at the age of 3, and then later if neurological disorders occur. b) Radiological and clinical monitoring of the spinal cord is particularly necessary during prepuberty. c) Examination of the lower limbs, and particularly of the plantar arch with a podoscope must be done regularly.

These regular consultations allow contacts between health care professionals and parents, and allow regular assessment of the expectations of each family and the problems of each child.

Errors to Avoid

Even if the list of medical concerns is long, we think that two errors must be avoided. 1) Children with Down syndrome must not be considered as patients; they are different from individuals with 46 chromosomes, some concerns are particular to them, but the fact of having three number 21 chromosomes is not an illness. 2) Any observed abnormality must not be systematically considered as being linked with Down syndrome; otherwise, this may prevent the screening for a possible independent pathology and lead to a failure to treat it.

At-Home Services

A health maintenance and special education service at home was created in St. Etienne, as in many other towns in France. It consists of a team of health care professionals working together. They work with children either at home, at school, or in a special place, which in our case is in a school where children attend special classes and share some activities with children without Down syndrome. They work together: the interdisciplinary team (teachers, physicians, psychologists, ancillary personnel) meet on a regular basis to discuss every child (once or twice a year) and to adapt management of each particular case according to the child's development. The conclusions of the meeting are then discussed with the parents and a definitive program of management is adopted until the next evaluation.

Our aim is to give every child the chance of developing in harmony according to his or her own pace, so that he or she can reach maximal autonomy. The physician has a role to play in planning and monitoring this program. It should be stressed that our health care service can only care for some of the children with Down syndrome in the region, but it is a reference center. Educators and paramedical staff with their own practices or who work in schools can contact the center and can ask for support and advice. The consulting physician is also the interface between all the people in charge of the management of children with Down syndrome.

Our methods vary according to the age of the child and include education, prevention of bad habits for younger ones, or rehabilitation and correction for older ones.

Early Management

Motor Development. We help the child attain the usual stages of motor development in order to avoid the onset of the classical morphotype and of serious disorders. It is mainly the physiotherapist who cares for motor concerns, aided by the psychomotrician although the rest of the team also plays a role. We work with usual rehabilitation and mobilization methods, but also with behavioral activities and games. We particularly pay attention to:

The cervical spine and scapular region. The usual posture of forward cervical projection needs to be prevented. The strengthening of the extensor cervical muscles is very important, given the abnormality of the occipitocer vical joint and ligamentous hyperelasticity. We teach the child correct posture with games such as ball throwing.

The shoulder girdle. Children with Down syndrome have a natural tendency to be round shouldered. Posterior muscles have to be strengthened. Specific exercises, such as games with antepulsion of the shoulders, are necessary to stabilize the shoulder girdle, particularly the median and inferior trapezius muscles.

The trunk. The frequency of pulmonary superinfection episodes is an indication for the development of the rib cage; respiratory exercises and development of pectoral muscles increase the amplitude of diaphragmatic movements and strengthen abdominal muscles as well as the latissimus dorsi and gluteus major, to prevent anterior flexion of the trunk.

The feet. Quite often, a flat plantar arch is observed. We advise walking exercises, on different sorts of ground, in bare feet if possible, trying to tiptoe. However, it is sometimes necessary to fit ortheses and/or adapted shoes.

The hands. This is one of the concerns that we consider to be of prime importance and we pay particular attention to it. Indeed, the hand is an essential tool of adaptation and sociabilization. Most often the child with Down syndrome presents with a weakness of the forearm rotator muscles (flexor and extensor digitorum), a decrease in discriminating sensitivity, and a coordination deficit, particularly for precise movements.

The education program must respect the stages of the child's growth and neurological maturation and be progressive. We work with games because they are accepted by the child. Management includes:

* physiotherapy to strengthen movements—particularly prehensile movements—including amplitude of gesture, precise movements, increase of tactile sensitivity, and coordination training
* occupational therapy with activities that interest the child: pottery, weaving, theater
* teaching graphism in order to prepare for handwriting.

Speech Education. We think that early speech education is useful and better than later rehabilitation, which is much more difficult and not always successful. Some difficulties particular to children with Down syndrome must be taken into account:

* motor difficulties of the bucco-facial region, due to hypotonia
* difficulties in linking and coordinating movements

- slowness to speak
- hypotonia of vocal cords
- hypotonia of soft palate, which gives the voice a rough and nasal sound.

Speech educators care for children individually or collectively to help them attain the appropriate stages of language development. Speech education is of prime importance for the future or these children, enabling them to have quality social contacts and therefore a reasonable level of autonomy.

Management Schedule

This is a fundamental issue: when should we begin the various stages of the management? Does early management mean management from birth? We think there is no fixed rule. It is important that the child find his place in the community and in his family without excessive medical attention.

The management of the child is made in accordance with parents. In the first few months, the role of parents is fundamental. The parents meet the medical team once every two weeks, so that they feel supported and can be shown useful movements for their child (particularly in motor development). Gradually, the management itself is started, adapted to the needs of the child. (Children with Down syndrome do not all have the same degree of hypotonicity.) In general, between 6 and 9 months we propose one session of physiotherapy per week, and at the end of the first year speech education is started.

CONCLUSION

We presently take care of 51 children; 19 receive preschool education in the nursery school of their district before the age of 6. Among the 32 children who attend school, 10 are placed in a special education class for children with Down syndrome, 10 attend a class attached to a teacher's training college, five are integrated in regular classrooms, and seven individually attend semiintegrated classes or regular classrooms.

60 children who had been seen during school years have left our medical center. They are aged 11 to 27. They did not all receive early management. Undoubtedly, the development of these 60 children is very different from what was observed before. Most of them have acquired satisfactory autonomy: they are able to have social contacts, take public transport, live outside their parent's home, and, for some of them, to be integrated into a regular workplace—in a hospital, bookshop, company, or workshop—but most of them work in a protected place.

However, the individuals who received early management generally live in a nearly normal environment, and their integration in a work place will probably be easier. This successful experience prompts us to continue and to improve the early management of children who are under our care.

Obesity and Nutrition in Children with Down Syndrome

Nancy J. Roizen, Amy Luke, Marjorie Sutton, and Dale A. Schoeller

In the general population, between 5% and 25% of children and adolescents are obese (Dietz, 1983; Gortmaker et al., 1987). In the population of individuals with mental retardation, the prevalence of obesity is similar (Burkart et al., 1985). Parents and health professionals caring for children with Down syndrome recognize that children with Down syndrome have a problem with obesity (Chumlea, 1981). Studies show that children with Down syndrome have a tendency to be overweight beginning in infancy (Chumlea and Cronk, 1981; Cronk, et al. 1985; Cronk, et al. 1988). Cronk et al.'s (1988) data on the growth of 730 children with Down syndrome from 1 month to 18 years of age indicated that the percentage of children with Down syndrome who were overweight increased to 50% of the girls by the third year of life and 50% of the boys by early childhood. The percentage of children with Down syndrome who were overweight fluctuated to 18 years of age but the percentage above the 85th percentile of weight per height always was greater than 30%. These studies document the early onset and persistence of obesity in children and adolescents with Down syndrome.

Obesity in children with Down syndrome is of concern because of its relation to social, developmental, and medical problems. Children with obesity are less sought after as playmates. Although not studied in children with Down syndrome, overweight is negatively associated with motor performance in normal children (Malina, 1980). Obesity can limit the capacity of children with Down syndrome to participate in sports and recreational activities, which are important for physical and emotional development. In the general population, obesity is associated with an increased risk of carbohydrate intolerance, diabetes mellitus, hyperlipidemia, hypertension, pulmonary and renal problems, and surgical complications (Kannel and Gordon, 1979; Bray, 1976; Van Itallie, 1979). In the general population, overweight during adolescence has important social and economic consequences (Gortmaker, et al., 1993).

Research has shown that the combination of inactivity and high caloric intake contribute to the development of obesity in most people. In studies done at the

University of Chicago, supported by the Down Syndrome Research Foundation, researchers have studied the relationship between energy expenditure and obesity in prepubescent children with Down syndrome as compared to controls matched for age, weight, and percent body fat. The researchers measured body composition, resting metabolic rate (RMR), and total energy expenditure using indirect calorimetry and the doubly labeled water method. Resting metabolic rate was significantly lower in the children with Down syndrome than in controls, whereas there were no significant differences in the total energy expenditure. Children with Down syndrome were just as active as control children when expressed as kcalories/kg body weight. As one would expect, lean children, both those with Down syndrome and their controls, tended to be more active than the obese children.

In the same study of energy expenditure and obesity, the dietary intake of the children with Down syndrome and the controls was measured using three-day dietary diaries recorded by the subjects' mothers. The three-day records were analyzed and compared to the 1989 Recommended Dietary Allowances (RDA). The proportions of carbohydrate, fat, and protein in the diet were comparable between the subject groups and to the proportions recommended by the American Heart Association (15% of kcalories from protein, 30% or less of kcalories from fat, and 55–60% of kcalories from carbohydrate). The reported caloric intake for children with Down syndrome was significantly less than the reported intake for controls: 86% of the RDA and 111%, respectively ($p = 0.05$). When reported intakes were compared to energy expenditures, as measured by the doubly labeled water method, over the same time period, it was found that parents overreported intake for both groups by 12%. Even with caloric and nutrient intakes being overreported, the majority of children with Down syndrome consumed less than 80% of the RDA for several nutrients, putting them at risk for deficiencies. These micronutrients include the minerals iron, calcium, zinc, and copper, and the vitamins A, C, E, and pantothenic acid. The diets of the nonobese children with Down syndrome were much more likely than the obese children to be low in several of the nutrients. In contrast, the diets of the majority of the control children met or exceeded the RDA for all nutrients except copper. The fact that the children with Down syndrome in this study who were not obese were those with low dietary intakes and increased risk of micronutrient deficiencies complicates the dietary management of obesity in Down syndrome. Lowering the caloric intake of children with Down syndrome to prevent or treat obesity is not the best option.

As with all obesity management programs, the prevention and treatment of obesity in children with Down syndrome includes behavior modification, diet, and exercise. In light of the low RMR found in children with Down syndrome, an exercise program should be emphasized more than for other individuals. Early in life, daily exercise should become part of the regimen of every child with Down syndrome. A daily walk is the simplest way to insure daily exercise in a young child. The other important part of dietary management of obesity in children with Down syndrome is to consider a daily vitamin–mineral supplement for any child with marginal total intake or limited variety in their diets. In summary, the management of obesity in children with Down syndrome is complicated by their low RMR and low dietary intake of individual nutrients. In the population of children with Down syndrome, exercise and the addition of a vitamin–mineral supplement are especially important.

REFERENCES

Bray GA (1976): "The Obese Patient." Philadelphia: Saunders.

Burkart JE, Fox RA, Rotatori AF (1985): Obesity of mentally retarded individuals: Prevalence, characteristics, and intervention. Am J Ment Defic 90:303–312.

Chumlea WC, Cronk CE (1981): Overweight among children with Trisomy 21. J Ment Defic Res 25:275–280.

Cronk CE, Chumlea WC, Roche AF (1985): Assessment of overweight children with Trisomy 21. Am J Ment Defic 89:433–436.

Cronk CE, Crocker AC, Pueschel SM, Shea AM, Zackai E, Pickens G, Reed RB (1988): Growth charts for children with Down syndrome: 1 month to 18 years of age. Pediatrics 81:102–110.

Dietz WH (1983): Childhood obesity: Susceptibility, cause, and management. J Pediatr 103:676–686.

Gortmaker SL, Dietz WH, Sobel AM, Wehler CA (1987): Increasing pediatric obesity in the United States. Am J Dis Child 141:535–540.

Gortmaker SL, Must A, Perrin JM, Sobol AM, Dietz WH (1993): Social and economic consequences of overweight in adolescence and young adulthood. New Engl J Med 329:1008–1012.

Kannel WB, Gordon T (1979): Physiological and medical concomitants of obesity: The Framingham study. In Bray GA (Ed.): "Obesity in America" (NIH Publication No. 79-359), pp. 125–163. Washington DC: Department of Health, Education, and Welfare.

Malina RM (1980): Growth, strength, and physical performance. In Stull GA (Ed.): "Encyclopedia of Physical Education, Fitness, and Sports." Salt Lake City: Brighton.

Van Itallie TB (1979): Obesity: Adverse effects on health and longevity. Am J Clin Nutr 32:Suppl:2723–2733.

Musculoskeletal Disorders in Persons with Down Syndrome

Siegfried M. Pueschel

INTRODUCTION

Although there are numerous musculoskeletal concerns and many bony structures in the person with Down syndrome are affected to some degree, it should be emphasized that the majority of individuals with this chromosome disorder are not motorically disabled. Actually, many persons with Down syndrome have very few complaints with regard to their musculoskeletal system and many individuals have become outstanding athletes. Participating in Special Olympics and involvement in the physical fitness movement are goals for many individuals with Down syndrome. We have heard of marathon runners, outstanding swimmers, skiers, and weight lifters, and there are numerous gold medal winners in various sports activities of Special Olympics, Inc. These are brilliant physical accomplishments. Why, then, should we be concerned with the musculoskeletal system in persons in Down syndrome since many of them are such successful athletes?

There are three main reasons why a discussion of this topic is of importance:

1. Due to the trisomic condition, we have observed that persons with Down syndrome are usually of short stature, their bone maturation is usually delayed, and there are numerous congenital abnormalities of various bony structures.
2. The ligaments and tendons that hold bones together and that connect muscles to the skeletal systems are often affected, and most children with Down syndrome have ligamentous laxity, which may result in musculoskeletal disorders.
3. There are specific musculoskeletal disorders such as atlantoaxial instability, hip dislocation, patellar subluxation, and others that deserve special attention.

STRUCTURAL BONE ABNORMALITIES
Skull

The head in children with Down syndrome has been described as brachycephalic, which is a shortening of the anteroposterior diameter with flattening of the occiput. Usually their head is smaller than in age-equivalent children who do not have Down syndrome, and, thus, the cranial capacity is reduced. In the neonatal period there is often an open sagittal suture and a widening in the parietal area, which is referred to as "false" fontanel. The nasal bones of the infant with Down syndrome are poorly developed and the maxilla as well as the sphenoid bones have been described as hypoplastic. Frequently, the palate is narrow and short which, together with the maxillary hypoplasia, results in a small oral cavity.

Thorax

Many children with Down syndrome have two ossification centers of the manubrium of the sternum. In addition, hypoplasia or absence of the twelfth rib has been described in several individuals with Down syndrome.

Pelvis

The pelvic bones of infants with Down syndrome usually show flattening of the acetabular angle, widening of the iliac wings, small ischial rami, and coxa valga of the femur. Prior to the availability of chromosome analysis, the measurements of the acetabular and iliac angles were often used in the diagnosis of children with Down syndrome.

Hands and Feet

The hands of children with Down syndrome are usually shortened due to the decreased length of the metacarpal bones and phalanges. Brachyclinodactyly of the fifth digit (a hypoplastic middle phalanx of the fifth digit) is seen in approximately 50–55% of children with Down syndrome. Unilateral partial adactyly has been described in some children with Down syndrome. The cause of this anomaly is unknown (Pueschel and O'Donnel, 1974).

The feet are usually short and broad. There is a wide separation between the first and second toes with an interdigital plantar furrow. It should be emphasized that the above-described skeletal abnormalities usually do not interfere with musculoskeletal functioning.

LIGAMENTOUS LAXITY

Most of the musculoskeletal abnormalities observed in individuals with Down syndrome are the result of ligamentous laxity, which will be discussed in detail in the subsequent section. It has been postulated that children with Down syndrome have an intrinsic defect of their connective tissue that is responsible for the observed general ligamentous laxity (Pueschel et al., 1981). Recently it has been shown that fetal heart collagen is encoded by two genes mapped on the distal part of the long arm of chromosome 21 (Duff et al., 1990). Apparently, these two genes encode for two chains of collagen Type VI molecule during human fetal heart development. It is conceivable that the collagen present in the ligaments of the musculoskeletal system is either encoded for by the same genes or by other genes on chromosome 21, which ultimately results in ligamentous laxity.

SPECIFIC SKELETAL DISORDERS

Atlantoaxial Instability

Atlantoaxial instability is primarily due to ligamentous laxity of the transverse ligaments that ordinarily hold the odontoid process close to the anterior arch of the atlas. Atlantoaxial instability is considered to be present when the atlanto–dens interval is 5 mm or more (Pueschel and Scola, 1987). In addition, the spinal canal width may be measured. A recent study indicated that the spinal canal width measurement is a better predictor of potential spinal cord compression than the atlanto–dens interval or the clivus–posterior odontoid process distance (White et al., 1993).

Atlantoaxial instability was first described in the early 1960s (Spitzer et al., 1961). Since then numerous case reports and large-scale studies have been published in the medical literature. The largest study involved 404 persons with Down syndrome (Pueschel and Scola, 1987). It was found that 14.6% of this population had atlantoaxial instability using the above-described criteria for this condition; 1.5% of the 404 children had symptomatic atlantoaxial instability, i.e., these individuals have significant neurologic symptoms and local findings in the neck area; and 13.1% had asymptomatic atlantoaxial instability, i.e., these children had pertinent radiologic findings but no abnormal neurologic signs.

It has been recommended that children with asymptomatic atlantoaxial instability not participate in those sports activities that potentially could result in an injury of the neck (Special Olympics Bulletin, 1983). Special Olympics, Inc. has developed a list of such sports activities that persons with Down syndrome who have atlantoaxial instability should avoid. These activities include gymnastics, diving, butterfly stroke in swimming, high jump, pentathalon, soccer, alpine skiing, and certain warmup exercises. The reason for avoiding these kind of sports activities is that there is a high risk for persons with Down syndrome injuring their neck and becoming neurologically symptomatic. In a previous review of patients with symptomatic atlantoaxial instability it was found that at least 17% of the 42 individuals with this disorder had sustained an injury to the cervical spine that either had caused atlantoaxial subluxation leading to neurologic symptoms or was in part a contributing factor augmenting the preexisting symptoms (Pueschel et al., 1984).

Children with Down syndrome and asymptomatic atlantoaxial instability should be followed closely by a physician knowledgeable about this condition. We usually recommend that parents report to the child's physician both local symptoms of the neck and neuromuscular dysfunction. These children should have neurologic examinations on a yearly basis or more frequently if symptoms become apparent. They also will require repeat radiological evaluations of the cervical spine. Children with asymptomatic atlantoaxial instability usually do not require surgical stabilization of the upper cervical spine. If, however, symptoms of spinal cord compressions are emerging, or if CT scan or magnetic resonance imaging reveals a significant abnormality within the spinal canal, then surgical intervention should be considered. The primary concern in persons with atlantoaxial instability is the identification of those individuals who are at a high risk of becoming symptomatic.

Recently we engaged in a longitudinal follow-up study of 141 persons with Down syndrome who had successive radiological examination of their cervical spine (Pueschel et al., 1992). When we analyzed the results of the atlanto–dens interval measurements of the X-rays we did not find any significant changes over time. The vast majority of persons had only minor changes of atlanto–dens interval measurements, compared with previous examinations. Thus, it was concluded that there is no need for frequent reexaminations of the cervical spine (Pueschel et al., 1992).

Usually, radiographs are obtained first at the age of 2½–3 years. It has been suggested that a repeat cervical spine X-ray be taken at about the age of 8–9 years, when many children enter Special Olympics or engage in potentially dangerous sports activities that may result in injuries of the neck. Some investigators also recommend a reexamination of the cervical spine radiologically during adolescence.

Occipitoatlantal Instability

Although there are numerous reports in the literature relating to atlantoaxial instability, there are only a few publications on occipitoatlantal instability in persons with Down syndrome. It has been estimated that, depending on the methodology used for identifying occipitoatlantal instability, 8–37% of children with Down syndrome have this condition. Although standardized radiographic criteria for the evaluation of occipitoatlantal joints have not been developed, it has been reported that the "Powers ratio" is the most reliable radiographic parameter for assessment of occipitoatlantal instability (Parfenchuck et al., 1994). It is assumed that occipitoatlantal instability is underreported and is probably as frequent in children with Down syndrome as atlantoaxial instability.

Skeletal Anomalies and Degenerative Changes of the Cervical Spine

A number of children with Down syndrome and atlantoaxial instability have been observed to have cervical spine anomalies involving the C1–C2 region (Pueschel et al., 1990). This suggests that these cervical spine anomalies may be a contributing factor to the pathogenesis of atlantoaxial instability.

Other cervical spine abnormalities include spondylosis which may cause cervical myelopathy. Therefore, close monitoring of neurologic function in these individuals is of significance. Flexion and extension radiographs of the cervical spine should be obtained not only to evaluate the occipitoatlantal and atlantoaxial relationships, but also to look for degenerative changes in the lower cervical spine. Degenerative changes often include osteophyte formation, subarticular sclerosis, cystic changes, fusion, and disk narrowing (Fidone, 1986).

Scoliosis

It has been estimated that nearly half of the Down syndrome population may have thoracic or lumbar scoliosis (Diamond et al., 1981). In our experience, scoliosis in children with Down syndrome occurs in about 6–8% and is often of a mild degree. Bracing is usually not successful in preventing progression of scoliosis. Only in rare instances, when a severe curve has developed, will surgical intervention be necessary.

Hip Dislocation

Because of the presence of a flattened roof of the acetabulum it is very rare to find congenital dislocation of the hip in newborns with Down syndrome. Later in life, however, hip dislocation has been found to occur at a higher frequency in individuals with Down syndrome than in the general population (Bennet et al., 1982). It has been reported that between the ages of 2–10 years the hip in children with Down syndrome can spontaneously dislocate. A sudden limp or reluctance to bear weight may be the only sign of hip dislocation. Therefore, a routine examination of the hips should be an essential part of the physical examination in persons with Down syndrome. If hip dislocation has been identified, the hip should be reduced under general anesthesia. Usually, closed reduction and immobilization in a spica cast will not be successful in preventing redislocation because of the presence of ligamentous laxity. Surgical intervention through tightening of the hip capsule has been shown to prevent future dislocations. Other surgical procedures are available to treat individuals with Down syndrome who have hip dislocation.

Patella Instability

Patella instability is a more common problem than hip instability in individuals with Down syndrome. It has been estimated that about 20% of persons with Down syndrome will have patella instability (Diamond et al., 1981). Fortunately, most persons with patella instability have full range of motion and can walk fairly well. There is some controversy as to whether individuals who have unstable patello-femoral joints should be treated surgically. Bracing may be attempted but it is often not very effective. In chronically dislocated joints, subsequent deformities are quite common.

Foot

Ligamentous laxity of the arch of the foot usually causes flat feet. Moderately flat feet that are painful may respond to treatment with orthotics. In young children with Down syndrome who just started walking, an ankle–foot orthosis may provide stability and assist with ambulation. Shoe inserts or custom foot orthoses with a well-molded heel can also be used in the older child. Sometimes severe symptomatic flat feet may require surgery. The importance of treatment of foot disorders is to ensure independent, comfortable ambulation. If not treated appropriately, impairment of walking will compromise activities of daily living and will restrict optimal functioning in the community.

Metatarsus primus varus with hallux valgus or hallux varus occur often in persons with Down syndrome. Particularly in the older person with Down syndrome, such moderate to severe foot deformities can give rise to shoe fitting problems. Some of these patients will require surgical intervention.

Arthropathy

Juvenile rheumatoid arthritis-like arthropathy has been reported in young persons with Down syndrome (Olson et al., 1990; Yancey et al., 1984). Some of these reports also indicate cervical spine abnormalities in individuals with juvenile rheumatoid arthritis. It was felt that the arthritic involvement in these children preceded the event of atlantoaxial instability. Subluxation of the joints of the hands and feet as well as the knees and hips have been observed in some people with Down syndrome and juvenile rheumatoid arthritis. It has been questioned whether the observed arthritis in persons with Down syndrome is a specific form of juvenile rheumatoid arthritis or whether this is a unique arthropathy only seen in patients with this chromosome disorder. Some investigators report a higher prevalence of arthropathy in persons with Down syndrome (Yancey et al., 1984).

If a person with Down syndrome has multiple joint involvements and complaints of intercurrent severe joint pain, it is important that one considers gout, since uric acid levels are known to be elevated in many individuals with Down syndrome. Reports have been published of significantly increased serum uric acid levels that caused gout (Dacre and Huskisson, 1988). Therefore, serum uric acid determination should be performed in persons with Down syndrome and coexisting arthritis.

SUMMARY

Although most persons with Down syndrome have an intact musculoskeletal system, physicians should be aware that there may be various skeletal disorders and orthopedic concerns that will need to be attended to. In particular, individuals who have extreme hyperflexibility due to ligamentous laxity, those who complain of neck discomfort and have pyramidal tract signs, those with hip, knee, or foot problems, as well as those with arthritic complaints should be carefully evaluated. It is well known that severe cervical spine pathology may have life-threatening consequences. Moreover, chronic instability of hips, knees, and other joints, as well as arthritis, may inhibit the individual's functioning and cause significant morbidity. Persons with Down syndrome who are found to have significant musculoskeletal disorders should be provided with optimal medical care and surgical intervention that will ultimately result in a better quality of life.

REFERENCES

Bennet GC, Rang M, Roye DP, Aprin H (1982): Dislocation of the hip in trisomy 21. J Bone Joint Surg 64:289–294.

Dacre JE, Huskisson EC (1988): Arthritis in Down's syndrome. Ann Rheum Dis 47:254–255.

Diamond LS, Lynne D, Sigman B (1981): Orthopedic disorders in patients with Down's syndrome. Orthoped Clin N Am 12:57–71.

Duff K, Williamson R, Richards SJ (1990): Expression of genes encoding two chains of the collagen type VI molecule during human fetal heart development. Int J Cardiol 27:128–129.

Fidone GS (1986): Degenerative cervical arthritis and Down syndrome. N E J Med 314:320.

Olson JC, Bender JC, Levinson JE, Oestreich A, Lovell DJ (1990): Arthropathy of Down syndrome. Pediatrics 86:931–936.

Parfenchuck TA, Bertrand SL, Powers MY, Drvaric DM, Pueschel SM, Roberts JM (1994): Posterior occipitoatlantal hypermodality in Down syndrome: An analysis of 199 patients. J Ped Orthoped 14:304–308.

Pueschel SM, O'Donnell P (1974): Unilateral partial adactyly in Down's syndrome. Pediatrics 54:466–469.

Pueschel SM, Scola FH (1987): Atlantoaxial instability in individuals with Down syndrome: Epidemiologic, radiographic, and clinical studies. Pediatrics 80:555–560.

Pueschel SM, Herndon JH, Gelch MM, Senft KE, Scola FH, Goldbert MJ (1984): Symptomatic atlantoaxial subluxation in persons with Down syndrome. J Ped Orthoped 4:682–688.

Pueschel SM, Scola FH, Perry CD, Pezzullo JC (1981): Atlantoaxial instability in children with Down syndrome. Ped Radiol 10:129–132.

Pueschel SM, Scola FH, Pezzullo JC (1992): A longitudinal study of atlantoaxial instability in individuals with Down syndrome. Pediatrics 89:1194–1198.

Pueschel SM, Scola FH, Tupper TB, Pezzullo JC (1990): Skeletal anomalies of the upper cervical spine in children with Down syndrome. J Ped Orthoped 10:607–611.

Special Olympics Bulletin (1993): Participation by individuals with Down syndrome who suffer from atlantoaxial dislocation condition. Washington, D.C., Special Olympics Inc., March 31.

Spitzer R, Rabinowich JY, Wybar KC (1961): A study of abnormalities of the skull, teeth, and lenses in mongolism. Can Med Assoc J 84:567–572.

White KS, Ball WS, Prenger EC, Patterson BJ, Kirks DR (1993): Evaluation of the craniocervical junction in Down syndrome: Correlation of measurements obtained with radiography and MR imaging. Radiology 186:373–382.

Yancey CL, Zmijewski C, Athreya BH, Doughty RA (1984): Arthropathy of Down's syndrome. Arth Rheum 27:929–934.

Neurological Problems Associated with Down Syndrome

Robert H. A. Haslam

Down syndrome is characteristically associated with generalized hypotonia, especially in the newborn period, and variable degrees of cognitive impairment. Less frequent, but important neurological problems related to Down syndrome include seizures, myelopathy secondary to atlantoaxial instability or anomalies of the occipitocervical region, and Down syndrome dementia. This chapter briefly reviews the unique aspects of epilepsy in Down syndrome and summarizes an approach to the management of atlantoaxial instability. Several treatable conditions that may present with dementia or loss of skills, and be confused with Alzheimer disease, will be highlighted in the discussion.

SEIZURES

Seizures occur more commonly in Down syndrome than in the general population, with an estimated frequency of 6–8% (Pueschel et al., 1991; Stafstrom et al., 1991). During childhood, a comprehensive history and examination with appropriate neurological studies will uncover specific causes for the seizures in about half of the cases. Congenital heart disease is a common finding in Down syndrome occurring in approximately 40% of infants. Occasionally, occlusion of the cerebral arteries or cerebral embolism complicates congenital heart disease, leading to infarction and seizures. However, with the current trend to early correction of heart defects, occlusion of the cerebrovascular system in Down syndrome seizures is much less of a problem. Moya moya disease is a progressive vascular occlusive disorder involving the carotid vessels and presents with acute strokes and seizures in children. The condition has been reported to occur with an increased frequency in children with Down syndrome (Pearson et al., 1985).

The immunological abnormalities common to Down syndrome render these children more susceptible to infections, including meningitis, which may present with a seizure, or result in epilepsy as a long-term sequela. The side-effects of leukemia therapy, a condition more common in Down syndrome than the general pediatric population, may lead to a chronic seizure disorder secondary to leukomalacia. Finally, seizures often herald the onset of Alzheimer disease (Down syndrome dementia), which will be discussed later in this section.

A cause for the remaining 50% of seizures is rarely found. These seizures are classified as idiopathic epilepsy. It is surprising that epilepsy is not more common in Down syndrome as several neurobiological abnormalities have been described that have been associated with epilepsy. These include dysgenesis of the dendritic spines (Becker et al., 1986), hyperexcitable neuronal membranes (Scott et al., 1982), alteration in membrane ionic channels, and a decrease in inhibitory motor neurons.

There are three seizure types that appear to be more common in children with Down syndrome: infantile spasms (Coriat and Fejerman, 1963; Pollock et al., 1978; Pueschel et al., 1991), myoclonic seizures (Wolcott and Chun, 1973) and reflex seizures (Gimenez-Roldan and Martin, 1980; Guerrini et al., 1990). Coleman (1971) first brought attention to the relationship between Down syndrome and infantile spasms. She reported the development of infantile spasms in 15% of 60 infants with Down syndrome and children during treatment with 5-hydroxytryptophan, which was used in a study to manage hypotonia and buccolingual dyskinesias. In five of nine children, the seizures disappeared by decreasing the drug; in the remaining four, the seizures persisted, following discontinuance of the 5-hydroxytryptophan.

Infantile spasms commonly appear between 4–6 months of age and are characterized by volleys of flexion or extension movements of the head and extremities, persisting for several minutes, often preceded by a cry. Occasionally the seizure consists of a mixture of flexion and extension movements. Infantile spasms may develop in a previously normal child, but may also be associated with tuberous sclerosis, congenital malformations of the brain, and a series of metabolic disorders. Although infantile spasms frequently respond favorably to parenteral ACTH or one of the benzodiazepines, the long-term prognosis for normal cognitive development, following control of the seizures, is limited to about 10% of cases. It has been my personal experience that children with Down syndrome with infantile spasms generally have a more favorable prognosis, with less likelihood of a detrimental effect on cognitive development, with cessation of the seizures.

Reflex seizures typically occur in patients with established epilepsy. They are characterized by a head nod or a fall to the floor and are triggered by a sudden noise (door slam, hand clap), a bright light stimulus, or tapping on the head or back. The electroencephalogram is nondiagnostic; the record may show polyspike wave discharges or sharp waves during a reflex seizure. Generally, reflex seizures are responsive to valproic acid or one of the benzodiazepines.

Investigation of seizures in a child with Down syndrome should include a thorough search for an underlying structural or vascular cause. Following a comprehensive history and physical examination, computed tomography or magnetic resonance imaging should be considered if an infarct or the side effects of cancer treatment are considered to be the cause of the seizure disorder. Cerebral angiography or magnetic resonance imaging with gadolinium are the procedures of choice if vascular lesion or moya moya disease is the likely cause. Prolonged electroencephalography and positron emission tomography (PET) may be useful in studying children with infantile spasms who have a focal abnormality on the routine electroencephalogram. A small number of these patients may be candidates for epilepsy surgery if unresponsive to anticonvulsant management.

ATLANTOAXIAL INSTABILITY AND MYELOPATHY

Atlantoaxial instability is common (10–20%) in people with Down syndrome, and is due to laxity of the transverse ligament, which holds the odontoid process of the axis against the atlas. Fortunately, compression of the spinal cord secondary to atlantoaxial instability is a relatively rare phenomenon in individuals with Down syndrome, occurring in less than 1%. The symptoms and signs of compressive myelopathy may be insidious or may have an abrupt onset, and are characterized by neck pain, urinary and fecal incontinence, head tilt, gait abnormalities, ataxia, hyperflexia, weakness, spasticity, and quadriplegia.

In 1984, the American Academy of Pediatrics published the following five recommendations:

1. All children with Down syndrome wishing to participate in sports that involve possible trauma to the head and neck should have lateral roentgenograms of the cervical region in the neutral, flexion, and extension positions.
2. If the distance between the odontoid process of the axis and the anterior arch of the atlas exceeds 4.5 mm, or the odontoid is abnormal (malformed, hypoplastic, or absent) participation in sports that involve trauma to the head and neck should be restricted and the patient should be observed at regular intervals.
3. Pending further research, repeated roentgenograms are not indicated for those previously found to be normal.
4. Persons with atlantoaxial subluxation or dislocation and neurological signs and symptoms should be restricted in all strenuous activities and operative stabilization considered.
5. Those who have no evidence of atlantoaxial instability may participate in all sports and follow-up is not required unless musculoskeletal or neurologic signs or symptoms develop.

These guidelines were subsequently followed rigorously by parents, physicians, and officials of Special Olympics Committees with the expectation that compressive myelopathy could be prevented in Down syndrome.

Recent reports have cast some doubt on the above recommendations. Burke et al. (1985) described a case of fatal C1–C2 dislocation during tumbling exercises in an 18-year-old who had a radiographically normal neck X-ray when 6 years of age. He retrospectively collected an additional 6 cases in which significant radiographic atlantoaxial instability became apparent during a 13-year-period, especially in males, despite normal radiographic measurements initially. On the basis of their study, Burke and colleagues recommended that all individuals with Down syndrome should be restricted from participating in high-risk events. Subsequently, a prospective longitudinal radiographic study of 141 individuals with Down syndrome reported only minor changes, between 1 and 1.5 mm, in the distance between the odontoid process and the atlas over a 13 year period in 92% of subjects, and there were no individuals who developed clinical symptoms during the study period (Pueschel et al., 1992). Others have highlighted the association of compressive myelopathy with procedures causing manipulation of the neck, particularly during intubation, and have recommended X-ray screening prior to an operation to identify those individuals at risk (Msall et al., 1990).

In a provocative report, Davidson (1988) noted that in excess of 500,000 individuals with Down syndrome had participated in the Special Olympics over a 17-year period without a single serious injury resulting from atlantoaxial instability. He reviewed the literature and identified 31 patients with Down syndrome with symptomatic atlantoaxial instability. In 90% of the cases, the patients had at least a one month history of symptoms of cord compression before neurological signs became apparent or irreversible. These findings suggest that the history and physical examination may be more predictive of impending spinal cord injury than the radiologic criteria currently recommended. In an attempt to improve upon the identification of individuals with Down syndrome at risk for compressive myelopathy, Pueschel et al. (1987) studied somatosensory evoked potentials (SSEP's) to determine whether subjects with asymptomatic atlantoaxial instability at risk for developing neurological symptoms and signs could be appropriate identified. The study showed no significant differences in the SSEP's between controls, asymptomatic, and symptomatic patients, but a high correspondence between SSEP latencies and odontoid-axis measurements.

A recent Dutch study has challenged the recommendations of the American Academy of Pediatrics (Cremers et al., 1993). In this study, children with Down syndrome who have atlantoaxial instability (defined as an atlantoaxial distance greater than 4 mm) were randomized into two groups. One cohort was restricted from participating in "high risk" sports and the other was not. These children were compared to a control group of similarly aged children with Down syndrome without atlantoaxial instability. One year later, there were no statistical differences in atlantoaxial distances or presence of neurological signs among the three groups. On the basis of these findings, the authors concluded that regular radiographic screening of the cervical column and restrictions from all sports was unwarranted.

The American Academy of Pediatrics defined atlantoaxial instability as a distance greater than 4.5 mm between the odontoid process of the axis and the anterior arch of the atlas. The majority of subjects (75%) in the Dutch study had an atlantoaxial distance between 4–5 mm. The mean atlantoaxial distance of the group of children with Down syndrome who were allowed to continue participating in all sports activities was 4.7 mm, a figure that would place almost half of the subjects in the nonatlantoaxial instability category, if the American Academy of Pediatrics radiographic criterion were utilized. Unfortunately, the study did not provide data as to which of the two study groups the children with atlantoaxial distances of 5–6.5 mm were randomized. Several longitudinal studies of children with Down syndrome have shown progressive widening of the atlantoaxial distance over a period of 10–15 years

(Burke et al., 1985; Pueschel et al., 1992) suggesting that a follow-up of greater than 1 year, particularly for the cohort with atlantoaxial distances greater than 5 mm, will be necessary to determine the long-term impact of "risky" sports on atlantoaxial instability in individuals with Down syndrome.

Until more precise screening methods become available to identify individuals with Down syndrome at risk for developing cord compression, the following recommendations are suggested:

1. Lateral X-ray films of the neck in the neutral, flexion, and extension positions at 3 periods of growth; 5–8 years, 10–12 years, and 18 years.
2. X-rays of the neck immediately preceding operative procedures or therapeutic programs that involve active neck movement or manipulation.
3. Parent and physician awareness of the symptoms and signs of cord compression.
4. Prompt investigation (neck X-rays, computed tomography, magnetic resonance imaging) and consideration of operative intervention, for patients with signs of myelopathy.

DOWN SYNDROME DEMENTIA

Down syndrome dementia (Alzheimer disease) has an average age of onset at 52–54 years, with as many as 75% affected by 60 years of age (Lai and Williams, 1989). Approximately 3% of the general population develop Alzheimer disease by 65 years of age and at 80 years of age, at least 8–9% have the disease. As an aging population lives longer, including those with Down syndrome, the incidence of Alzheimer disease will continue to increase. The neuropathological changes of Alzheimer disease (cortical atrophy, neurofibrillary tangles, and neuritic plaques in the hippocampus and amygdala) are present in most individuals with Down syndrome by the age of 40 years, but clinical symptoms and signs of Down syndrome dementia may remain quiescent for a decade or longer and, in some cases, dementia never becomes evident, in spite of the presence of classical neuropathological changes of Alzheimer disease. An early onset form of familial Alzheimer disease in the general population, inherited in an autosomal dominant fashion, characteristically begins in the early 50's, similar to Down syndrome dementia. It is of interest that the gene for this condition has been mapped to the long arm of chromosome 21 (St. George-Hyslop et al., 1987).

The early changes of Down syndrome dementia include personality changes, which may be manifested by apathy, social withdrawal, and day time sleepiness, followed by loss of self-help skills. Later, findings consist of deterioration of gait, speech, and memory. The onset of myoclonic seizures, on a background of significantly personality changes coupled with alterations in gait (rigidity, bradykinesia) or loss of speech and memory, is highly suggestive of Down syndrome dementia.

There are several treatable conditions common to Down syndrome which may mimic Alzheimer disease. Many of the personality changes associated with Alzheimer disease are prominent in depressed patients. Depression is not uncommon in middle age, especially in Down syndrome, as unemployment, separation from friends, and loneliness are particularly common among this population. Hypothyroidism must always be considered in the differential diagnosis of Down syndrome dementia. The prevalence of congenital hypothyroidism in Down syndrome neonates has been reported to be 28 times greater than in normal neonates (Fort et al., 1984) and autoimmune thyroiditis is more common in adolescents with Down syndrome. Hearing loss may be mistaken for dementia, due to inattentiveness, disinterest, withdrawal, and apparent loss of speech. Individuals with Down syndrome are particularly liable to develop conductive hearing loss due to stenotic ear canals, a small nasopharynx and, in children, dysfunctional eustachian tubes and adenoid and tonsil hypertrophy. In a recent study of children with Down syndrome, 66% were found to have either conductive, mixed, or sensorineural hearing losses (unilateral 28%, bilateral 38%) (Roizen et al., 1993). Similar findings have been reported in adults with Down syndrome (Keiser et al., 1981). Finally, cataracts and keratoconus are more common in adults with Down syndrome than in the general population. These disorders of the visual system may result in disinterest, withdrawal from social activities, and a loss of certain self-help skills.

With the advent of medical checklists for individuals with Down syndrome and routine screening for hypothyroidism and hearing problems, these conditions can be identified early and treated appropriately. Unfortunately, the adult with Down syndrome is less likely to be followed as closely as the child or adolescent and, therefore, treatable conditions that may mimic Alzheimer disease may be missed or overlooked. It is imperative that every physician who treats individuals with Down syndrome should be aware of those treatable conditions that may be confused with Down syndrome dementia.

REFERENCES

American Academy of Pediatrics, Committee on Sports Medicine (1984): Atlantoaxial instability in Down syndrome. Pediatrics 74:152–154.

Becker LE, Armstrong DL, Chan F (1986): Dendritic atrophy in children with Down's syndrome. Ann Neurol 20:520–526.

Burke SW, French HG, Roberts JM, Johnston CE, Whitecloud TS, Edmunds Jr OE (1985): Chronic atlantoaxial instability in Down syndrome. J Bone Joint Surg Am 67-A:1356–1360.

Coleman M (1971): Infantile spasms associated with 5-hydroxytryptophan administration in patients with Down's syndrome. Neurology 21:911–919.

Coriat LF, Fejerman N (1963): Infantile spasms in children with trisomy 21. Semin Med Pediatr 15:493–500.

Cremers MJG, Bol E, deRoos F, van Gijn J (1993): Risk of sports activities in children with Down's syndrome and atlantoaxial instability. Lancet 342:511–514.

Davidson RG (1988): Atlantoaxial instability in individuals with Down syndrome: a fresh look at the evidence. Pediatrics 81(6):857–865.

Fort P, Lifshitz F, Bellisario R, Davis J, Lanes R, Pigliese M, Richman R, Pest EM, David R (1984): Abnormalities of thyroid function in infants with Down syndrome. J Pediatr 104:545–549.

Gimenez-Roldan S, Martin M (1980): Startle epilepsy complicating Down syndrome during adulthood. Ann Neurol 7:78–80.

Guerrini R, Genton P, Bureau M, Dravet C, Roger J (1990): Reflex seizures are frequent in patients with Down syndrome and epilepsy. Epilepsia 31(4):406–417.

Keiser H, Montaque J, Wold D, Maune S, Pattison D (1981): Hearing loss of Down syndrome adults. Am J Ment Defic 85:467–472.

Lai F, Williams RS (1989): A prospective study of Alzheimer disease in Down syndrome. Arch Neurol 46:849–853.

Msall ME, Reese ME, DiGaudio K, Griswold K, Granger CV, Cooke RE (1990): Symptomatic atlantoaxial instability associated with medical and rehabilitative procedures in children with Down syndrome. Pediatrics 85:447–449.

Pearson E, Lenn NJ, Cail WS (1985): Moya moya and other causes of stroke in patients with Down syndrome. Pediatr Neurol 1:174–179.

Pollock MA, Golden GS, Schmidt R, Davis JA, Leeds N (1978): Infantile spasms in Down syndrome, a report of five cases and review of the literature. Ann Neurol 3:406–408.

Pueschel SM, Findley TW, Furia J, Gallagher PL, Scola FH, Pezzullo JC (1987): Atlantoaxial instability in Down syndrome: roentgenographic, neurologic, and somatosensory evoked potential studies. J Pediatr 110:515–521.

Pueschel SM, Louis S, McKnight P (1991): Seizure disorders in Down syndrome. Arch Neurol 48:318–320.

Pueschel SM, Scola FH, Pezzullo JC (1992): A longitudinal study of atlanto–dens relationships in asymptomatic individuals with Down syndrome. Pediatrics 89(6):1194–1198.

Roizen NJ, Walters C, Nicol T, Blondes TA (1993): Hearing loss in children with Down syndrome. J Pediatr 123:S9–S12.

St. George-Hyslop PH, Tanzi RE, Polinsky RJ, Haines JL, Nee L, Watkins PC, Myers RH, Feldman RG, Pollen D, Drackman D, Growden J, Bruni A, Fonan J-F, Salmon D, Frommett P, Amaducci L, Sorbi S, Piacentini S, Stewart GD, Hobbs WJ, Conneally PM, Gusella JF (1987): The genetic defect causing familiar Alzheimer's disease maps on chromosome 21. Science 235:885–889.

Scott BS, Petit TL, Becker LE, Edwards BAV (1982): Abnormal electric membrane properties of Down's syndrome DRG neurons in cell culture. Dev Brain Res 2:257–270.

Strafstrom CE, Patxot OF, Gilmore HE, Wisniewski KE (1991): Seizures in children with Down syndrome: Etiology, characteristics and outcome. Dev Med Child Neurol 33:191–200.

Wolcott GJ, Chun RWM (1973): Myclonic seizures in Down's syndrome. Dev Med Child Neurol 15:805–808.

Adolescence and Young Adulthood:
Issues in Medical Care, Sexuality, and Community Living

William E. Schwab

Adolescence is a time of dramatic physical and emotional change. During this stage of life young people typically experience sexual maturation, explore intimate relationships, and seek to establish their independence from their parents. For youth with Down syndrome, adolescence is a particularly important time because the presence of cognitive and other disabilities can significantly alter the natural progression to autonomy. Thoughtful, highly individualized planning is necessary to assure a successful transition from childhood to adulthood in such individuals.

MEDICAL CARE

As children with Down syndrome enter their teens, they require the same ongoing health care that their peers without Down syndrome receive. This includes treatment for acute illnesses, attention to immunization, and appropriate education about critical issues such as safety, substance abuse, depression, exercise, weight control, and sexuality. Routine check-ups with a primary care physician, nurse practitioner, or physician assistant are an important time for offering guidance about these topics and for building rapport so that the medical office becomes a place that teens feel comfortable turning to for information and advice. Youth with Down syndrome may require some adaptation in the content and format of this type of education. Coordination among the primary care provider, school personnel, and family members can facilitate the development of an independent relationship between the child with Down syndrome and his or her physician and is essential to assuring that health education is conveyed in a coherent manner.

In addition, health care providers need to continue their routine monitoring of thyroid status, auditory ability, cardiac function, and other conditions known to occur with increased frequency in individuals with Down syndrome. Radiographic cervical spine evaluation to detect atlantoaxial instability should have been performed initially earlier in childhood. There is considerable controversy about whether follow-up X-rays are necessary, but currently most protocols recommend re-screening every ten years, with more frequent X-ray assessment reserved for those whose results have been in the borderline range or who have developed symptoms. A neurologic examination should be repeatedly annually to assess for signs of cord compression as well. As skeletal maturation occurs, some of the other orthopedic problems associated with Down syndrome, such as pes planus, patello-femoral syndrome, and scoliosis, can become more significant. These may require more active intervention.

The timing of puberty and the sequence of sexual maturation are comparable to that of the general population. Some males with Down syndrome may experience the onset of pubertal changes at a slightly older age than their peers without Down syndrome, but this is extremely variable in both populations. Similarly, there have been studies that have suggested that testicular volume and penile size may be slightly decreased in males with Down syndrome, but this too is subject to considerable variability between individuals and cannot be considered characteristic of trisomy 21. Other researchers have not demonstrated this finding. It has been consistently noted that absence of testicular descent is more common in Down syndrome, occurring in more than 25% of boys.

Menstruation is quite variable in its age of occurrence in females with and without Down syndrome. No specific differences have been noted in its character or in the evolution of secondary sex characteristics, though girls who are hypothyroid or who have chronic medical problems, such as heart disease, are more likely to be delayed in their pubertal development. Most young women with Down syndrome will have regular menstrual periods after menstruation has become established. Painful menses is an occasional problem that responds well to treatment with nonsteroidal and antiinflammatory medications. This therapy is most effective when it is initiated prior to the onset of menses and is continued for at least the first three days of the menstrual period. Changes in mood, behavior, learning ability, and even motor function can occur due to cramping and other perimenstrual symptoms. Heavy menstrual bleeding and irregular periods can be a problem in women who are obese or hypothyroid. This can usually be managed with appropriate hormonal therapy.

Fertility is clearly markedly reduced in males with Down syndrome. This is thought to be due to a combination of oligospermia and chromosomal abnormalities, but this has not been well studied. There is at least one well-documented report in the medical literature of paternity involving a man with Down syndrome. The offspring in that case was genetically normal.

Women with Down syndrome are much more likely to be fertile than men. Up to 40% have a normal cyclical ovulatory pattern, while another 30% ovulate on a less predictable basis. The data on pregnancy outcomes is scant, but those studies that have been published suggest that at least one-third of offspring will have Down syndrome and that other developmental problems may be common, though it is not clear whether this is due to genetic or social factors. There is no evidence that the timing or character of menopause is different in women with Down syndrome, but this too occurs within a broad age range for all women. Some clinicians have observed that those women with Down syndrome who demonstrate evidence of premature aging are more likely to experience early menopause.

Routine health maintenance care for young men with Down syndrome should include periodic testicular palpation, as well as instruction in testicular self-examination when possible. Tumors, particularly of germ cell origin, have been reported in men with Down syndrome. It remains unclear if the true incidence is higher than in the general population. Testicular cancer is known to be markedly increased when cryptorchidism is present, so closer monitoring is indicated when an individual has an undescended testicle.

Young women should receive routine gynecological care beginning at about age eighteen, unless they become sexually active before then. Pap smears for cervical cancer screening should be done every one to three years for women who are or have been sexually active. Because cervical cancer is extremely rare in women who have not had intercourse, visual inspection and cellular sampling of the cervix is not a requisite part of their routine health care. Given that unreported sexual abuse or unacknowledged intimate relationships can occur, medical practitioners should exercise careful judgment before concluding that a specific patient does not require a pap smear. A speculum examination of the vagina and cervix, even if a pap smear is not going to be performed, remains useful for detecting the presence of infection or, rarely, of other anatomic problems. However, these conditions will usually be symptomatic. The bi-manual component of the gynecological exam is intended to detect asymptomatic uterine and ovarian abnormalities. Fibroid tumors and benign cysts are certainly possible in women with Down syndrome, though these conditions will generally produce symptoms if they become significant. Cancers have also been reported, but they most commonly occur later in life. Early detection of these tumors is desirable. There are no data to suggest any particular difference in the risk of developing these conditions.

Many women with Down syndrome will readily undergo a gynecologic examination if they are sensitively prepared for it. Anticipatory information, the presence of a familiar support person, and the establishment of a trusting relationship with the health care provider who will perform the procedure will enhance comfort and success. Modifications in the usual sequence of the gynecological evaluation may also be indicated. The speculum examination can be omitted or held until the end of the procedure if it will be unduly invasive for the woman, especially when there have been no specific problems with vaginal discharge, unusual bleeding, or past abnormal pap smears. The pap smear can be obtained with the guidance of digital palpation of the cervix rather than visual inspection if this will be better tolerated. Similarly, a bi-manual examination may be best performed with a single digit if the hymen is intact or the introitusis stenotic. Acceptance of internal examination may be improved by positioning the woman in the frog leg position and standing next to her instead of the usual lithotomy approach. It is always important to reassure the woman that this is a necessary part of her health care as a young adult and to reinforce education about sexual abuse by indicating that contact with her genitals is appropriate in this context because it is for medical reasons. With patience and sensitivity, this important aspect of routine health care can be assured without difficulty for most women with Down syndrome.

Other approaches to the pelvic examination in women with significant cognitive impairments have also been described. These include performing an examination during anesthesia for dental care or other procedures, or obtaining a pelvic ultrasound to assess for uterine and ovarian pathology. Protocols for the use of short-acting hypnotic agents, such as midazolam or ketamine, in outpatient settings where this can be safely accomplished, have also been developed. While this may be necessary at times, especially when a more thorough evaluation is essential for the assessment of bleeding, pain, or discharge, the small risk of respiratory complications that this approach entails and its impact on the woman's sense of personal control should always be thoughtfully weighed against the benefits of the examination. The use of oral benzodiazapines at anxiolytic rather than sedative doses may be successful for some women, but can often have a paradoxical effect by further impairing the woman's cognitive ability to understand what is taking place.

Annual breast examination by an experienced medical provider is another important component of routine health screening for women and should begin in young adulthood. This too will be best accomplished when there has been appropriate preparation and planning. Instruction in monthly breast self-examination is recommended when possible. Involving parents or caregivers in home breast assessment is controversial. It should only be done when there is continuing education about sexual issues, including protective behaviors. Mammography is recommended annually or biannually in all women over age 50 and in younger women known to be at increased risk due to their family history. There is no current evidence that the presence of trisomy 21 impacts on the risk of breast cancer.

SEXUALITY

As community living in more independent settings becomes more common for adolescents and young adults with Down syndrome, opportunities for the development of intimate relationships increase as well. Sexuality encompasses an individual's self-esteem, interpersonal interactions, and social experiences related to dating, marriage, and the physical aspects of sex. Sexual feelings are an intrinsic element of human emotion, and self-exploration, which leads to personal awareness of physical pleasure, is a normal part of human development. Individual sexual expression is highly influenced by family values, cultural norms, and peer-group behavior.

While most people would agree that a goal for all adolescents and young adults is entry into emotionally nurturing and physically satisfying sexual relationships as well as the avoidance of exploitation, abusive interactions, and undesired pregnancy, this does not always occur in our society. Parents and professionals who work with young people with Down syndrome must consider whether they intend to severely truncate personal independence in all spheres of life in an attempt to eliminate any possibility of intimate relationships, or whether they want to acknowledge the existence of sexual feelings and work together to foster responsible decision making.

Open discussion and accurate information are essential to facilitating positive sexual development. For youth with Down syndrome, this means tailoring educational efforts to the particular learning style of the individual. Didactic lectures or published materials may not be optimal ways to communicate. Talking about sex with family members and peers is likely to be more successful. In addition to assuring that factual material about reproduction is presented, commenting on intimate relationships as they are portrayed in the media can also be a very effective way of facilitating personal understanding.

A number of excellent formal curricula about sexuality that are specifically designed for individuals who have cognitive impairments have been written. Key educational goals in these materials are improved understanding of the nature of different types of personal relationships, development of social interaction skills, awareness of sexual feelings, knowledge of human reproduction, and facilitation of assertiveness in personal encounters, including teaching about protective behaviors to prevent undesired sexual contact. These topics can be presented as part of school materials, religious education, social group activities, or community agency programming. They can also be addressed informally within the home if desired. Health care providers, community based professionals, and parents must work together to assure the availability of this type of education.

Information about contraception is an essential part of discussions about sexuality. Individuals with Down syndrome can use all available forms of contraception. The choice must be individualized based on personal preference and ability to assure appropriate use. Barrier methods may be difficult for women with Down syndrome, because they require a high level of planning and motivation for successful use and because they must be properly inserted prior to every sexual contact. Oral contraceptive pills are generally safe and can be taken as part of a daily routine either independently or with supervision. There is increasing interest in the use of long acting progestational agents such as Depo-Provera® injections every three months or subcutaneous Norplant®, which is inserted by a minor surgical procedure and remains effective for up to five years. While these methods are not highly user dependent, they can cause troubling side effects such as menstrual irregularity, weight gain, bloating, skin changes, jaundice, and depression. Many practitioners suggest a trial of a progesterone-only contraceptive pill or an injectable preparation prior to proceeding with Norplant® insertion in order to assess the intensity of side effects, though this approach may not be fully predictive of an individual's ultimate response. Intrauterine devices are similarly less user dependent but do require self-checking to assure that they are in place. They are known to substantially increase the risk of serious pelvic infection.

Permanent sterilization is another option that individuals with Down syndrome and their families can consider. This must be done in the context of laws that may limit access to this procedure in the United States because of past abuses.

Discussion about the prevention of sexually transmitted diseases is also an essential component of sexuality education. Teaching about condom use is most effective when it includes very direct information about the proper technique for putting a condom on and removing it. Women may need assistance, usually through role playing, in learning how to insist that a condom be used. Easy access to condoms is important for all sexually active young people.

Learning about contraceptive options typically comes within a broader discussion of decision making about relationships, marriage, and childbearing. Though still unimaginable to some people, an increasing number of individuals with cognitive disabilities are choosing to marry and to parent. It is imperative that young people with Down syndrome receive the information necessary to make responsible choices. Men with Down syndrome need to be aware of their reduced fertility and to also understand that this does not mean that they and their partners can forego contraception with absolute certainty or that they do not have to consider sexually transmitted disease prevention. Women with Down syndrome need to learn about the possibility that their children could have Down syndrome or other developmental problems so that they can make an informed decision about pregnancy. Men and women need the opportunity to very seriously consider the intense responsibility that intimate relationships and having children entails, and to develop a realistic understanding of the amount of support they might need from others.

COMMUNITY LIVING

The physical changes of puberty are often what triggers consideration of important adolescent issues in families. Sexuality is just one area that requires attention. Substance abuse is another issue that is all too often neglected. Studies have shown that smoking, alcoholism, and abuse of prescription and illicit drugs are greatly underrecognized in people with disabilities. Individuals may initially experiment with these agents in response to peer modeling or pressure and to their perception of societal expectations. Isolation, low self-esteem, and emotional stress may contribute to continued use, which can lead to addiction. Substance abuse, especially when it is surreptitious, frequently leads to significant social problems and can complicate therapy for medical conditions. Treatment programs often find it difficult to adapt their approaches to meet the needs of people with developmental disabilities. Adolescents with Down syndrome should have the opportunity to participate in educational programs on this topic with other teenagers. Family members and professionals need to maintain an awareness of substance abuse issues as they work with young adults with Down syndrome in the community.

For youth with Down syndrome, active efforts may be required to promote the development of positive self-esteem and accurate self-identity. These allow the adolescent to appreciate him- or herself as a whole person with a unique combination of strengths and limitations. This understanding is necessary before the adolescent can assume greater independence and self-direction. Every attempt must be made to assure that the teenager with Down syndrome is able to exercise as much personal choice and control as possible under the guidance of family, friends, and professionals in preparation for adult life. This includes acceptance of the fact that making mistakes can be an important part of the learning process.

Future planning is a crucial activity during the adolescent years. This involves setting realistic goals for adult life and assuring that the educational, social, and medical services being received by a child with Down syndrome will support the attainment of these goals. Such transition planning usually requires multidisciplinary discussion and action. In the United States, this is a mandated component of special education services. Ultimately, future opportunities are defined by a combination of community resources, family values, and individual preferences and abilities.

In a recent survey, primary care physicians indicated a substantial interest in working in partnership with families and community-based professions to comprehensively meet the needs of individuals with cognitive impairments. They also identified a need for technical assistance so that they can expand their own knowledge bases about appropriate health care of specific conditions, including Down syndrome. Issues like sexuality and substance abuse require a coordinated approach if they are to be successfully addressed. People with Down syndrome will be best served by active collaboration among all of the people in their lives. This is particularly important during the adolescent years.

SUGGESTED READINGS

Bovicelli L, et al. (1982): Reproduction in Down syndrome. Obstet Gynecol 59(6)(supplement):13S–17S.

Cohen WI (1992): "Down Syndrome Preventive Medical Check List." Pittsburgh: Ohio/Western Pennsylvania Down Syndrome Network.

Cooley WC, Graham Jr, JM (1991): Common syndromes and management issues for primary care physicians. Clin Pediat 30(4):233–253.

Dexeus FH, et al. (1988): Genetic abnormalities in men with germ cell tumors. J Urol 140:80–84.

Elkins TE (1992): Gynecologic care. In Pueschel SM, Pueschel JK (Eds.): "Biomedical Concerns in Persons with Down Syndrome," pp. 139–146. Baltimore: Brookes.

Elkins TE, et al. (1988): A clinical observation of a program to accomplish pelvic exams in difficulty-to-manage patients with mental retardation. Adolesc Pediatr Gynecol 1:195–198.

Heighway S, Kidd Webster S, Shaw M (Eds.) (1988): "STARS: Skills Training for Assertiveness, Relationship-Building, and Sexual Awareness." Madison, WI: Waisman Center.

Minihan PM, Dean DH, Lyons CM (1993): Managing the care of patients with mental retardation: A survey of physicians. Ment Retard 31(4):239–246.

Patterson PM (1991): "Doubly Silenced: Sexuality, Sexual Abuse, and People with Developmental Disabilities." Madison, WI: Wisconsin Council on Developmental Disabilities.

Pueschel SM, et al. (1985): Adolescent development in males with Down Syndrome. AJDC 139:236–238.

Pueschel SM, Blaymore Bier J (1992): Endocrinologic aspects. In Pueschel SM, Pueschel JK (Eds.): "Biomedical Concerns in Persons with Down Syndrome," pp. 259–272. Baltimore: Brookes.

Schwab WE (1992): Sexuality and community living. In Lott It, McCoy EE (Eds.): "Down Syndrome: Advances in Medical Care," pp. 157–166. New York: Wiley-Liss.

Schwab WE (1992): Substance abuse in patients with physical and cognitive disabilities. In Fleming MF, Barry BL (Eds.): "Addictive Disorders," pp. 287–2990. St. Louis: Mosby Year Book.

Sheridan R, et al. (1989): Fertility in a male with trisomy 21. J Med Genet 26:294–298.

Sobsey D, et al. (Eds.) (1991): "Disability, Sexuality, and Abuse: An Annotated Bibliography." Baltimore: Brookes.

Summers JA (Ed.) (1986): "The Right to Grow Up." Baltimore: Brookes.

Turnbull HR, et al. (1989): "Disability and the Family: A Guide to Decisions for Adulthood." Baltimore: Brookes.

United States Department of Health and Human Services Public Health Service, Health Resources and Services Administration, Maternal and Child Health Bureau (1992): "Moving On: Transition from Child-Centered to Adult Health Care for Youth with Disabilities." Washington, DC: U.S. Government Printing Office.

United States Preventive Services Task Force, Lawrence RS (1989): "Guide to Clinical Preventive Services." Baltimore: Williams and Wilkins.

Clinical Follow-up of Adolescents and Adults with Down Syndrome

Alberto Rasore-Quartino and Marco Cominetti

INTRODUCTION

Progress in medical care and early rehabilitation have led to a general normalization of the life of children with Down syndrome. They can attend normal school, participate in sports, and enjoy their lives like their normal peers. After school age, increasing health problems are encountered. Even as social inclusion is becoming a current reality, good medical treatment is not yet available for adolescents and adults with Down syndrome.

Life expectancy for persons with Down syndrome is approaching that of the general population (Table 1). The number of adults has increased over the years and the trend is expected to continue in the near future (Baird and Sadovnick, 1988) (Table 2). Accurate knowledge of the most frequently observed diseases in this age range is required and subsequent measures have to be taken in order to ensure a good quality of life. The main difficulties found in the follow-up of adults with Down syndrome result from the reduced interest about health problems among the patients' relatives, the atypical presentation and lack of clear-cut symptoms of the diseases and the low compliance of the patients and their families towards the therapies.

Medical controls must have a multidisciplinary character, concerning a number of clinical specialities, although with coordinated programs (Carey, 1992). A schematic protocol for the follow-up of adolescents and adults is proposed, based on yearly controls (Table 3). The rationale for the periodic controls listed above will be explained in detail, pointing out the peculiar presentation and increased frequency of some diseases.

GENERAL GUIDELINES FOR THE FOLLOW-UP

For adults with Down syndrome, medical and neuropsychiatric examinations should be made every year, in order to assess the patient's well-being. An important concern is the necessity of avoiding overdoctoring; it therefore seems reasonable not to emphasize the medical approach. It is also important to have specialists' examina-

238

Table 1. Life Expectancy of Persons with Down Syndrome

Year	Life expectancy
1929	9 years
1947	12 years
1970	55.3 years (male)
	52.7 years (female)

tions for sensory defects, which can greatly reduce the acquisition of mental abilities, even if appropriate rehabilitation programs are established.

Ocular abnormalities are frequent and emphasis should be laid on strabismus and refractive efforts that can impair correct vision, thereby adding an organic defect to the mental disability. Cataracts and keratoconus can develop with advancing age. Every impairment of vision is dangerous for the maintenance of physical and mental abilities. Corrections, either prothesic or surgical, must be taken into consideration. Yearly examinations are advised.

Up to 70% of persons with Down syndrome have some hearing defect, most of which are of the conductive type, due to repeated middle ear infections, developing chiefly in childhood. Treatment of ear infections seldom is completed, because symptoms, like pain and discharge, are of short duration, and chronicity often ensues. Underlying anatomical malformations, even minor ones, like narrowing of the Eustachian tubes, are factors that can add to the auditory defects, worsening them. Partial hearing defects are often not diagnosed in childhood if the child is alert and shows progress in rehabilitation programs. Their effects can be more severe in middle age, causing the patient to become withdrawn. Specific therapies and surgical options should be available, and hearing aids, if tolerated, are very useful.

Orthopedic disorders in Down syndrome are chiefly the consequence of ligamentous laxity. Pes planus, subluxing patella, hip dysplasia, slipped capital femoral epiphysis, and scoliosis are frequently observed. A recently focused problem is atlantoaxial instability. It can be observed in 10–15% of persons with Down syn-

Table 2. Increased Survival Rate of Persons with Down Syndrome

Year	Survival rate
1944–55	60% dead before 10 years
1963	25% surviving to the age of 30 years
	4% surviving to the age of 50–55 years
1970	71% alive at 30 years
	79% alive at 30 years (without heart disease)

Table 3. Guidelines for the Clinical Follow-up of Adolescents and Adults with Down Syndrome

Procedure	Frequency
Clinical examination	once a year
Neurologic and psychiatric examination	once a year
Nutritional and dietary counseling	once a year
Orthopedic control	once a year
Dental control	once a year
Audiometric control	once a year
Ophthalmologic control	once a year
Gynecologic control	once a year
Serologic tests for thyroid disorders, autoimmune disorders, intestinal malabsorption, immunologic deficiencies, etc.	once a year

drome. It is generally asymptomatic, but it can lead to luxation, causing cord compression, whose consequences can be very severe: sensory disturbances, abnormal gait, torticollis, and, in rare instances, even death (Pueschel and Scola, 1987). Persons at risk can be detected by lateral cervical radiographs in flexion, extension, and neutral positions. If the distance between the posterior margin of the anterior arch of the atlas and the odontoid process of the axis is more than 5 mm, there is positive risk of luxation upon minor trauma. High resolution CT scan or Magnetic Resonance Imaging are also diagnostic; the real significance of the radiographs in diagnosing atlantoaxial instability has been questioned, due to the lack of correspondence between the imaging and the clinical symptoms.

Accurate neurological examinations are important for the diagnosis of the initial symptoms. In any case, a correct assessment of the instability should be performed in adolescents and young adults engaging in sports particularly dangerous for articulation, including tumbling, boxing, diving, etc.

Dental anomalies constitute a well-known problem that is generally underestimated given the actual difficulties encountered in the management of mentally handicapped people. Unusual dental and oral anatomy, developmental anomalies, and malocclusions are common in Down syndrome, while dental caries is less frequent than in normal people. When oral hygiene is poor, it leads to gingivitis, subsequent periodontal disease, and early and total tooth loss. Dental examinations should therefore be performed not only in childhood, but also in adulthood. Orthodontic help should be available at any age, so as to avoid the disruptive consequences of progressive dental decay (Lowe, 1990).

Pulmonary hypoplasia and immunological impairment are major causes of the increased frequency of respiratory infections in Down syndrome. Even today, mortality from respiratory infections is prevalent in persons with Down syndrome. Congenital heart defects, if not corrected, can lead to pulmonary artery hypertension, a facilitating background for recurrent respiratory infections. They can also lead to the secondary development of pulmonary vascular obstructive disease, a very severe, life-threatening condition (Spicer, 1984). A striking, unexpected decreased incidence of bronchial asthma has recently been found in a study of more than 500 children and adults with Down syndrome in our center; no explanation has been given up to now (Forni et al., 1990).

Although congenital heart defects in Down syndrome have always been stressed, because of their frequency and of the devastating consequences on development and life itself, less data are available on cardiac status in adults with Down syndrome, compared to children. From recent literature records, it becomes evident that adults also have cardiac problems other than congenital defects. The most frequent anomalies found in asymptomatic adults are mitral valve prolapse (MVP) and aortic regurgitation (AR) with a prevalence of about 70%. These defects seem to occur only in adults, since they have never been detected in children (Goldhaber et al., 1987). MVP has been associated with disorders characterized by laxity of connective tissue, such as Marfan's or Ehlers-Danlos Syndromes, so the connective tissue abnormalities that are almost constant in Down syndrome might explain the increased frequency of these cardiac defects. Accurate cardiac diagnostic investigations are therefore recommended in young adults, especially before dental and surgical procedures, for the presence of valve defects. Antibiotic prophylaxis for endocarditis should also be taken into consideration.

With increasing age, the reduced immunological competence of Down syndrome is responsible for increased infectious episodes, particularly of the skin. Autoimmune disorders, with protean clinical manifestations, are most frequently observed: hypothyroidism, diabetes mellitus, alopecia, chronic active hepatitis, and autoimmune thrombocytopenia are the most common.

Neurologic problems become more prevalent with increasing age, including seizures. There is, moreover, a constant, though slow and variable, decline of intelligence. A reduction in thought elaboration ability, in particular abstract thought and logical performance, both inductive and deductive, is likely to occur shortly after the age of 30. Dementia is also characteristic of aging in Down syndrome, showing striking similarities with Alzheimer disease. At present there is no procedure able to slow down this pathologic process. It is noteworthy that persons with Down syndrome for whom early rehabilitation has been available are just now reaching adulthood. It is possible that intensive stimulation and social inclusion will prove to be beneficial in slowing down precocious aging and mental deterioration. Recent research, mapping the gene for Alzheimer disease to the long arm of chromosome 21, has brought to light the problem of presenile dementia, awakening new interest in its relationships with Down syndrome (St. George-Hyslop et al., 1987).

HYPOTHYROIDISM

Since the first descriptions of Down syndrome almost a century ago, hypothyroidism was considered a constant feature of the syndrome. When laboratory tests for thyroid function became available, it was evident that most persons with Down syndrome are actually euthyroid. Nevertheless, it was also demonstrated that a higher incidence of thyroid disorders, mainly hypothyroidism, is characteristic of Down syndrome. According to the literature, congenital hypothyroidism in Down syndrome varies from 0.7–10%, whereas in the general population it varies from 0.015–0.020%. Figures for acquired hypothyroidism are also largely variable (13–54% versus 0.8–1.1%) (Fort et al., 1984).

Two forms of hypothyroidism can be distinguished. The most frequent one, the so-called compensated hypothyroidism, shows only increased levels of TSH, with T_3 and T_4 values within normal limits. Strictly speaking, it shouldn't even be called hypothyroidism, since thyroid function is still normal. It can represent only a temporary phase preceding a probable hypofunctional condition. Increased TSH represents a central response to the reduction of functional thyroid tissue and is followed by a progressive decrease of T_3 and T_4 levels. Although this is generally the course of the disease, in Down syndrome TSH values often fluctuate without any modification of thyroid function. These transient thyroid neuroregulatory dysfunctions are possibly related to inappropriate secretion of TSH or to insensitivity to TSH.

In our center, the thyroid function of 254 persons with Down syndrome aged 1–40 years has been studied. Among them there were 62 adolescents or adults (age range 13–40 years). 58 patients with TSH values above normal (5 µU/ml) were found (22.8%)—21 in the older age group (33.85%). In all, there were 21 individuals with T_3, T_3 uptake, and T_4 values at the hypothyroid level (8.2%), 12 of whom were adolescents or adults (19%) (Table 4). An increased frequency of thyroid antibodies has also been found. In particular, antimicrosomial antibodies were more frequently associated with high TSH (Table 5). Clinically, only one patient showed any sign of hypothyroidism, mainly in behavioral terms. The only clinically positive subject had a history of unexplained increasing weight over a period of several months before being examined. He had developed an evident goiter and was clearly mixedematous. According to his parents, he had become lazy, was easily fatigued, and was always drowsy.

Substitute therapy with levothyroxine was started in all the hypothyroid subjects, irrespective of their clinical status, at the lowest dosage sufficient to bring the circulating hormones to normal levels. Significantly lower IQs were found in persons with Down syndrome having both abnormal TSH and T_4 values, compared to persons with only elevated TSH levels.

In our study, there were no differences between the two groups; it is possible that

Table 4. Hypothyroidism in Down Syndrome (254 cases)

Measure	Number of cases
High TSH/normal T_3, T_4	58 (22.8%)
High TSH/low T_3, T_4	21 (8.2%)

Table 5. Thyroid Antibodies in Down Syndrome (117 cases)

MsAb (IU/ml)	*n*	TSH (μU/ml)
<50	108	3.06
>50	9	10.9
TgAb (IU/ml)	*n*	TSH (μU/ml)
<50	83	3.053
>50	34	5.3

the absence of any effect on IQ, as well as the absence of clinical features we found in our hypothyroid population, can be related to the early diagnosis. Actually, the only patient for whom the diagnosis was delayed exhibited clear features of hypothyroidism, albeit we didn't have comparative IQs at different stages. The results of our investigations confirm that persons with Down syndrome are at increased risk of developing hypothyroidism at any age. One person with Down syndrome out of 12 has either compensated or subclinical hypothyroidism. Since untreated hypothyroidism may interfere with normal neuronal function, causing decreased intellectual abilities, appropriate substitutive therapy is strongly recommended.

Generally in Down syndrome hypothyroidism is the consequence of autoimmune destruction of functioning thyroid tissue and a subsequent reduced synthesis of hormone.

Initially, only increased TSH values are detected, then hormone deficiency develops (reduced T_3 and T_4). With progression of the disease, clinical symptoms appear. Unfortunately they may go unrecognized or be mistaken for the features of the syndrome itself (dullness, increased fatigability, loss of attention, etc.), chiefly in adolescents and adults. Periodical controls of thyroid function are therefore mandatory in childhood and during the whole lifespan, in order to detect decreased activity in time and to start a suitable treatment.

CELIAC DISEASE

Only recently the relationship between Down syndrome and celiac disease has been demonstrated, with a frequency well above that of the general population, in the still partially explored field of the association between Down syndrome and autoimmune disorders.

Celiac disease, or gluten intolerance, in its typical form, is a rather uncommon severe disease developing in early childhood, after the introduction of gluten into the diet. It manifests with diarrhea, bulky stools, prominent abdomen, and poor thriving.

At present, more frequent atypical or moderate forms are found, appearing in late childhood or adolescence and showing scarce or absent intestinal symptoms, hypovitaminosis, anemia, and stunted growth. IgG and IgA gliadin antibodies have been considered a reliable and simple screening test to detect subjects eligible for intestinal biopsy, substituting for the more common xylose test.

The first observation of gliadin antibodies (AGAs) in persons with Down syndrome clearly showed an excess of positive results not confirmed by the bioptic results. IgA AGAs, which are more specific, are positive in about 30% of subjects, whereas IgG AGAs, less specific but more sensitive, are even more often positive (Storm, 1990). A more reliable, highly specific screening test for celiac disease seems to be the antiendomysium immunofluorescence test, whose only drawback is its high cost.

In order to evaluate the sensitivity and specificity of the different tests for celiac disease, we studied 169 persons with Down syndrome ranging in age from 1–50 years. IgG AGAs were determined in 128 and were found to be positive in 65 (50.8%). IgA AGAs were determined in 169 and positive in 34 (20.1%), while antiendomysium antibodies (AEAs) were determined in 108 subjects and positive in 6 (3.5%).

Intestinal biopsies (duodenal–jejunal biopsies) were performed in 11 persons for whom informal consent had been obtained. The only three positive biopsies, that is with flattening of the intestinal mucosa, were from one child and two adults with both positive IgA AGAs and AEAs. The remaining eight individuals all had positive IgA AGAs, but negative AEAs (performed in only four persons). Three of them showed an aspecific inflammatory pattern of the intestinal mucosa; the remaining five were definitely normal. As for the three patients with positive biopsies, two were asymptomatic; only one, a 30-year-old obese woman, had long-lasting diarrhea, iron deficiency anemia, and hypotension. When she was put on a gluten-free diet, a marked improvement of her health status occurred, along with the cessation of her diarrhea, although her compliance became poor after a short time. Later she developed hypothyroidism. As for the remaining two patients, there was a debate on the necessity of introducing a gluten-free diet, because of the absence of significant intestinal disorders or of any sign referable to gluten intolerance. Finally, it was decided to begin with it, due to the dangers of late complications like intestinal malignancies, or the possible occurrence of the consequences of global malabsorption.

The pathogenesis of celiac disease is still controversial: recent studies attribute the mucosal damage an abnormal immune response to gliadin (Marsh, 1992).

CONCLUSIONS

If a somewhat effective program of specific controls has been provided for the child with Down syndrome, this is not true yet for the adult. The diseases affecting this population are often misdiagnosed or underestimated.

The main difficulties of obtaining thorough knowledge of the pathological problems of these persons have been due to the relatively low number reaching adult age and, more often, the lack of relatives caring for them, thus rendering very difficult an effective clinical follow-up.

In this context, programs of periodical clinical controls have been proposed, taking into consideration the peculiar aspects of the different ages and, therefore, the different demands. It is our opinion that every program should be flexible enough, in order to avoid medical dependence. It is also important that general suggestions of specific controls be readily available for those who care for persons with Down syndrome of whatever age, from infancy to adulthood, to prevent the secondary disabilities we know to occur with increased frequency and that actually can hinder successful rehabilitation or social integration and, consequently, a better quality of life.

REFERENCES

Baird PA, Sadovnick AD (1988): Life expectancy in Down syndrome adults. Lancet ii:1354–1356.

Carey JC (1992): Health supervision and anticipatory guidance for children with genetic disorders (including specific recommendations for trisomy 21, trisomy 18 and Neurofibromatosis I). Pediat Clin N Am 39:25–53.

Forni GL, Rasore-Quartino A, Acutis MS, Strigini P (1990): Incidence of bronchial asthma in Down syndrome. J Pediat 116:487 (letter).

Fort P, Lifschitz F, Bellisario R, Davis J, Lanes R, Pugliese M, Richman R, Post EM, David R (1984): Abnormalities of thyroid function in infants with Down syndrome. J Pediat 104:545–549.

Goldhaber SZ, Brown WD, St. John Shutton MG (1987): High frequency of mitral valve prolapse and aortic regurgitation among asymptomatic adults with Down's syndrome. JAMA 258:1793–1795.

Lowe O (1990): Dental problems. In: Van Dyke DC, Lang DJ, Heide F, Van Duyne S, Soucek MG (Eds.): "Clinical perspectives in the management of Down syndrome," pp. 72–79. New York: Springer-Verlag.

Marsh MN (1992): Gluten, major hystocompatibility complex and the small intestine. A molecular and immunobiologic approach to the spectrum of gluten sensitivity ("celiac sprue"). Gastroenterol 102:330–354.

Pueschel SM, Scola FH (1987): Atlantoaxial instability in individuals with Down syndrome: Epidemiologic, radiographic and clinical studies. Pediatrics 80:555–560.

St. George-Hyslop PH, Tanzi RE, Polinsky RJ, Haines JL, Nee JL, Watkins C, Myers RH, Feldman RG, Pollen D, Drachman D, Growdon J, Bruni A, Foncin JF, Salmon D, Frommelt P, Amaducci L, Sorbi S, Piacentini S, Stewart D, Hobbs WJ, Conneally PM, Gusella JF (1987): The genetic defect causing familial Alzheimer's disease maps on chromosome 21. Science 235:885–890.

Spicer RL (1984): Cardiovascular disease in Down syndrome. Pediat Clin N Am 31:1331–1343.

Storm W (1990): Prevalence and diagnostic significance of gliadin antibodies in children with Down syndrome. Eur J Pediatr 149:833–834.

VII. Community Participation

Perspective

Mitchell Levitz

My name is Mitchell Levitz. I am 22 years old and live in Westchester County, near New York City. I attended my local schools and had both regular education and special education for students with disabilities. I graduated with a high school diploma. I think that students with disabilities should be able to be included in regular education with other students so that they can make friends and have the same opportunity as all other students. I always felt a part of my community and participated in scouts, competitive soccer league, summer camps, and religious education related to my bar mitzvah. Now I serve on the ritual committee of my synagogue.

I have learned from personal experience that it makes a lot of sense for young people with Down syndrome to begin early having experiences with jobs so that they can have a chance to prepare for careers in today's society. I learned about different kinds of job skills when I was in school by having volunteer work experiences and paid employment.

After finishing high school, I worked as a teller at a bank and now I am working 4 days a week as an office assistant at the Peekskill Chamber of Commerce. I take public transportation to work. I am being trained on the computer and I use the fax machine, the copier and do filing. I have prepared mailings and special projects. And I answer the phones and provide information. I also help walk-in customers with directions or events in our community. What I like most about this job is when I go to the bank, post office, city hall, and do all the business for the office staff. I meet people I know who live and work in town. When I am with my friends and family, I like water skiing, downhill skiing, tennis, and ping pong. I enjoy travelling, eating pizza, watching basketball, and wrestling. Every day I read the newspaper so that I know what is happening in the world.

Now I am serving on the governmental affairs committee of the New York State ARC and a community action committee for my local school district. I will be helping with geopolitical campaigns, taking a course at Westchester Community College, and joining advocacy groups.

After high school, I lived in a traditional apartment and learned to cook, clean, shop, and budget my money. Next month, I'll be moving into a house, living independently and sharing the rent with a few other people.

Something very exciting for me and my friend, Jason Kingsley, was writing our book. It's called, "Count Us In: Growing up with Down Syndrome." It is published by Harcourt Brace & Co. We have been on a national book tour and are doing public appearances.

My career goals are being in politics and government. Part of this is to help other people like myself. I believe that it is important to talk to people and listen to their concerns. Being an advocate allows you to speak for yourself and for others on issues that affect people with disabilities, including health care and equal rights for all individuals and laws to prevent discrimination in schools, the community, and employment opportunities. It is important for us to make sure that the leaders of our country are informed about these and other issues. This happens by getting parents, professionals, people with disabilities, and the community together to work out solutions.

My message to all of you is to keep your minds open to the idea that we should be able to make our own choices. If young people with Down syndrome are given opportunities to have many experiences in life, we will be better prepared to make decisions for ourselves. My advice to you is to encourage children and young adults with Down syndrome to have dreams and goals and to believe that success comes from belief in ourselves.

Living in the Community:
Beyond the Continuum

Steven J. Taylor

Recent years have seen the emergence of new approaches to supporting people with Down syndrome and other developmental disabilities to live in the community. Referred to as "supported living" or "housing and supports," these approaches represent a radical departure from the traditional continuum of residential services. This chapter provides a critique of the traditional least restrictive environment (LRE) continuum and describes the characteristics of a supported living approach.

THE RESIDENTIAL CONTINUUM

Since its earliest conceptualization, the LRE principle has been defined operationally in terms of a continuum, an ordered sequence of placements that vary according to the degree of restrictiveness. A common way of representing the LRE continuum is a straight line running from the most to the least restrictive alternative or, alternatively, a hierarchical cascade of placement options (see Hitzing, 1980; Reynolds, 1962; Schalock, 1983). The most restrictive placements are also the most segregated and offer the most intensive services; the least restrictive placements are the most integrated and independent and offer the least intensive services. The assumption is that every person with a developmental disability can be located somewhere along this continuum based on individual needs.

The residential continuum runs from institutions (the most restrictive environment) to independent living (the least restrictive environment). Between these extremes are nursing homes and private institutions, community intermediate care facilities for the mentally retarded, community residences or group homes, foster care, and semiindependent living or transitional apartments. Figure 1 depicts a traditional continuum model of residential services.

The residential continuum assumes that people with developmental disabilities will move progressively to less and less restrictive environments and, ideally, to independent living. A common justification of institutions is that they prepare people with developmental disabilities, especially those with severe disabilities, to live in

THE RESIDENTIAL CONTINUUM

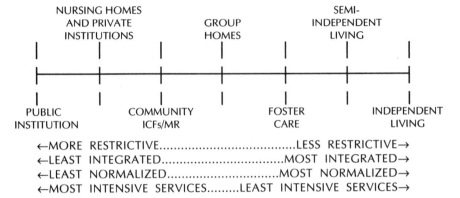

Fig. 1. The traditional residential continuum model.

less restrictive environments (see Crissey and Rosen, 1986; Walsh and McCalion, 1987).

THE NEW COMMUNITY-BASED CONTINUUM

A failure to examine critically the principle of the least restrictive environment has led to the creation of a new "community-based" continuum. Critiques of the traditional continuum rightfully reject the most restrictive and segregated environments and the assumption that segregated settings prepare people to function in integrated settings (Bronston, 1980; Galloway, 1980; Haring and Hansen, 1981; Hitzing, 1980, 1987). Yet these critiques stop short of rejecting the LRE principle itself, which underlies the continuum concept. A community-based continuum is emerging as a guiding principle for the design of services for people with developmental disabilities and their families. Like the traditional continuum, this new continuum envisions a series of options varying in restrictiveness, integration, and normalization, with a preference—but not a mandate—for the least restrictive and most integrated and normalized settings. It is also generally assumed that people with the most severe disabilities will be found in the more restrictive and less integrated environments. In contrast to the traditional continuum, the community-based continuum eliminates totally segregated environments located at the most restrictive end of the scale. The range of acceptable options is confined to settings "in the community" that provide for at least some degree of interaction with nondisabled people.

The community-based residential continuum includes settings that range from group living arrangements on the most restrictive end to independent living on the least restrictive end. Specific residential programs found in the community-based continuum include small community-based intermediate care facilities for the mentally retarded, community residents or group homes, three- to four-person "minigroup homes," apartment clusters, supervised apartments, and "semiindependent living situations" (Halpern, Close, and Nelson, 1986). As in the case of the traditional continuum, it is assumed that people with severe disabilities will be served in the more restrictive congregate settings, albeit small by institutional standards, and people with mild disabilities will live in less restrictive, smaller apartments.

PITFALLS IN THE LRE PRINCIPLE

Outside of discussions of its legal and constitutional dimensions (Burgdorf, 1980; Turnbull, 1981), the LRE principle, as a policy direction, has received relatively little critical analysis in the field of developmental disabilities. The soundness of the principle generally has been assumed. While books, articles, and policies have been written on living and learning in the least restrictive environment (Bruininks and Lakin, 1985), the meaning and implications of the principle as a foundation upon which to build services have not been thoroughly and critically explored.

It is difficult to arrive at a precise definition of LRE, because the term is used so diversely by people in the field. However, out of the many usages a common meaning can be identified. The principles of LRE for residential, educational, vocational, and other services may be defined as follows: services for people with developmental disabilities should be designed according to a range of program options varying in terms of restrictiveness, normalization, independence, and integration, with a presumption in favor of environments that are least restrictive and most normalized, independent, and integrated. The LRE principle and associated continuum model are characterized by seven serious conceptual and philosophical flaws (Taylor, 1988).

1. *The LRE principle legitimates restrictive environments.* A principle that contains a presumption in favor of the least restrictive environment implies that there are circumstances under which the most restrictive environment would be appropriate. In other words, to conceptualize services in terms of restrictiveness is to legitimate more restrictive settings. As long as services are conceptualized in this manner, some people will end up in restrictive environments. In most cases, they will be people with severe disabilities.

2. *The LRE principle confuses segregation and integration, on the one hand, with intensity of services, on the other.* As represented by the continuum, LRE equates segregation with the most intensive services and integration with the least intensive services. The principle assumes that the least restrictive, most integrated settings are incapable of providing the intensive services needed by people with severe disabilities.

When viewed from this perspective, it follows that people with severe disabilities will require the most restrictive and segregated settings. However, segregation and integration on the one hand and intensity of services on the other, are separate dimensions. In fact, some of the most segregated settings have provided the least effective services (Blatt and Kaplan, 1966; Blatt et al., 1979; Center on Human Policy, 1979).

3. *The LRE principle is based on a "readiness model."* Implicit in LRE is the assumption that people with developmental disabilities must earn the right to move to the least restrictive environment. In other words, the person must "get ready" or "be prepared" to live, work, or go to school in integrated settings, with many residential and vocational programs designed to be "transitional."

The irony is that the most restrictive placements do not prepare people for the least restrictive placements. Institutions do not prepare people for community living, segregated day programs do not prepare people for competitive work, and segregated schooling does not prepare students for integrated schooling.

4. *The LRE principle supports the primacy of professional decision making.* Integration is ultimately a moral and philosophical issue, not a professional one. Yet LRE invariably is framed in terms of professional judgments regarding "individual needs." The phrase "least restrictive environment" is almost always qualified with words such as "appropriate," "necessary," "feasible," and "possible" (and never with "desired" or "wanted"). Professionals are left to determine what is appropriate, possible, feasible, or necessary for any particular individual.

5. *The LRE principle sanctions infringements on people's rights.* LRE is a seductive concept; government should act in a manner that least restricts the rights and liberties of individuals. When applied categorically to people with developmental disabilities, however, the LRE principle sanctions infringements on basic rights to freedom and community participation beyond those imposed on nondisabled people. The question implied by LRE is not whether people with developmental disabilities should be restricted, but to what extent (Turnbull, 1981, p. 17).

6. *The LRE principle implies that people must move as they develop and change.* As LRE is commonly conceptualized, people with developmental disabilities are expected to move toward increasingly less restrictive environments. Schalock (1983) writes: "The existence of a functioning system of community services would provide a range of living and training environments that facilitate client movement along a series of continua" (p. 22).

Even if people moved smoothly through a continuum, their lives would be a series of stops between transitional placements. People with developmental disabilities sometimes move to "less restrictive environments" only because new programs open up or space is needed to accommodate people with more severe disabilities. This can destroy any sense of home and may disrupt relationships with roommates, neighbors, and friends.

7. *The LRE principle directs attention to physical settings rather than to the services and supports people need to be integrated into the community.* As Gunnar Dybwad (personal communication, February, 1985) has stated, "Every time we identify a need in this field, we build a building." By its nature, the principle of the least restrictive environment emphasizes facilities and environments designed specifically for people with developmental disabilities. The field of developmental disabilities has defined the mission in terms of creating "facilities," first large ones

and now smaller ones, and "programs," rather than providing the services and supports to enable people with developmental disabilities to participate in the same settings used by other people.

HOMES, NOT FACILITIES

In contrast to the LRE continuum model, a supported living approach focuses on the person, not the facility or the program. As developed by agencies like Options in Community Living in Wisconsin, Centennial Developmental Services in Colorado, and others (Taylor et al., 1991; also see O'Brien, 1994), this approach has the following characteristics.

1. *Separation of housing and support services.* In traditional residential programs, a single agency both owns or rents the facility and provides the staff services and supports needed by the people living there. In a supported living approach, people with disabilities or their families own or rent their homes; agencies coordinate or provide the services people need to live successfully in the community. Since people are not guests in someone else's residence, they have maximum control over their personal living space. They do not have to fit into an existing program.

2. *Choice in living arrangements.* Such matters as the location of people's homes and the selection of roommates are based on personal preferences and choices, rather than being predetermined by agency policies. While some people may choose to live alone, supported living should not be equated with one person per home.

3. *Flexible services.* Under the continuum approach, people were expected to leave their residence as their service needs changed. If they required less intensive services, they moved to a less restrictive setting; if they required more intensive services, they moved to a more restrictive setting. Since a supported living approach separates housing and supports, people can receive more or less intensive services while remaining in their homes. The services can range from live-in support to various forms of part-time or drop-in assistance. This support or assistance can be provided by paid roommates, neighbors, and personal-assistance aides as well as regular agency staff.

4. *Increased control over services.* Traditionally, people with developmental disabilities have had little or no say over who provided support for them. Many supported living agencies are attempting to involve people in the selection and supervision of support staff or personal-assistance aides. For example, at Wisconsin's Options in Community Living, the agency helps many of the people it supports to find and hire personal-assistance aides.

5. *Emphasis on personal relationships.* Supported living should not be viewed as a "model" or "program," but a different philosophy of helping people with developmental disabilities to enjoy meaningful lives in the community. Central to this philosophy is an emphasis on personal relationships between people with developmental disabilities and friends, family members, and nondisabled community members. Some supported-living agencies employ "community builders" or include this role in the job descriptions of all staff. Friendships and unpaid relationships are not intended to replace paid staff, but to assist people in becoming part of the community (Bogdan and Taylor, 1987).

CONCLUSION

The principle of the least restrictive environment was extremely forward-looking for its time. It emerged in an era in which people with developmental disabilities and their families were offered segregation or nothing at all. As a legal concept and policy direction, LRE helped to create options and alternatives.

It is now time to find new ideas, concepts, and principles to guide us. The LRE principle defined the challenge in terms of creating less restrictive and more integrated and normalized environments and programs. Now we must define the challenge in terms of helping people with developmental disabilities to live successfully in their own homes in the community.

ACKNOWLEDGMENTS

This chapter was prepared with partial support of the Research and Training Center on Community Integration, Center on Human Policy, School of Education, Syracuse University, supported by the U.S. Department of Education, Office of Special Education and Rehabilitative Services, National Institute on Disability and Rehabilitation Research, through Cooperative Agreement H133B00003-90. No endorsement by the U.S. Department of Education of the opinions expressed herein should be inferred.

REFERENCES

Blatt B, Kaplan F (1966): "Christmas in Purgatory." Boston: Allyn & Bacon.

Blatt B, Ozolins A, McNally J (1979): "The Family Papers." New York: Longman.

Bogdan R, Taylor SJ (1987): Conclusion: The next wave. In Taylor SJ, Biklen D, Knoll J (Eds.): "Community Integration for People with Severe Disabilities," pp. 209–213. New York: Teachers College Press.

Bronston W (1980): Matters of design. In Apolloni T, Cappuccilli J, Cooke TP (Eds.): "Towards Excellence: Achievements in Residential Services for Persons with Disabilities," pp. 1–17. Baltimore: University Park Press.

Bruininks RH, Lakin KC (Eds.) (1985): "Living and Learning in the Least Restrictive Environment." Baltimore: Brookes.

Burgdorf RL (Ed.) (1980): "The Legal Rights of Handicapped Persons: Cases, Materials, and Text." Baltimore: Brookes.

Center on Human Policy (1979): "The Community Imperative." Syracuse, NY: Author.

Crissey MS, Rosen M (Eds.) (1986): "Institutions for the Mentally Retarded." Austin: Pro-Ed.

Galloway C (1980): The "Continuum" and the Need for Caution. Unpublished manuscript.

Halpern AS, Close DW, Nelson DJ (1986): "On My Own." Baltimore: Brookes.

Haring NG, Hansen CL (1981): Perspectives in communitization. In Hansen CL (Ed.): "Severely Handicapped Persons In the Community," pp. 1–27. Seattle: Program Development Assistance System.

Hitzing W (1980): ENCOR and beyond. In Apolloni T, Cappuccilli J, Cooke TP (Eds.): "Towards Excellence: Achievements in Residential Services for Persons with Disabilities," pp. 71–93. Baltimore: University Park Press.

Hitzing W (1987): Community living alternatives for persons with autism and severe behavior problems. In Cohen DJ, Donnellan A (Eds.): "Handbook of Autism and Pervasive Developmental Disorders," pp. 396–410. New York: John Wiley.

O'Brien J (1994): Down stairs that are never your own: Supporting people with developmental disabilities in their own homes. Ment Retard 32(1):1–6.

Reynolds M (1962): A framework for considering some issues in special education. Exceptional Children 28:367–370.

Schalock RL (1983): "Services for Developmentally Disabled Adults." Baltimore: University Park Press.

Taylor SJ (1988): Caught in the continuum: A critical analysis of the principle of the last restrictive environment. J Assoc Persons Severe Handicaps 13(1):41–53.

Taylor SJ, Bogdan R, Racino JA (Eds.) (1991): "Life in the Community: Case Studies of Organizations Supporting People with Disabilities." Baltimore: Paul H. Brookes Publishing Co.

Turnbull R, with Ellis JW, Boggs EM, Brookes PO, Biklen DP (Eds.) (1981): "Least Restrictive Alternatives: Principles and Practices." Washington, DC: American Association on Mental Deficiency.

Walsh KK, McCallion P (1987): The role of the small institution in the community services continuum. In Antonak RF, Mulick JA (Eds.): "Transitions in Mental Retardation, Volume 3: The Community Imperative Revisited," pp. 216–236. Norwood, NJ: Ablex.

Innovation in the Way People with Disabilities Can Be Supported to Live and Participate in Community Life

Gillian Chernets

This is the story of the development of a number of housing cooperatives and an organization that supports people with special needs to live, participate, and be members of both the cooperative communities and the broader community in Metropolitan Toronto. It is a story about creating intentional communities.

I am the parent of three daughters. Two of them have been labeled disabled. As a parent, I listen to my children's dreams for their futures. It is apparent to me that the service system as it exists at present cannot possibly provide what my children dream about.

I am also a professional and an activist. My work has always focused on relationships. I am the Executive Coordinator of Extend-a-Family Toronto. Extend-a-Family is a nonprofit community service that assists individuals with handicaps to enter into relationships with their fellow citizens. I helped start Citizen Advocacy in Toronto. Citizen Advocacy also helps people develop relationships that will enable them to achieve the kind of life they hope for.

THE EXCLUSION SYSTEM

As a parent and through my work, I know that people with disabilities, including those with Down syndrome, are frequently controlled by the human service system. The majority of their activities and, more appropriately, their inactivities are determined by the system. This system has grown and developed out of people's weaknesses. It sees people as a collection of needs to be met, rather than individuals with dreams to be fulfilled. It is a system that tests, labels, and categorizes, then determines who will get what support, from whom, where, and when.

In Toronto, Canada, the system offers little choice in terms of where and how people with disabilities live. There are group homes for four to twelve people. For those deemed "more able," there are supported living apartments. In both, the service agency controls the home and decides who will live where and with whom. People

256

who share similar needs, from the perspective of the agency, generally live together. People who are nonverbal are in one home, and people with behavior problems live in "the behavior house." Their disability labels make individuals who are quite different from one another into "them."

These residential services require people to have day programs—somewhere to go from eight in the morning to three in the afternoon every day. One young man I know refused to go to such a day-wasting program. They locked him out of his home. He had to stay in the carport. This happened every day for three months until he learned to be compliant.

In all of this, parents must relinquish their role as primary supporter. The agency takes over. Ties to family and community are made to suffer.

This system keeps people apart from community. The community is taught to think that the needs of people with disabilities can only be met by trained professionals. People are only able to live in licensed, fire-regulated residences. These places are called "homes." They are not. "Home-like" is like "life-like"—not good enough.

In this environment, it is less and less likely that ordinary citizens will experience the gifts and contributions of these individuals, or develop relationships with individuals as individuals.

MY DAUGHTER SPEAKS HER MIND

My daughter Kerrie did not want to be controlled or excluded. She had a lot to say about what she wanted: 1) She wanted to choose where she lived, and it had to be in our neighborhood. 2) She wanted her own place. She wanted control over that place. She wanted to live there as long as she liked. 3) She did not want to live only with other people who have been labeled disabled. 4) She needed affordable housing. 5) She wanted to know the people who lived around her. She wanted to be able to help other people.

Kerrie's list is probably the same list most of us would produce when making a choice of where to live. For many ordinary people in Toronto, there are places where you can check off everything on the list. For Kerrie, there was no place in the system that would let her check off anything on the list.

HOUSING COOPERATIVES—DECENT, AFFORDABLE, COMMUNITY

About thirty years ago, I was instrumental in developing a ski cooperative in Australia. "A cooperative society is an enterprise formed and directed by an association of users, applying within itself the rules of democracy and directly intended to serve both its own members and the community as a whole" (Paul Lambert, *Studies in the Social Philosophy of Co-operation*). It seemed to me that the cooperative model could meet some of my daughter's desires. A housing cooperative, in fact, could be the basis for developing an intentional community. The principles of housing cooperatives are consistent with what we are looking for (see Fig. 1).

A housing cooperative is started by a group of people who form themselves into a nonprofit board. They work through the myriad of government bureaucratic hoops

1. OPEN AND VOLUNTARY MEMBERSHIP
   Membership of a cooperative society should be voluntary and available without artificial restriction or any social, political, or religious discrimination to all persons who can make use of its services and are willing to accept the responsibilities of membership.
2. DEMOCRATIC CONTROL
   Cooperative societies are democratic organizations. Their affairs should be administered by persons elected or appointed in a manner agreed upon by the members and accountable to them. Members of primary societies should enjoy equal rights of voting (one member, one vote) and participation in decisions affecting their societies. In other than primary societies, the administration should be conducted on a democratic basis in a suitable form.
3. LIMITED INTEREST ON SHARES
   Share capital should only receive a strictly limited rate of interest, if any.
4. RETURN OF SURPLUS TO MEMBERS
   Surplus or savings, if any, arising out of the operations of a society belong to the members of that society and should be distributed in such a manner as would avoid one member gaining at the expense of others. This may be done by decision of the members as follows:
   a. by provision for development of the business of the cooperative
   b. by provision of common services
   c. by distribution among the members in proportion to their transaction with the society
5. COOPERATIVE EDUCATION
   All cooperative societies should make provisions for the education of their members, officers and employees, and of the general public in the principles and techniques of cooperation, both economic and democratic.
6. COOPERATION AMONG COOPERATIVES
   All cooperative organizations, in order to best serve the interests of their members and their communities, should actively cooperate in every practical way with other cooperatives at local, national, and international levels.

Fig. 1. The Essential Principles of Cooperative Organizations as Approved by the International Co-operative Alliance, September 1966.

to either build or renovate the housing that will meet their needs and those of like-minded people. The members of the co-op collectively manage and control their housing.

In Canada, cooperative housing is supported by the federal and provincial governments. Support is available for both construction and to subsidize the rents of people with lower incomes.

In a cooperative housing model, my daughter is able to have and afford a one bedroom apartment of her own. The housing subsidy makes this possible.

Everyone who lives in a co-op participates in the running and management of their

NABORS stands for Neighbours Allied for Better Opportunities in Residential Support. It is a nonprofit organization incorporated in 1984 in Toronto, Canada.

NABORS is committed to assisting up to 12 individuals with disabilities to live as valued and contributing members of either Courtyard Housing Cooperative or CHORD Housing Cooperative.

With funding from the Ministry of Housing, the Board of Directors of CHORD is constructing an apartment/townhouse development in the Jane/Eglinton neighborhood consisting of 136 units.

The Board of Directors of the Courtyard Co-op is completing a 35 unit project as part of a Cityhome Development in the Yonge/Eglinton neighborhood.

Both co-op communities are committed to the creation of welcoming, inclusive, supportive communities representing people of various ages, income levels, abilities, and cultural origin.

CHORD and Courtyard are planning intentional supportive communities. Both communities want to welcome and include people with disabilities. There are 5 people who have expressed a desire to live in the Courtyard Co-op who will require paid supports in order to ensure their participation.

As a separate organization NABORS Inc. will work in conjunction with CHORD and Courtyard Co-ops to create a supportive community.

NABORS philosophy is based on the following five principles:

- Individualization. Availability of appropriate personal support at a level required to ensure each individual's full participation, based on an individual's particular needs.
- Social Support. Building mutually supportive relationships among all members of both cooperative communities.
- Self-determination. Assuring that individuals with disabilities have control over their own support managements, with access to both technical advice and advocacy as appropriate to their needs and preferences.
- Participation. Enabling members with disabilities to have full and active involvement in the life of the cooperatives and the surrounding community.
- Nondiscrimination. Inclusion of all members and provision of the support needed, regardless of the nature of the physical or developmental disability or whatever other label has been previously acquired.

Required support services will include: attendant care, paid companion, homemaker assistance and facilitation of experiences, activities, and working relationships typical of community living. What is required through NABORS will be planned and negotiated with each individual and/or his/her family or other advocates.

NABORS is a unique and innovative model of supportive housing for people with disabilities. Not only will it blend the principles of cooperative living with social integration for people with a variety of disabilities, but will also demonstrate how to cultivate and nurture mutually supportive relationships within an intentional community.

Fig. 2. Overview of NABORS, Inc.

housing. My daughter Kerrie has work to do around the co-op and a valued role in the co-op. As people work together and make decisions, Kerrie also has a chance to meet and get to know her neighbors. Kerrie is now living in Courtyard Co-op.

As we developed these new initiatives, people heard about our plans and asked for assistance. We now have four housing co-op projects with a total of 465 units under development in the Greater Toronto Area. Two are built and recently occupied. The two others will come on-stream over the next eight months. The CHORD Co-op was my first project, and it has yet to be completed. Sometimes planning approvals hold the projects up for months and years.

KERRIE NEEDS SOME SUPPORT

Kerrie is significantly challenged. Her verbal skills are pretty limited and she does not appear to read. Kerrie needs a bit of assistance if she is going to live on her own. So, the question was how to do this.

In 1987 I initiated a nonprofit organization called NABORS (see Fig. 2). Through NABORS we requested government funding to support 12 people we knew. The 12 people have a variety of abilities and disabilities. They are challenging in different ways.

The government was stumped. They could not figure out which department should respond to our proposal. Funding is based on the type and level of disability and our group was integrated and variously challenged. In the end, the funding came.

The funding is controlled by each of the individuals and their support circles. The support circles include family and friends. They tell NABORS how they want the money used, and whether they want to hire their own staff or want NABORS to assist. The support is intended to enable a person to participate in the co-op and the wider community.

The paid support people are trained to encourage and nurture relationships, and avoid creating barriers to participation or friendship. For Kerrie, support will probably fade out over the next few months. As relationships within the co-op develop, her support circle and co-op neighbors will probably be able to provide the support that currently comes from paid people.

Joe also lives in the co-op. He has cerebral palsy and needs personal care and assistance with eating. Recently, however, Joe used his Bliss Board to tell his attendant to call Mike, a co-op neighbor, to ask him if he wanted to go out for a beer. This stands in marked contrast to the life Joe had in the chronic care hospital he lived in before moving to Courtyard!

THE MAGIC INGREDIENT

So now we have a housing co-op and NABORS to support people. There is a third ingredient to our approach—intentional community. Housing cooperatives and support to individuals, we believe, will increase the likelihood that people with disabilities will enter into new and supportive relationships. I wanted to increase the opportunities for relationships even more. I wanted people with disabilities to be seen and appreciated for their gifts and the valued roles they could play in the life of communities.

Housing co-ops are based on working together to run the co-op. I wanted the co-op members to also be committed to nurturing one another. I decided we needed people to live in the co-ops because they were committed to being good neighbors. Mutual, neighborly acts would be seen as central to the life of the co-op.

This has taken time and training to achieve. We have had retreats, parties, and get-togethers on a regular basis to draw more and more families together. Over time, people have come together to plan and develop a neighborly, supportive community for everyone.

This approach to intentional community depends on a partnership involving 1) the individual, family, and support circle; 2) NABORS as the support organization; and 3) the housing cooperative as both a place to live and a group of people who depend on one another.

I was nervous through all of this. I did not know if our talk about intentional community in co-op housing would scare people away. In fact, that happened in a few situations. It was probably for the best. Now, we have families calling almost every day asking if they can be put on the waiting list to move into a co-op.

So, Kerrie has a home of her own with the supports tailored to meet her particular lifestyle, her needs, and dreams. She is already a valued member of the co-op. It is her home. She furnished it. She chose the colors. She decides when and what to eat. She decides when not to bother about the dishes. She walks her dog every night with the young guy down the hall.

She is in the same neighborhood in which she grew up. She can walk home to visit her sister and me any time. She has held on to the community connections she already had. She also has renewed some old connections as people she knows have also moved into the co-op.

Thirty five people in the co-op know Kerrie's name. They greet her and expect her to participate in the co-op. I called her last night. She said she had invited a couple

---

THE MODEL—SHARED COMMITMENT

NABORS   THE COOPERATIVES

• Responsible for support (in partnership   • Responsible for the community
  with individual and circle)

SHARED COMMITMENT TO THE INTENTION OF MUTUAL SUPPORT

   • The people are the center
   • Friendship, mutuality, participation, inclusion, neighborliness, security

Fig. 3.

The founders of Courtyard Cooperative state our purpose as follows:

To create a housing cooperative where members have chosen to foster a community spirit. This spirit is based on neighborliness, mutual respect, and helpfulness, with people of all ages, backgrounds, and abilities making commitments to one another. Including people with special needs and ensuring that they will have support to be fully active members of the cooperative will be central to life in this community.

Through living and working together for the mutual benefit of the co-op we intend to foster lasting personal relationships for people who have been isolated because of their disabilities.

The cooperative recognizes that each member has unique ideas and skills to offer and must play a valued role in the management and day-to-day life of the community.

We strive to create an environment where members will feel comfortable and secure. We will not tolerate acts of physical violence, intimidation, or discrimination based on age, gender, ethnicity, sexual orientation, or disability.

The cooperative will maintain an agreement with NABORS, a unique and innovative model of support for people with disabilities. NABORS will provide the formal support services as required by some members in order to enable them to live in this community (e.g., attendant care, homemaker assistance, etc.).

The co-op recognizes the responsibility of promoting:

- good citizenship within the neighborhood of North Toronto and the City of Toronto;
- cooperation with other members of the broader cooperative movement.

Fig. 4. Courtyard Cooperative—vision statement.

who live on the fourth floor for supper on Monday. On Saturday, she was going shopping for blinds with Hugh who lives on the third floor.

I am a happy parent. My daughter is a valued member of a community. We have found a way to enable some people with disabilities to offer their gifts to the community. No one in the co-op is independent. They are interdependent members of a community where each counts on the others, and the others count on each member.

Supported Employment for People with Disabilities:
What Progress Has Been Made?

Paul Wehman

There was a time in the not too distant past when people with Down syndrome did not participate in the nation's competitive labor force. Those that did were traditionally involved in sheltered workshops, adult activity centers, or assumed lengthy stays in prevocational training programs. Previous thinking reflected the view that people labeled with disabilities such as Down syndrome, severe mental retardation, autism, severe cerebral palsy, and deaf–blindness could not possibly work in competitive employment. Real work seemed to be outside the range of possibility for tens of thousands of people who remained at home, lived in institutions, or sat in large segregated day programs of which there are, even today, over 7,000 in the United States. It was not unusual as little as two decades ago for families of people with Down syndrome to think that real work was a total impossibility. Beginning in the 1970s behavioral training technologies emerged, however, and began to show a way that vocational competence could be achieved by people with severe intellectual disabilities. Pioneering researchers such as Marc Gold and Tom Bellamy were able to consistently show that intellectually and behaviorally challenged individuals who were nonambulatory were able to complete challenging vocational tasks such as putting together electronic circuit boards when given systematic training and instruction.

As this behavioral technology developed, a new group of researchers began to investigate how to expand the range of involvement in the competitive workplace for people with intellectual and physical disabilities. This was an important change in thinking, since in the 1970s the emphasis was clearly upon vocational training, not placement followed by training. Early on, it was clear that a nonverbal individual with an IQ of 25 or a person with a high rate of head banging who was labeled autistic could not be put into a workplace alone. This persons would obviously fail. In fact, such thinking had never been seriously considered because, on face value, it appeared to be ridiculous.

However, beginning in the 1980s a new way of providing services began to emerge called supported employment. This service technology was as complicated to implement as it was simple in principle. The basic notion involved the use of a trained staff person who would accompany the person with a disability into a paid placement in the workplace. There was no negative outcry from business and industry and, in fact, parents and individuals with disabilities welcomed the opportunity to try a real job. The most challenging efforts, as this technology spread, were to encourage service providers and local programs in the community to critically reexamine their practices and reevaluate what they were doing. It became increasingly clear that many of the dollars that were going to support services for people in segregated day programs would need to be reallocated into supporting job coaches who work with people in the community.

WHAT HAS BEEN ACCOMPLISHED?

It is important for those of us who work with people who have Down syndrome and other intellectual disabilities to look carefully at what has been accomplished in improving employment possibilities over the past 10 years. The gold standard of service 1–2 decades ago was for a person with Down syndrome to enter some type of adult day program; that is, to get off of a waiting list and gain day services. With the rapid change of philosophy towards placement into competitive employment, however, there is a new gold standard, one that could not have occurred without a supported employment technology. This standard is to have a real job with decent pay and benefits and good working conditions. As Rebecca McDonald, Board member of the Association for Persons in Supported Employment, noted in her testimony to Congressman Major Owens' Subcommittee on Select Education, more and more parents of disabled young people are requesting not only integrated classroom opportunities but active transition planning for competitive employment (McDonald, March 6, 1992). In the 1985–1986 period, the United States Department of Education, under the leadership of then Assistant Secretary Madelene Will, allotted money for 27 sates to revamp their adult service system so as to open doors for more people with severe disabilities to enter supported employment. We moved from a series of university based and other isolated demonstrations of supported employment to a nation that would begin to build supported employment capacity across all 50 states. The groundwork that was laid for these five-year systems change grants provided a blueprint for what would happen in the 1990s, particularly in the event that a severe recession would occur. It is important to remember that through the 1980s the United States was essentially in an economic boom period, and supported employment programs that depend on business hiring new workers were able to prosper. Proponents of supported employment always wondered how well these programs would fare during an economic downturn.

What do the present and future hold? First, it is clear that in a very short period of time a new gold standard has been established for adult services. No longer is simply entering and receiving day program services sufficient. Families, individuals with Down syndrome, and their advocates alike are rightfully asking for more. They want better jobs, better fringe benefits, and more working hours. Simply put, they want what people without disabilities want from a job.

The second area where tremendous progress has been made is the amount of participation that has occurred over the short period 1985–1990. This period has witnessed a growth from less than 10,000 people with disabilities in supported employment to over 75,000 (Shafer et al., 1990).

A third area of growth and progress that we can look back upon favorably is that all 50 states have now established supported employment programs. Families also have a greater likelihood than they did 5–10 years ago of helping their adult child with severe disability gain a real job. Typically, the federal/state vocational rehabilitation program provides and monitors oversight, in accordance with regulations established in the Rehabilitation Act Amendments of 1992.

Finally, there continues to be a growing level of interest and greater calls for participation, particularly from those people with traumatic brain injury, sensory impairment, and physical disabilities, as well as those families of young people who are leaving school and are looking for a job for the first time. Also included in this request for services are minorities with disabilities, perhaps the most underserved group of all.

What follows is a detailed review of articles, most of which generated some form of quantitative data related to supported employment within the past 13 years. This review is divided into several categories of literature and is followed by an analysis of needs which remain.

DEVELOPMENT AND IMPLEMENTATION OF INDIVIDUAL CLIENT INTERVENTIONS

The first category of literature to be reviewed is by far the most substantial. Many papers and articles have been written since the late 1970s about how to provide supported employment intervention for people with disabilities. In developing this review, primarily papers that provided data were included, and they are presented, for the most part, in a chronological sequence.

Sowers et al. (1979) developed a Food Service Vocational Training Program at the University of Washington. This program demonstrated clearly that with intensive job training and extensive on-the-job monitoring many persons with mental retardation, including those with Down syndrome, who were currently in workshops, could successfully work in competitive employment. In addition, these results showed that financial savings to society are overwhelming when adults with mental retardation are removed from workshops, trained, and placed in the competitive workforce.

The outcome data from this program indicated that not all of the trainees who entered the program were trained and placed successfully. The authors indicate that this raises the issue of identification of those individuals who are most likely to succeed in a "training for placement" program. They indicate that the issue is complex, since a multitude of variables are involved, including living environment, family support, past work and training experience, etc. Their data showed that measured intelligence (IQ) was not a useful indicator of success for those whose IQs were above 40 and that "poor attitude" behaviors were more important. This report did not indicate success with people with mental retardation whose IQs were less than 40. Sowers et al. do note, however, that it appears that the reason for the failure with this group lies more with inadequate training skills than with the person.

Concurrent with the Sowers et al. study, Wehman et al. (1979) reported a demonstration project called Project Employability, which was a job placement and training program initially funded by the Virginia Department of Rehabilitative Services. This paper describes three case studies of individuals with developmental disabilities, two of whom had Down syndrome. None of these individuals had worked competitively before, and they were selected for competitive employment because it was believed that they would provide a true picture of the planning requirements, observation, and intervention difficulties involved in competitive employment.

It is in this early paper that the concept of a "trainer–advocate" being regularly available was outlined as a helpful intervention. In addition to this paper, Wehman and Hill edited a multi-article volume that reported a number of demonstrations and studies involved with helping put people with severe developmental disabilities into competitive employment using supported employment. The Wehman and Hill (1980) volume focused extensively on a place, train, and follow along approach.

Brickey et al. (1982) also reported job placement histories of 73 sheltered workshop employees placed in projects with industry. Competitive jobs were examined during a 30 month period, with 48% of the total people placed into competitive employment. Brickey et al. indicate that job variables such as training structure at the job site appear to be more important to job success than employee demographic variables such as IQ. Also at this time Krauss and MacEachron (1982) reported a program to place persons with mental retardation into competitive employment. The program was initiated as a pilot in 1979 and the authors were interested in investigating the viability of competitive placement. The results indicated that clients' work behavior, ability to meet the skill requirements for the jobs, and employment reinforcement were predictors of successful competitive employment. The placement rate was reported as being 50%.

Also in 1982, Wehman et al. (1982) published one of the first definitive papers documenting three-year outcomes of a supported employment program that focused exclusively on individual placements. This paper described a training and advocacy approach—supported employment to placement that involved client training by the staff at the job site. Staff advocacy took place with coworkers and employers and all clients were paid by employers as part of the regular workforce. A total of 63 clients were placed with 42 working at the time of the report for a placement rate of 67%. Wehman et al. report that $265,000 was earned by these clients and over $26,000 paid in state and federal taxes. The significance of this paper is that it is the first large study that described the follow along approach of supported employment with clients who have been viewed by professionals and parents alike as "realistically unemployable."

Three years later Wehman et al. (1985) published a follow-up paper of individuals with mental retardation who had been working competitively for a six-year period. A total of 167 clients with a median IQ of 49 were placed into competitive employment using the identical model as described in the Wehman et al. (1982) paper. Over one million dollars were earned through the six-year period by clients, with the average length of time on a job for all clients being 19 months. For most clients this was their first real job.

In another approach, Rhoades and Velenta (1985) reported one of the first data-based approaches to industry-based supported employment using a group approach, in this case, the industrial enclave. This article describes a program model that provides ongoing supported employment within a normal industrial setting to six persons who were previously judged to have severe mental retardation. After one year these employees had dramatically increased earnings and productivity, and public cost had declined to one-third that of alternative state programs.

In another study involving the teaching of janitorial skills in a competitive work setting, Test et al. (1988) examined the use of supported employment for training competitive work experiences to a 19-year-old student with severe retardation. The job involved complex janitorial skills, and training consisted of a combination of total-task presentation and an individualized prompting hierarchy. A multiple base-line of cross-behavior design was employed across the three sets of behaviors—emptying trash cans, detail cleaning, and daily cleaning. The use of supported employment as a means of providing competitive work experience for young adults with severe disabilities was discussed. In yet another report of persons with severe retardation, Wehman et al. (1987) reported the competitive employment experiences of 21 individuals with IQs of under 40, approximately one-third of whom had Down syndrome. Over an eight-year period from 1978 to 1986, 21 persons were competitively employed, with ongoing or intermittent job experiences. A cumulative total of over $230,000 of wages was earned. Significant vocational problems included slow work rate and lack of appropriate social skills, e.g., behavior problems. While this report extends the competitive employment literature to persons with more severe intellectual handicaps, more work needs to be done with this group.

It was in this general time frame of 1985 to 1990 that more sophisticated work began to emerge. For example, Nisbet and Hagner (1988) examined the importance of natural supports in the workplace. They strongly suggested that less-intrusive ways of supporting clients at the job should be created; that is, the use of agency sponsored job coaches should not be viewed as the exclusive or primary mode of providing support. Berg et al. (1990) wrote extensively on generalization and maintenance of work behavior, particularly in the context of supported employment. In similar fashion to the Nisbet and Hagner (1988) paper, Buckley et al. (1990) also began, in greater detail, to talk about the varied types of support strategies. They noted that support strategies could be separated into three categories. The first includes structurally oriented strategies that directly involve the individual with disabilities. The second is aimed at increasing coworker and supervisor involvement. The third is directed toward parent, advocate, and other service providers.

As a follow-up to the earlier Wehman et al., article on looking at outcomes for people with severe retardation, Wehman and Kregel (1990) undertook a much larger analysis of 109 persons with severe mental retardation, with about one-quarter having

Down syndrome. The mean age of the group was 28 years old and mean intelligence (Stanford-Binet) was 32. The data were drawn from over 90 local community programs in the United States and results indicated that all persons were in supervised residential situations. A total of 93% were competitively employed, with a mean wage of $3.63 per hour and an average of 22 hours of weekly employment. After 12 months of placement 81.5% of the clients were still employed. These data provided a much brighter picture of the capabilities and involvement of people with severe and profound retardation in supported employment.

Kregel et al. (1989) undertook an investigation of the characteristics of over 1,400 individuals with severe and profound disabilities who were involved in supported employment in eight states. Results indicated that individuals currently participating in supported employment possessed very limited previous employment experience, yet did not possess functional characteristics indicative of individuals with severe disabilities. Persons with severe/profound disabilities were found to be minimally represented in current supported employment efforts, representing less than 8% of all individuals investigated. When one begins to carefully look at the supported employment outcomes for persons with severe retardation, it becomes abundantly clear that actual participation level in supported employment is much lower than it might be. Undoubtedly, this reflects the greater skills required on the part of job coaches to place individuals with severe and profound mental retardation as well as the substantial cost that is involved.

The late 1980s also showed an increasing interest in studying social integration and the role of coworkers. For example, McNair and Rusch (1991) developed a coworker instrument to assess levels of friendship and helping in the workplace. At the same time Parent (1992) and her colleagues were validating a Vocational Integration Index.

Finally, several investigators looked at the impact of supported employment in different states. For example, Ellis et al. (1990) evaluated supported employment outcomes in Illinois. The authors indicate that supported employment has been implemented throughout the state of Illinois and that hundreds of individuals are now participating in supported employment that previously wouldn't have been. Kregel et al. (1990) also reported supported employment outcomes in Virginia. They provided outcomes related to level of participation, level of severity, hours of work per week for supported employment clients, the types of models that used, and the nature of supported employment job retention. Additionally, Vogelsburg (1990) reported 24 months of supported employment implementation in the state of Pennsylvania. Major sections of this paper identify service-development issues, challenges for long-term funding, and ways to expand the initial two years of state implementation.

The above papers, for the most part, do not provide stringent experimental controls or even control groups. They are aggregate demonstrations with a heavy reliance on descriptive data presentation. Generally speaking, the sample sizes are small and, subsequently, the ability to make definitive extrapolations is not good. On the other hand, the population that has participated in these supported employment programs historically has never been in a competitive employment and has only been in sheltered workshops, day care programs, or on waiting lists. It is reasonable to assume that with such a large number of demonstrations, even with the inability to carefully document replicable procedures and the incumbent subject selection bias, supported employment has made a significant difference in the lives of people who traditionally would not be in an integrated workplace.

The outcome data from these aggregate reports clearly provide a basis and challenge for more sophisticated research to occur in the 1990s, as well as for more specific questions to be asked concerning differential effects of service-delivery models, best ways to predict outcomes, and other related matters such as benefits and costs. It is this category that our literature review will turn to next.

BENEFITS AND COSTS ASSOCIATED WITH SUPPORTED EMPLOYMENT PROGRAMS

A common question frequently asked about supported employment is: What will it cost? From the beginning of the development of supported employment programs this has always been a frequent question and even criticism. Although the benefits, monetary and otherwise, have been readily acknowledged by many, the costs involved in developing supported employment programs have varied considerably. There have been, however, some studies that have looked specifically at costs and benefits.

In one of the early studies Hill and Wehman (1983) presented an analysis of cost incurred and tax money saved over an approximately four-year period through the implementation of an ongoing supported employment program. The focus of this analysis was on the amount of money saved rather than on the wages earned by workers with moderate and severe mental retardation. Factors in the cost analysis included the number of months a client had been working, the amount of staff hours expended on the client at the job site, the amount of funds expended proportionally to each client, SSI income saved and the estimated cost of day programming for the client if no job placement had been made. Since initiation of the program, Hill and Wehman reported that the clients cumulative earnings were over half a million dollars.

An extension of this analysis to 8 years was reported by Hill et al. in 1987. It was found that the positive financial consequences accruing to the public was over one million dollars. Since the study extended over 8 years, all figures were corrected for inflation and discounted to 1986 dollars. Individual analysis revealed that all clients served benefited financially from the program and that results show substantial savings to taxpayers with the utilization of a supported employment model.

Echoing the positive benefits associated with supported employment is a telling paper by Noble and Conley (1987). They indicated that evidence about benefits and costs of supported employment were growing rapidly. Their biggest caveat was that there was a lack of definitive data collected in controlled experimental studies. Beale et al. (1989) also noted various methodological pitfalls of cost/benefit analysis for supported employment programs, including concerns about the logic of the analyses and omission of data. Heal et al. (1989) reported data from Illinois indicating similar conclusions to Hill et al. (1987), but reduced certainty that taxpayers would definitively benefit from supported employment programming.

Another article with similar methodology published by Thornton (1992) indicates that a critical but often overlooked aspect of cost/benefit analysis is an assessment of the uncertainty inherent in all program evaluation. The level of uncertainty is highest for evaluations of new prototype programs such as supported employment and decreases as the programs are replicated in a number of settings. An understanding of the causes and magnitudes of uncertainty is essential for interpreting and using cost/benefit analysis. This is illustrated, according to Thornton, in the literature that pertains to benefits and costs of transitional and supported employment.

In related papers associated with cost, Kregel et al. (1988) did an in-depth analysis of employment specialist intervention time for first jobs of 51 clients with moderate and severe retardation. This important analysis focused on the amount of staff intervention time provided as a percentage of the total number of hours worked by the client each week and a comparison of the amount of intervention time provided to two subsamples. Results from this study indicated that clients previously classified moderately to severely mentally retarded did not require significantly greater amounts of intervention time than those who were previously classified as borderline or mildly retarded during the first year of employment.

The reader will recall that one of the studies noted earlier (Sowers, et al.) suggested that persons with low IQs would not be able to work competitively or would require tremendous amounts of time. The Kregel et al. paper provides an 8-year empirical analysis that provides clear information to the contrary.

West et al. (1990), studied the likelihood of clients in supported employment receiving fringe benefits; their study indicated that only 64% of supported employees received fringe benefits. Most recently Sale et al. (1992) report supported employment fiscal activities from 50 states. Data from a survey of fiscal year 1990 related to supported employment fiscal activity across the U.S. are presented and sources of different funds are compared to previous years surveys. Supported employment expenditures grew approximately 19% from 1989 to 1990, with nonvocational rehabilitation dollars accounting for over two-thirds of the total state dollars going into supported employment.

It would appear, as we move ahead into the 1990s, that more program-oriented cost/benefit analyses will be necessary on a larger scale in order to determine the cost of intervention and, equally important, the relative importance of benefits and gain versus costs incurred. On a similar level of analysis, it is essential to look within state and across state fiscal aggregates of funds expended for supported employment and, even more importantly, to consider the source of funding. Our research plan clearly reflects this need for more reliable and better-quality information.

NATIONAL SURVEY DATA AND POLICY ANALYSIS

The third and final area of this literature review involves a brief discussion of a number of policy analysis and national survey data papers that have begun to emerge as a result of the national implementation of supported employment programs. One of the earliest papers in this regard, by Kregel et al. (1989), reported that supported employment for persons with developmental and other severe disabilities has moved rapidly from university-based demonstration projects to the development of comprehensive statewide service delivery systems. This article reported a survey of 27 states that receive major systems-change grants from the U.S. Department of Education to convert traditional day activity programs to supported employment. This paper reported outcome data from fiscal year 1986 to 1988 in which vocational rehabilitation expenditures approached $75 million and obligations from mental health and mental retardation agencies increased by 460%. Collectively, over $214 million had been obligated by federal and state agencies for supported employment when this report was published. This amount of money and effort is remarkable, indeed, considering that less than 10 years ago supported employment was nothing more than a handful of isolated demonstrations scattered around the country.

A follow-up paper by Shafer et al. (1990) showed that 27 states had received federally supported employment grants. There was an increase of 150% (10,000 to 25,000) during a three-year period of time. Furthermore, over 1,400 programs of supported employment were authorized by state agencies during this time. Individual placement options remain prevalent, as did the fact that the beneficiaries of these services were predominantly people with mental retardation. Similarly, Shafer, Revell and Isbister (1991) reported that over a 3-year period, 32,000 people were receiving supported employment.

In one of the few published papers that examined states' technical assistance needs, Mank et al. (1991) present an extremely helpful table of how 23 states view their needs. More specific information is reported in the Needs part of the Training section.

At the same time that these studies were occurring, Kiernan et al. (1991) reported a wide-ranging and comprehensive survey of day programs for people with disability in the United States. The Kiernan et al. studies looked carefully at the service and closure activity associated with vocational rehabilitation systems for persons with mental retardation and related conditions. They indicated that by far the largest percentage of people receiving services were labeled as having mild or moderate mental retardation. They further indicated that the addition of supported employment appears to have reduced utilization of sheltered employment as a closure option for those with disabilities.

In another paper that looked at national outcome data, West et al. (1992) showed that in the time period 1986–1990 a total of 74,657 supported employment participants were reported by over 2600 state provider agencies. While persons with mental retardation continued to be the primary service group there has been a dramatic increase in the proportion of supported employment participants with mental illness. The availability of extended services funding was found to be limited across a number of disability groups. The limitations in funding, particularly extended-services funding, will also be a major focus of policy analysis for this R&T Center over the next five years. It is clearly the overriding policy issue for supported employment service providers as they seek to improve and expand their programs.

SUPPORTED EMPLOYMENT: WHAT ARE THE MAJOR AREAS OF NEED FOR THE 1990s?

First, fewer than 10% of all individuals currently participating in supported employment have physical disabilities, traumatic brain injury, autism, or sensory impairment, and yet there is a tremendous interest and need for services among many of these people. Therefore, expanding opportunities for underserved or unserved populations with severe disabilities is one very definite need. We must learn better ways to modify supported employment models to accommodate the vast range of needs presented by the many different disabilities. We must study and disseminate ways to provide better types of jobs for people with Down syndrome and other disabilities who have high vocational aspirations.

A second area of need that must be addressed is the expansion of alliances with business and industry, particularly in light of the implementation of ADA and the greater responsibilities that business will need to take in establishing reasonable accommodation and nondiscriminatory hiring practices. The opportunity for job coach liaison with natural business support is stronger than ever. We view this as a very important issue, since the need for providing natural support for people with disabilities who have been hired will be more easily met with strong business alliances. The recently passed Rehabilitation Act Amendments of 1992 include natural supports as a vehicle for extended services.

A third area, which was much discussed in the late 1980s, but in which very little progress has been made to date, is long-term funding. The nemesis of many well-established programs that prevents more people with disabilities from gaining access to services is the lack of ongoing funding to help maintain the covenant that is made with business upon the initial hiring. The long-term funding area will need continued legislative and administrative policy attention at state and federal levels.

Fourth, there continues to be an ongoing need to improve supported employment technology and the efficiencies with which this technology is delivered. We need to know more about how to help people with the most severe disabilities enter the workforce. We need to know how to help people who have been supported for a number of years progressively reduce the amount of support they require and/or move up into more competitive, better paying positions. We also need to know how to integrate the use of assistive technology advances in robotics, computers, and electronics to empower the job coach and consumer when working at the job site.

Fifth, we must continue to improve our ways of delivering technical assistance to those local programs converting to supported employment, recruiting and training new job coaches, or who need help with new populations. Training and technical assistance is very high on future issues needs, since the technology is of little value if it cannot be broadly delivered. Consider comments made at the National Conference of State Legislatures by the Task Force on Developmental Disabilities (February, 1991):

> Despite the advantages of supported employment, the bulk of state employment funds for persons with disabilities still goes to sheltered work-

shops and other segregated settings. In 1988, federal and state governments spent between $385 and $582 million to place 109,899 people with developmental disabilities in sheltered workshops at a per capita rate between $3,500 and $5,300. In the same year, only $62 million was spent on 16,458 people in supported employment, at a per capita rate of $3,767. The challenge facing state legislators is to develop methods to transfer people currently in day programs and sheltered workshops into the competitive work force successfully. (p. 28)

Sixth, and finally, we must reach out to the consumers and their families to study choice and self-determination processes in the context of vocational planning. The need for informal choice in supported employment programs on the part of consumers is a paramount concern. People with Down syndrome must be encouraged to develop a career path and have the opportunity to make many vocational choices.

REFERENCES

Berg WK, Wacker DP, Flynn TH (1990): Teaching generalization and maintenance of work behavior. In Rusch FR (ed.): "Supported Employment: Models, Methods, and Issues." Baltimore: Brookes.

Brickey M, Browning L, Campbell K (1982): Vocational histories of sheltered workshop employees placed in Projects with Industry and competitive jobs. Ment Retard 20(2):52–57.

Buckley J, Mank D, Sandow D (1990): Developing and implementing support strategies. In Rusch FR (ed.): "Supported Employment: Models, Methods, and Issues." Baltimore: Brookes.

Ellis WK, Rusch FR, Tu J, McCaughrin W (1990): Supported employment in Illinois. In Rusch FR (ed.),"Supported Employment: Models, Methods, and Issues." Baltimore: Brookes.

Heal LW, McCaughrin WB, Tines JJ (1989): Methodological nuances and pitfalls of benefit–cost analysis: A critique. Res Dev Disabil 10:201–202.

Hill M, Wehman P (1983): Cost-benefit analysis of placing moderately and severely handicapped individuals into competitive employment. J Assoc Persons Severe Handicaps 8(1):30–38.

Hill ML, Wehman PH, Kregel J, Banks PD, Metzler HMD (1987): Employment outcomes for people with moderate and severe disabilities: An eight-year longitudinal analysis of supported competitive employment. J Assoc Persons Severe Handicaps 12(3):182–189.

Kiernan WE, McGaughey MJ, Lynch SA, Schalock RL, McNally LC (December 1991): "National Survey of Day and Employment Programs: Results from State VR Agencies." Boston: Children's Hospital, Training and Research Institute for People with Disabilities.

Krauss MW, MacEachron AE (1982): Competitive employment training for mentally retarded adults: The supported work model. Am J Ment Defic 86(6):650–653.

Kregel J, Hill M, Banks PD (1988): Analysis of employment specialist intervention time in supported competitive employment. Am J Ment Retard 93(2):200–208.

Kregel J, Wehman P, Revell WG, Hill M (1990): Supported employment in Virginia. In Rusch FR (ed.): "Supported Employment: Models, Methods, and Issues," pp. 15–29. Sycamore, IL: Sycamore.

Kregel J, Wehman P, Banks D (1989): Effects of consumer characteristics and type of employment model of individual outcomes in supported employment. J Appl Behav Anal 22:407–415.

Mank DM, Buckley J, Rhodes LE (1991): Systems change to supported employment: new approaches to improvement. J Voc Rehab 1(1):59–68.

McNair J, Rusch FR (1991): Parent involvement in transition programs. Ment Retard 29(2):93–101.

Nisbet J, Hagner D (1988): Natural supports in the workplace: A reexamination of supported employment. J Assoc Persons Severe Handicaps 13(4):260–267.

Noble JH, Conley RW (1987): Accumulating evidence on the benefits and costs of supported and transitional employment for individuals with severe disabilities. J Assoc Persons Severe Handicaps 12:163–174.

Parent WS, Kregel J, Wehman P (1992): "The Vocational Integration Index: A Guide for Rehabilitation Professionals." Stoneham, MA: Andover Medical.

Rehabilitation Act Amendments of 1992, Public Law 102-569. Title 29, U.S.C. 701 Section 101[c].

Rhoades L, Valenta L (1985): Industry-based supported employment: An enclave approach. J Assoc Persons Severe Handicaps 10(1):12–20.

Sale P, Revell G, West M, Kregel J (1992): Achievements and challenges II: An analysis of 1990 supported employment expenditures. J Assoc Persons Severe Handicaps 17(4):236–246.

Shafer M, Revell G, Isbister F (1991): The national supported employment initiative: A three-year longitudinal analysis of 50 states. J Voc Rehab 1(1):9–18.

Shafer M, Wehman P, Kregel J, West M (1990): The national supported employment initiative: A preliminary analysis. Am J Ment Retard 95(3):316–327.

Sowers J, Thompson LE, Connis RT (1979): The Food Service Vocational Training Program: A model for training and placement of the mentally retarded. In Bellamy GT, O'Connor G, Karan OC (eds.): "Vocational Rehabilitation of Severely Handicapped Persons." Baltimore: University Park Press.

Test DW, Grossi T, Keul P (1988): A functional analysis of the acquisition and maintenance of janitorial skills in a competitive work setting. J Assoc Persons Severe Handicaps 13(1):1–7.

Thornton C (1992): Uncertainty in benefit-cost analysis of supported employment. J Voc Rehab 2(2):62–72.

Vogelsberg RT (1990): Supported employment in Pennsylvania. In Rusch FR (ed.): "Supported Employment: Models, Methods, and Issues." Baltimore: Brookes.

Wehman P, Hill M (eds.) (1980): "Vocational Training and Placement of Severely Disabled Persons: Project Employability, Volume 2, 1980." Richmond, VA: Virginia Commonwealth University.

Wehman P, Hill J, Koehler F (1979): Placement of developmentally disabled individuals into competitive employment: Three case studies. Ed Train Ment Retard 14(4):269–276.

Wehman P, Hill M, Hill J, Brooke V, Ponder C, Pentecost J, Pendleton P, Britt C (1985): Competitive employment for persons with mental retardation: A follow-up six years later. Ment Retard 23(6):274–281.

Wehman P, Hill M, Goodall P, Cleveland P, Brooke V, Pentecost J (1982): Job placement and follow-up of moderately and severely handicapped individuals after three years. J Assoc Severely Handicapped 7(2):5–16.

Wehman P, Hill J, Wood W, Parent W (1987): A report on competitive employment histories of persons labeled severely mentally retarded. J Assoc Persons Severe Handicaps 12(1):11–17.

Wehman P, Kregel J (1990): Supported employment for persons with severe and profound mental retardation: A critical analysis. Int J Rehab Res 13:93–107.

Wehman P, Kregel J, Shafer M (eds.) (1989): "Emerging Trends in the National Supported Employment Initiative: A Preliminary Twenty-seven State Analysis." Richmond, VA: Virginia Commonwealth University, Rehabilitation Research and Training Center on Supported Employment.

West M, Kregel J, Banks PD (1990): Fringe benefits available to supported employment participants. Rehab Couns Bull 34(2):126–138.

West M, Revell WG, Wehman P (1992): Achievements and challenges I: A five-year report on consumer and system outcomes from the supported employment initiative. J Assoc Persons Severe Handicaps 17(4):227–235.

West M, Wehman P, Kregel J, Kreutzer J, Sherron P, Zasler N (1991): Costs of operating a supported work program for traumatically brain-injured individuals. Arch Phys Med Rehab 72(2):127–131.

Creative Job Options:
A Chance to Work

William E. Kiernan

Over the past 10 years there has been a growing realization that employment for people with Down syndrome can be a realistic option. On-site training and support, technology in the workplace, job redesign and accommodation, and the involvement of coworkers and supervisors as both trainers and support resources are strategies that have been effectively utilized to assist persons with severe disabilities in realizing their employment goals.

The acknowledgment of the role a community may play in assisting a person with a disability has grown with a movement toward consumer empowerment, consumer choice, and consumer-driven service delivery systems (Bradley, 1992; Schalock and Kiernan, 1990). A change in the perception of the role of the individual with a disability from one of dependence to independence, inability to ability, and passivity to active involvement will influence how services are developed, operated, and evaluated (Halpern, 1993; Schalock and Kiernan, 1990). Such a change in perception is noticeable in the development of service options such as inclusive education, supported employment, home ownership for persons with disabilities, personal assistance services, and integrated leisure and recreation services (McDonnell, et al., 1991; Kiernan et al., 1991; Rusch, 1990; Sailor, et al., 1991; Wehman and Moon, 1988). For persons with disabilities it is not presence in the community but membership in the community that is the focus. As a member of the community, those resources and supports inherent in that community can assist the individual with the disability in realizing personal goals and aspirations.

There is a growing recognition that the process of obtaining a job is one that requires an identification of the vision and desires of the individual with the disability and a matching of that vision to the work and social requirements of the job. The role of both paid and natural supports are emerging. Finally, there is an evolving acknowledgment that outcomes must be viewed in terms of changes in the quality of life of the individual rather than solely by the more quantitative variables such as job title held, dollars earned, or type of employment and living environments (Halpern, 1993; Schalock, 1990).

IDENTIFYING THE VISION

The process of identifying a vision of adult life that meets the personal interest and choices of an individual with a disability is referred to as whole-life planning (Butterworth and Hagner, 1993). Such planning encourages the participation of family and friends in establishing and achieving personal goals. Social relationships and supports both within and outside the work setting play a key role in facilitating the personal and social adjustment of persons with and without disabilities.

A whole-life plan should provide a clear definition of those outcomes that are desired by the individual in work, social relationships, living conditions and leisure and reaction. This planning approach reflects:

1. An emphasis on the preferences, talents, and dreams of the individual rather than needs or limitations.
2. Participation by the person with the disability and significant others from their life in an ongoing group planning process.
3 Defining a vision of the lifestyle that individual would like to attain and the requirements needed to attain that goal.
4. Identifying the support and/or services an individual needs to reach his or her goals.
5. Organizing resources and supports for the individuals that are as local, informal, and generic or nonprofessional as possible to implement the plan.

Organizing a whole-life planning process involves recognizing the need for planning to take place in partnership with an individual and their family or friends, identifying a structure and format for meetings that work for everyone involved, and recruiting participants. A whole-life planning process is a strategy for placing other plans such as the individual education plan (IEP) or the individual transition plan (ITP) into the life-cycle context for the individual.

Critical to the success of a whole-life planning process is the careful identification of those individuals whom the person with the disability feels should be included in the planning process: family and friends, professionals, neighbors, or individuals who the person with the disability has come to know through local business or community activities. Active incorporation of the person with the disability and identification of who should attend, what tasks the attendees are to perform, and where the meeting should be located is critical. A whole-life planning process is a dynamic and evolving process that may lead in some instances to observations that do not have measurable outcomes or may not be possible to achieve due to constraints from the service-provider agency.

A product of the whole-life planning process is the development of a personal profile. This profile is a comprehensive inventory of places, people, and activities in the person's life. This process seeks a deeper understanding of the individual's preferences, dislikes, and choices. Typically, the personal profile section of the whole-life planning process is organized around the major life activities of the individual, including home life, work and work experiences, school, and social and leisure activities. The whole-life planning process provides an opportunity for the person with the disability as well as those selected by the individual to come together and think through personal dreams, wishes, and aspirations over the next several years. This personal profile provides information that will lead into the discussion about the major life-domain areas and a personal vision.

The development of a personal vision requires that the team merge the information in the profile into a coherent set of comments that define what is important to the individual. This step also requires using that information to create a vision in each of the major life areas for the person that makes sense and that is not constrained by a service system. The more thorough discussion of what is available ought to occur in the last part of the whole-life planning process—the development of the action steps or the action plan.

Along with the vision comes the necessity to become more active and action oriented. It is necessary to look beyond the vision and to begin to identify what steps must be taken in order to accomplish the elements of the vision and to identify what needs to be done and who will be involved in the completion of these tasks. The question of what should be done next requires the identification of persons, resources, and activities that might help in realizing the vision of the individual.

The whole-life planning process develops a vision of the future reflecting what the individual wants and what others hope could be developed. The next section examines how employment options can be developed once the interests of the individual are identified. This section will review job development and placement strategies and the role that natural supports may play in employment for persons with disabilities.

JOB DEVELOPMENT OPTIONS IN NATURAL SUPPORTS

Job Development

A number of approaches through vocational training have emerged during the past 20 years. Specific-skill training and retraining remain the approaches most often used by the public vocational rehabilitation agencies. For persons with more severe disabilities an on-site training approach has evolved (Wehman and Moon, 1988; Kiernan and Stark, 1986). School systems have, over the past 10 years, placed an increasing emphasis on the development of programs that provide real work experiences for students prior to the transition from school to adult life (Hasazi, et al., 1985). There has been a greater emphasis on the establishment of functional curricula at the secondary level directed at developing work-related skills and abilities for students with disabilities.

With the development of supported employment, there is a growing recognition of the role that on-site supports play in the success of the person with severe disabilities on the job. For such persons pretraining or readiness training strategies are being replaced by direct placement, as in the case of supported employment (Kiernan and Schalock, 1989). The matching of the individual needs to the job requirement rather than the fitting of the individual into the job duties is now the approach that is most frequently utilized by community rehabilitation programs. The methods for accessing jobs continue to depend heavily upon formal and informal mechanisms. Structured employment and job-placement services through the state vocational-rehabilitation agencies, nonprofit community based rehabilitation programs, school-to-work transition services through local school systems, and the public employment services are resources for job identification.

In addition to the above-noted job-placement resources, the more informal family/friend networks have been shown to be effective mechanisms in identifying job options. This network is the one that persons without disabilities rely upon in their job searches. The family/friend network can work with the more formal supports in the identification of job leads and employment options for persons with disabilities. This network relies on the involvement of persons who are knowledgeable about the interest and skills of the individual with the disability and can use that information to seek resources through their personal connections. The family/friend network can emerge from the whole-life planning process presented above.

Managing Jobs and People

A variety of approaches have emerged with an increased emphasis upon placement of persons with severe disabilities in integrated work settings. In some instances, a specific job will be obtained through one of the networks noted above, the tasks identified, and the placement made. In other instances, though the job is identified, there are elements of the job that must be adapted if the individual is to be successfully placed. An ecological approach to job placement calls for the matching of the individual's interests and skills to the specific job demands. This approach looks at several ways of reducing the mismatch of the individual to the job. In some instances, there is a need to provide specific skill training for the applicant. In others, there can be a redesign of the job duties or the use of assistive technologies, while in some others, on-site supports from employment training specialists (ETS), co-workers, and/or supervisors may be accessed.

The matching of the individual to the job differs from the previous approaches to job placement where the focus of the placement effort was on fixing the individual. An ecological approach recognizes that there are several methods available to strengthen the fit between the individual and the specific job. Adapting the workplace, the individual, or both requires that time be spent in clarifying job tasks and individual skills, identifying problems related to the accomplishment of the tasks, and the developing a plan to remove barriers.

In some instances, where the interest of the individual is very specific and there is a level of disability requiring considerable redesign, a job creation approach will be used. When significant individual accommodations are necessary, it will be unlikely that a specific job responding to the expressed interests and abilities of the individual will be found. In these cases, job development strategies may reflect a restructuring of a number of jobs such that an entirely new job position is created. Such job creation efforts require considerable time and the willingness of the employer to look at several different jobs or functions performed in the company. Some of the most successful job creation efforts have been realized where there are many persons performing similar tasks and a specific element of the job can be isolated and combined into a single position, as in the case of opening mail in an insurance company, entering invoice numbers into a computer, or sorting materials prior to delivery. In other instances, there may be a need but no current job function exists, as in the case of the delivery service for a restaurant in a local shopping mall, the preassembly of a component part, or the development of a mailing list for posting. Job creation is not the first step in the identification of a job for all individuals with severe disabilities, since it does take considerable time and effort on the part of many. It is, however, a strategy that can respond to a unique interest expressed by an individual with a very severe disability.

Job Supports

The development of additional skills and abilities can be accomplished through the use of an employment training specialist, who provides on-site instruction such that the individual can learn skills in the environment in which they will be used. The place-and-train approach of supported employment was developed around the concept of on-site training and assistance in the development of the individual's capacity to complete the required tasks of the job. Task analysis, systematic training, and the reduction of the training support provided are some of the functions of the ETS.

There has been a growing awareness that there is a need to support not just the skill-development aspects of the job but the social skill development as well. The task of the ETS has evolved from one of on-site trainer to on-site support resource, advocate, and job redesign specialist. Initially, the ETS was viewed as the primary trainer of the individual; however, there has been a growing interest in the ETS providing a support function to the supervisor and coworkers as they provide the specific skill training for the individual. Coworker training approaches have been explored over the past several years and have shown that coworkers can serve as on-site trainers (Curl and Chisholm, 1991; Rusch, 1990).

The nature of the on-site support provided, as in the case of the key functions of the ETS, is changing. The need to integrate the individual with severe disabilities into the work setting has called into question the role of the ETS as the primary trainer. The recognition of the natural support of the work setting has stimulated considerable debate about the need to consider not only the task performed by the individual but the culture of the workplace and the role natural supports can play in assisting the individual in the work setting. The following section examines the issue of natural supports more closely, considering the definition and nature of such supports in facilitating the adjustment of the individual to the job.

NATURAL SUPPORTS

As in whole-life planning, natural support is not just an approach but rather a process or mind set (Kiernan et al., 1993). The purpose of accessing natural supports is to develop a capacity to respond in a timely and efficient fashion to the needs of individuals utilizing those resources that are available within the community setting (Hagner et al., 1992; Nisbet and Hagner, 1988). There are a number of assumptions that I make regarding natural supports including:

1. Support networks are available in all life domains (including community living, recreation, school, employment, and health and wellness).
2. Specific strategies for accessing natural supports may vary depending on external factors such as geographic location (urban versus rural), cultural groupings and orientation of the individual, internal culture of an environment, and the specific life domain being accessed.
3. The use of naturally occurring supports will drive the delivery of services toward a more inclusive and integrated outcome for the individual with the disability.

Issues in the Utilization of Natural Supports in Employment

The cornerstones of integrated employment reflect: clarification of the aspirations and dreams of the individual, identification of the job opportunities that respond to those dreams and aspirations, and matching of the individual's needs, abilities, and interests to the job demands, duties, and work environment expectations; the provision of on-site training and ongoing supports; and the fading of those supports as the individual becomes more proficient on the job (Halpern, 1993; Kiernan et al., 1993). Effective employment placement is a planning, resource identification, and evaluation process that includes the individual with the disability, family members and friends, professionals, and other community members.

The considerable reliance on the job coach and the potential for ignoring or excluding more naturally occurring support in the work setting as well as the level of social integration being achieved by those in supported employment is a growing concern (Agosta et al., 1993; Hughes et al., 1990; Kiernan et al., 1993; Nisbet and Hagner, 1988). To date, the primary approach to assisting persons with disabilities, particularly those for whom supported employment is appropriate, has been through the use of a job coach (Powell et al., 1991; Wehman and Moon, 1988). The job coach can also play a key role in identifying and accessing naturally occurring support. However, in some instances, the presence of a job coach may serve to inhibit accessing natural supports and developing relationships (Nisbet and Hagner, 1988). Furthermore, the presence of a job coach in a workplace for an extended period can actually serve to distance the individual with disabilities from coworkers, create an aura of separate status with respect to the individual, and interfere with spontaneous and naturally occurring social interactions in the workplace (Curl and Chisholm, 1991; Nisbet and Hagner, 1988).

In the case of the use of natural supports, the potential for accessing employment through the use of integrated employment (supportive, transitional, and competitive) strategies is not in question. The issue of assuring inclusion of the worker with the disability into the culture of the workplace; the need to maximize the perceptions of separate, special, or different; the need to remove barriers through natural and spontaneous social interactions; and, ultimately, the need to be as cost-effective as possible while providing quality of services in the work setting are the issues that need to be addressed. The obvious direction to take in responding to these concerns is the development of strategies to enhance access to those networks and associated support services that are available within the workplace for all workers.

Definition of Natural Supports in Employment

Natural support has been defined as "those strategies and resources that promote the interest and cause of individuals with and without disability by enabling such persons to access information, resources, and the relationships inherent in the integrated workplace and community, resulting in a valued and satisfied employee." A central element of this definition is the declaration of the purpose of natural supports to "promote the interest and cause of individuals with and without disabilities." This element of the definition clearly indicates that service, supports, and opportunities for persons with disabilities should be the same or similar to those available to persons who are not disabled. The concept of separateness is thus contrary to the developing principles of natural supports.

A second key aspect of this definition is the identification and location of the elements of natural supports. Natural supports include the accessing of "information, resources, and relationships inherent in the integrated workplace and the community." This aspect of the definition acknowledges that natural supports include not just on-site job supports but resources, information, and social opportunities that may occur in or outside the work setting.

The final element of the definition addresses the issue of outcomes or results. Here again the focus is on the needs and interests of the individual. As a result of accessing natural supports, the individual should be better suited to meet the requirements of the workplace (both production and social) and thus be viewed by others as a valued employee. The elements of natural supports, that is, the information, resources, and relationship access should lead to the maintenance or enhancement of the employee level of satisfaction. The accessing of natural supports must result "in a valued and satisfied employee."

This definition of natural supports reflects a belief that these supports are diverse, individually focused, and common, thus available to all employees. The networks within which natural supports are found can be varied and reflect a wide variety of organizations, individuals, and environments. The outcome of natural supports is one of increased interaction, inclusion, and appreciation of the employee by both management and fellow employees, thereby generating an increased level of employee satisfaction.

The Process for Identifying Natural Support

The place to begin in developing natural supports in a community or workplace setting is the identification of the environmental arrangement or changes that will be needed in a given context to enable the individual with disability to accomplish his or her defined role with success and dignity. The steps used include:

1. Identifying the need.
2. Establishing the life activity or areas impacted.
3. Identifying the extant networks of support.
4. Examining the natural support resources available within those networks.
5. Enabling a decision to be made as to whether existing resources will resolve the need.
6. Putting a support plan in place.
7. Evaluating the outcome of the support activities.

In the accessing of natural supports, it is important for the individual with the disability to be actively involved in all of the steps of the process. Additional other persons (friends, relatives, or interested parties) may be involved in the various steps.

The Role of Supports

The role of external supports, i.e. job coach or employment training specialist (ETS), has evolved over the past decade. Initially, in supported employment the ETS role was one of job analysis, on-site training, and ongoing support. Implicit in the design of the ETS role was the concept that the supports for the individual would be reduced as the tasks relating to the job were mastered. What has evolved, however, is a more structured and ongoing on-site role for the ETS. Nisbet and Hagner (1988) have offered a number of alternatives to the more traditional role of the ETS, noting that this external support can serve as a mentor or training consultant and thus support the individual, the employer and coworkers (See Table 1). As such, the ETS becomes a resource to the individual and all of the employees and can assist in orientation of workers and supervisors through the worker with the disability, serve as a training resource to the supervisors and the coworkers, or assist in job redesign and restructuring through the use of technology and/or job-task modification.

In the implementation of whole-life planning goals there is a role for both internal or natural supports and external or paid support resources. Recognition of both and a clear understanding of the role that these supports can play will facilitate the inclusion of the individual into the specific community setting. Exclusive reliance on either internal or external supports may limit the adjustment of the individual with the disability. In some instances, the role of the external supports will be minimal and reflect a consultative or indirect relationship to the individual. In other instances, the on-site training by the ETS will be critical to the success of the individual in mastering the task required. The issue of support resources is not an either/or issue but a both/and issue. It is important, however, to first look at those supports that are inherent to the workplace as the first option, with the paid or external supports utilized when no appropriate natural supports are available.

Accessing needed supports within various environments requires both new thinking and different staff-utilization patterns. The new thinking focuses on the "naturalness" and potential effectiveness of natural supports; the new staff-utilization patterns focus on a support or resource manager/advocate who looks to the utilization of those supports that are available to all individuals in a specific setting. Assisting in the

Table 1. Community Employment Support Options[a]

| Option | Support/Person Role | | Responsible to | Agency Role |
	Internal	Ongoing		
Job Coach	Job coach training	Coach fades: worker is presumed independent	Agency	Direct: Training and follow-up
Mentor	Job coach trains: supervision is transferred to mentor	Mentor remains on-site providing support and supervision	Company	Indirect: Matching and support for mentor
Training Consultant	Job coach trains with the coworkers and supervisors	Coworkers and supervisor provide support, supervision, and additional training	Company	Indirect: Consultation and stipend
Job sharing	Job coach identifies job sharer, then trains and assists	Job sharer remains on-site	Agency and company	Indirect: Matching— support for job sharer, stipend
Attendant	Attendant trains and assists (may need some assistance from job coach)	Attendant remains on-site at worker's discretion	Worker	Possibly initial training: afterward little or no intervention

[a]Adapted from Nisbet and Hagner (1988)

development of the person's whole-life goals, completing an inventory of supports, conducting a discrepancy analysis between the person's needed and available internal and external supports, and accessing needed support form the conceptual framework of whole-life planning and natural supports in employment. It is now appropriate to consider how the employment process should be evaluated.

EVALUATION OF EMPLOYMENT IN A QUALITATIVE PERSPECTIVE

The concept of quality of life is not new but has been discussed for several years (Andrews, 1986; Edgerton, 1990). However, the application of quality of life as a measurement tool to document changes and outcomes for persons with disabilities is new (Goode, 1990; Rosen, 1986; Schalock, 1990; Walker and Calkins, 1986). It has only been in the last decade that an interest in assessing consumer outcomes reflecting qualitative variables has emerged.

Halpern (1993) has advocated the utilization of quality of life as a measure of the transition process. His model suggests that there is a need to differentiate personal and societal perspectives of quality of life. From a personal perspective, personal choice is the underlying principle. From a societal perspective, social norms are the most meaningful form of reference. Social norms identify socially desirable goals of groups of people as a whole while acknowledging that such norms may not be appropriate for every individual within that group (Halpern, 1993). Halpern suggests three specific content dimensions when looking at quality of life: 1) physical and material well-being; 2) performance in a variety of adult goals; and 3) a sense of personal performance. Within these there are 15 subcategories of basic outcomes. Halpern's approach provides some guidance toward a normative way of evaluating quality of life outcomes.

When identifying key factors in quality of life it is important also to look at what values and significant factors are perceived by persons with mental retardation and other developmental disabilities. People on the Go, a self-advocacy group sponsored by the Arc of Maryland, has developed a list of statements that they refer to as the litmus test for measuring quality of life (Maryland, 1992) (See Table 2). The answers to these questions provide data on levels of quality according to members of this self-advocacy group.

O'Brien (1987) suggests that the assessment of quality of life must reflect community presence, community participation, choice, respect, competence, and satisfaction. These guiding principals along with some proposed natural support standards provide the basis upon which the qualitative assessment of employment can be initiated.

Within the context of quality of life it is important to understand how we evaluate the effect and impact of employment. Habilitation services are currently being influenced by many significant factors including strong forces advocating for greater consumer empowerment and self-outcomes. The combination of these will sub-

Table 2. Litmus Test Questions. A Consumer's Perspective on Quality of Life

---

Did you ask me?
Can I change my mind?
Can I say "no" and still receive services?
Will I be safe?
Is my health protected?
Do I have privacy?
Are my rights, dignity, and individuality respected?
Am I spending time the way I choose and with the people I choose?
Can you give me what you promise?
Will you help me learn how to be a part of the community?
Are you providing me the opportunities that support my choices?
Does the service make sense?
Can I get the service if I move?
Would I want it?
Does the service increase my opportunities?
Does the service help me look good to others?

---

sequently lead to an increased quality of life for the consumer. Obviously, what is central to the measurement of quality is a clear identification of the goals and outcomes which are person-specific and related to the needs of the individual. We have moved from the number of persons placed and dollars earned to individual satisfaction and increased levels of choice and inclusion in all community settings.

SUMMARY

Creating meaningful employment options for persons with Down syndrome and other developmental disabilities begins with the identification of the interests and aspirations of the individual, the involvement of both paid and natural supports in the identification and establishment of the job, and an evaluation of the impact through the documentation of changes in the quality of life. For certain individuals, the strategies for finding a job are similar to those used by most job seekers, that is, developing skills, identifying employers who employ persons with such skills, and seeking a job with those employers. For the individual with more severe disabilities, successful employment may require creating a job that matches the individual skills of the person, modifying existing jobs through task restructuring or using technology to reduce the discrepancy between the limitations of the individual and the demands of the job. Regardless of the job placement or support approach used, the need to access natural support resources through the job setting is evident.

The family and friend network has proved to be one of the most effective strategies in identifying employment opportunities not only for persons with disabilities but all people. This is a network that is utilized most effectively by many job seekers. It is the accessing of the customary and typical resources available to all persons, those inherent to the setting or naturally occurring, which can and do play a significant role in creating job options for persons with Down syndrome.

REFERENCES

Agosta J, Brown L, Melda K (1993): Job Coaching in Supported Employment. Present Conditions and Emerging Directions: National survey results. Salem, Oregon: Human Services Research Institute.

Andrews FM (Ed.) (1986): "Research on the Quality of Life." Ann Arbor: The University of Michigan, Institute for Social Research.

Bradley V (1992): The Paradigm Shift. Cambridge, MA: Human Services Resources Institute.

Butterworth J, Hagner D (1993): "Whole Life Planning: A Guide for Organizers and Facilitators." Boston: University of Massachusetts, Training and Research Institute for People with Disabilities (UAP), Graduate College of Education.

Curl R, Chisholm LA (1991): "Unlocking Co-Worker Potential in Competitive Employment: Keys to a Cooperative Approach." Unpublished manuscript.

Edgerton R (1990): Quality of life from a longitudinal perspective. In Schalock R, Begab M (Eds.), "Quality of Life: Perspectives and Issues," pp. 149–160. Washington, DC: American Association on Mental Retardation.

Goode D (1990): Thinking about and discussing quality of life. In Schalock R, Begab M (Eds.), "Quality of Life: Perspectives and Issues," pp. 41–58. Washington, DC: American Association on Mental Retardation.

Goode DA (1989): Quality of life and quality of work life. In Kiernan WE, Schalock RL (Eds.), "Economics, Industry, and Disability: A Look Ahead." Baltimore: Brookes.

Hagner D, Rogan P, Murphy S (1992): Facilitating natural supports in the workplace: Strategies for support consultants. J Rehab 58:29–34.

Halpern AS (1993): Quality of life as a conceptual framework for evaluating transition outcomes. Exceptional Children 59:486–498.

Hasazi SB, Gordon LR, Roe CA (1985): Factors associated with the employment status of handicapped youths exiting high school from 1979 to 1983. Exceptional Children 51:455–469.

Hughes C, Rusch FR & Curl RM (1990): Extending individual competence, developing natural support, and promoting social acceptance. In Rusch FR (Ed.), "Supported Employment: Models, Methods, and Issues," pp. 181–197. Sycamore, IL: Sycamore.

Kiernan WE, Schalock R (Eds.) (1989): "Economics, Industry, and Disability: A Look Ahead." Baltimore: Brookes.

Kiernan WE, Stark J (Eds.) (1986): "Pathways to Employment for Adults with Developmental Disabilities." Baltimore: Brookes.

Kiernan WE, Schalock RL, McGaughey MJ, Lynch SA, McNally LC (1991): "National Survey of State Information Systems Related to Day and Employment Programs." Boston: Training and Research Institute for People with Disabilities, The Children's Hospital.

Kiernan WE, Schalock RL, Butterworth J, Sailor W (1993): "Enhancing the Use of Natural Supports for People with Severe Disabilities." Boston: Training and Research Institute for People with Disabilities, Children's Hospital.

McDonnell J, Wilcox B, Hardman M (1991): "Secondary Programs for Students with Developmental Disabilities." Boston: Allyn and Bacon.

Nisbet J, Hagner D (1988): Natural supports in the work place: a reexamination of supported employment. JASH 13(4):260–267.

O'Brien J (1987): A guide to life-style planning: Using The Activities Catalog to integrate services and natural support systems. in Wilcox B, Bellamy GT (Eds.), "A Comprehensive Guide to the Activities Catalog: An Alternative Curriculum for Youth and Adults with Severe Disabilities," pp. 175–189. Baltimore: Brookes.

Powell TH, Panscofar EL, Steers DE, Butterworth J, Itzkowitz JS, Rainforth B (1991): "Supported Employment: Providing Integrated Employment Opportunities for Persons with Disabilities." New York: Longman.

Rosen M (1986): Quality of life for persons with mental retardation: A question of entitlement. MR 24:365–366.

Rusch FR (1990): "Supported Employment: Models, Methods, and Issues." Sycamore, IL: Sycamore.

Sailor W, Gerry M, Wilson WC (1991): Disability and school integration. In. Husen T, Postlethwaite TN (Eds.), "International Encyclopedia of Education: Research and Studies" (2nd suppl.), pp. 159–163. Oxford, England: Pergamon Press.

Schalock RL (1990): "Quality of Life: Perspectives and Issues." Washington, DC: American Association on Mental Retardation.

Schalock RL, Kiernan WE (1990): "Habilitation Planning for Adults with Disabilities." New York: Springer-Verlag.

Walker H, Calkins C (1986): The role of social competence in the community adjustment of persons with developmental disabilities: Processes and outcomes. J Remed Special Ed 7:46–53.

Wehman P, Moon MS (Eds.) (1988): "Vocational Rehabilitation and Supported Employment." Baltimore: Brookes.

Index